THE NOURISHED
SPROUT

therapeutic recipes for a vibrant pregnancy

Anise Thorogood | Dr. Carrie Mitchell
The Nourished Sprout

Copyright © 2023 by Anise Thorogood
First Edition

ISBN 978-1-7381081-1-4

All rights reserved.
No part of this book may be reproduced in any form or by any electronic or mechanical means, including information storage and retrieval systems, without written permission from the author, except for the use of brief quotations in a book review.

The content is not intended to diagnose or treat any diseases. Always consult with your primary care physician or licensed healthcare provider for all diagnosis and treatment of any diseases or conditions, for medications or medical advice as well as before changing your health care regimen.

Cover photo: Anise Thorogood

THE NOURISHED SPROUT

therapeutic recipes for a vibrant pregnancy

Anise Thorogood

Certified Holistic Nutritionist

with Dr. Carrie Mitchell, *Naturopathic Doctor*

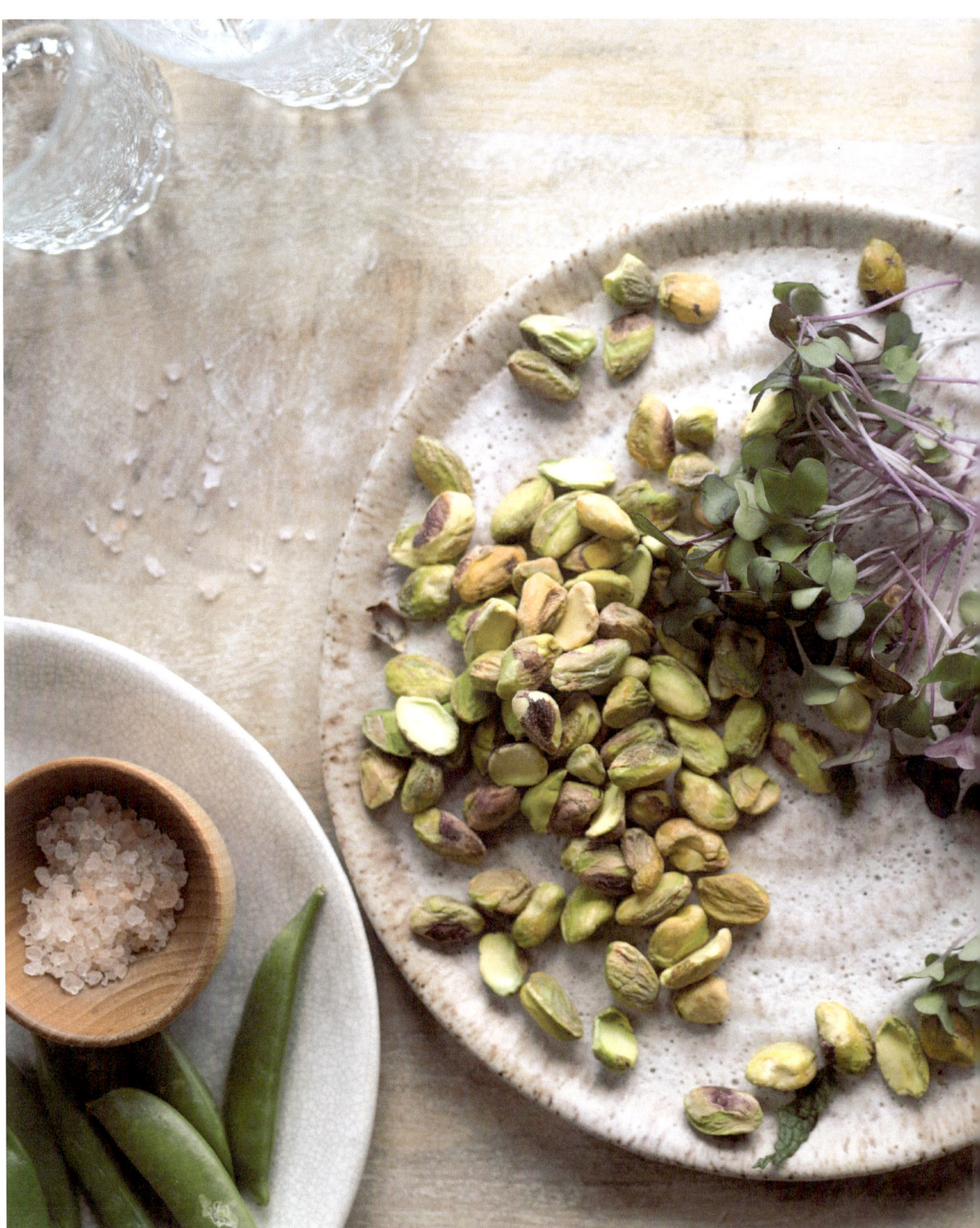

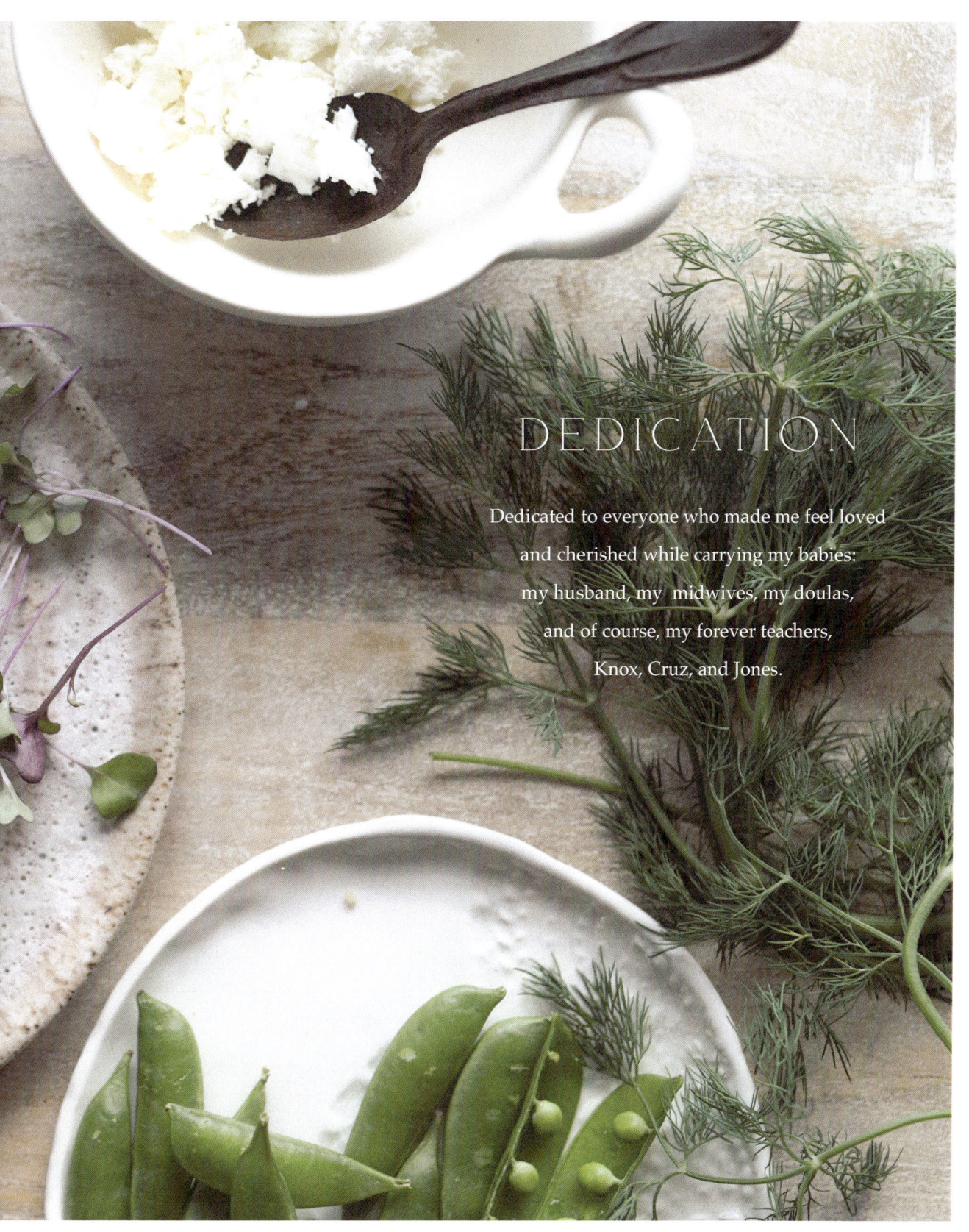

DEDICATION

Dedicated to everyone who made me feel loved and cherished while carrying my babies: my husband, my midwives, my doulas, and of course, my forever teachers, Knox, Cruz, and Jones.

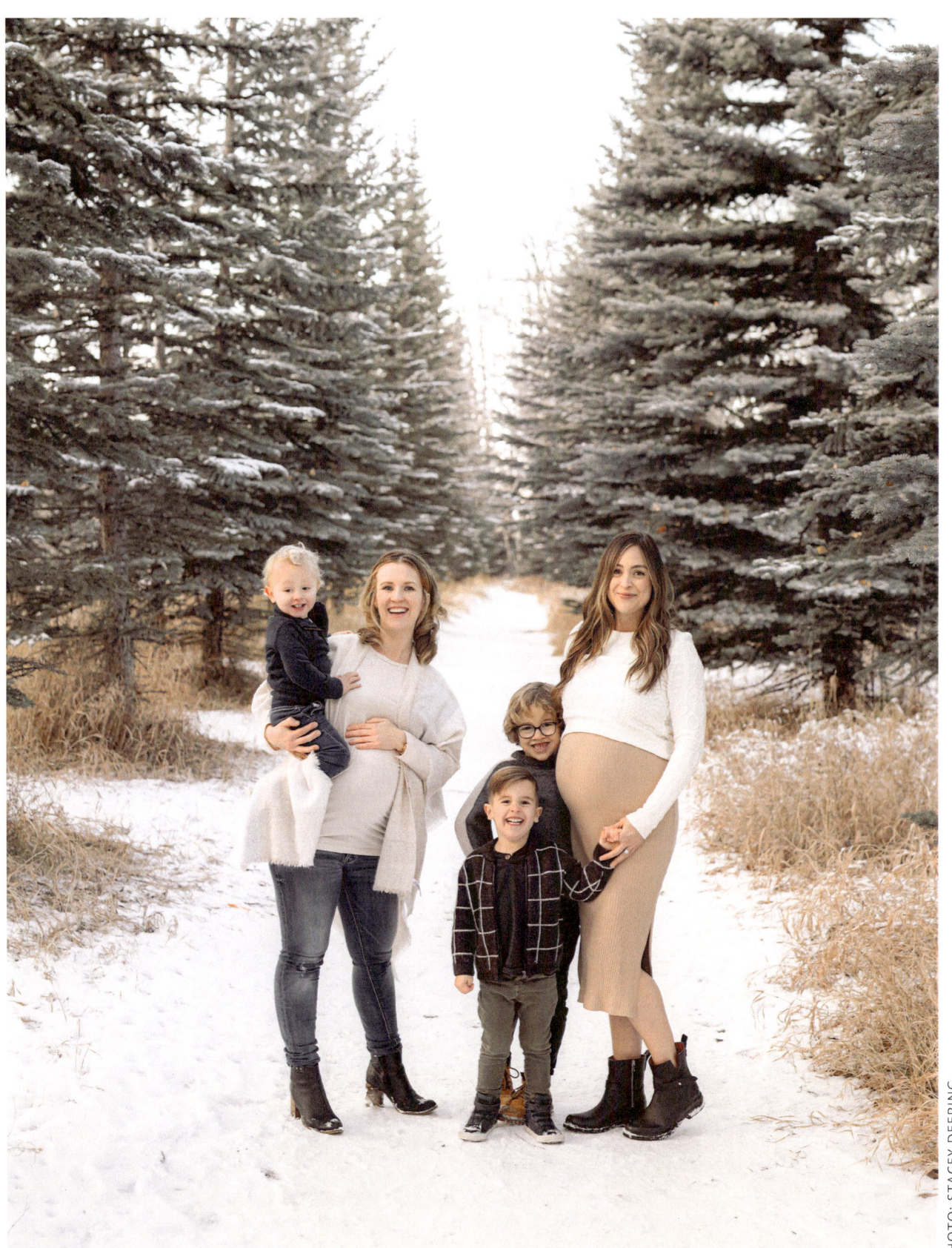

PHOTO: STACEY DEERING

INTRODUCTION

Pregnancy, labour, and childbirth are some of the most beautiful and important life events a person can experience. The magical journey through pregnancy is not only a huge shift but a beautiful metamorphosis. While evolution from bump to babe can sometimes be challenging, mamas can feel great during their pregnancies, nourishing the mind, body, soul, and sprouting babe. Our wish is to empower families to choose vibrant, simple, and delicious whole-food meals to get them through these monumental nine months and beyond.

This cookbook provides the tools to super-charge your diet and provide abundant nutrition to increase energy, reduce some irritating symptoms of pregnancy, and ensure you are getting everything you and the growing babe need. We believe food should be a joy to prepare and eat.

As mothers and friends, we bring different expertise to the table. Anise is a certified holistic nutritionist and holistic home chef who is a natural in the kitchen. Dr. Carrie Mitchell has been a naturopathic doctor in Calgary, Alberta for over 12 years, specializing in women's health, fertility, pregnancy, and postpartum. We share a passion for health, holistic wellness, pregnancy, and postpartum care. As mothers ourselves, we know what a powerful role nutrition plays during these phases of life. The goal of this cookbook is to blend a pregnancy-specific, therapeutic eating plan with delicious and fresh recipes. We want you to feel proud of your pregnancy diet, and to experience its health and wellness benefits.

While writing this cookbook, we have juggled pregnancies, babies, busy lives, and crazy times. We know this stage of life can be hard, and we want to provide the meals to get you through it. And while this book often refers to mamas, women, and breastfeeding, it acknowledges and speaks to all pregnant people who are nurturing a babe and themselves, no matter how they identify.

With specifically chosen whole foods, you can support your amazing body throughout this sacred and precious journey of pregnancy.

Love your babe, your body, and your health!

xoxo

Anise and Dr. Carrie

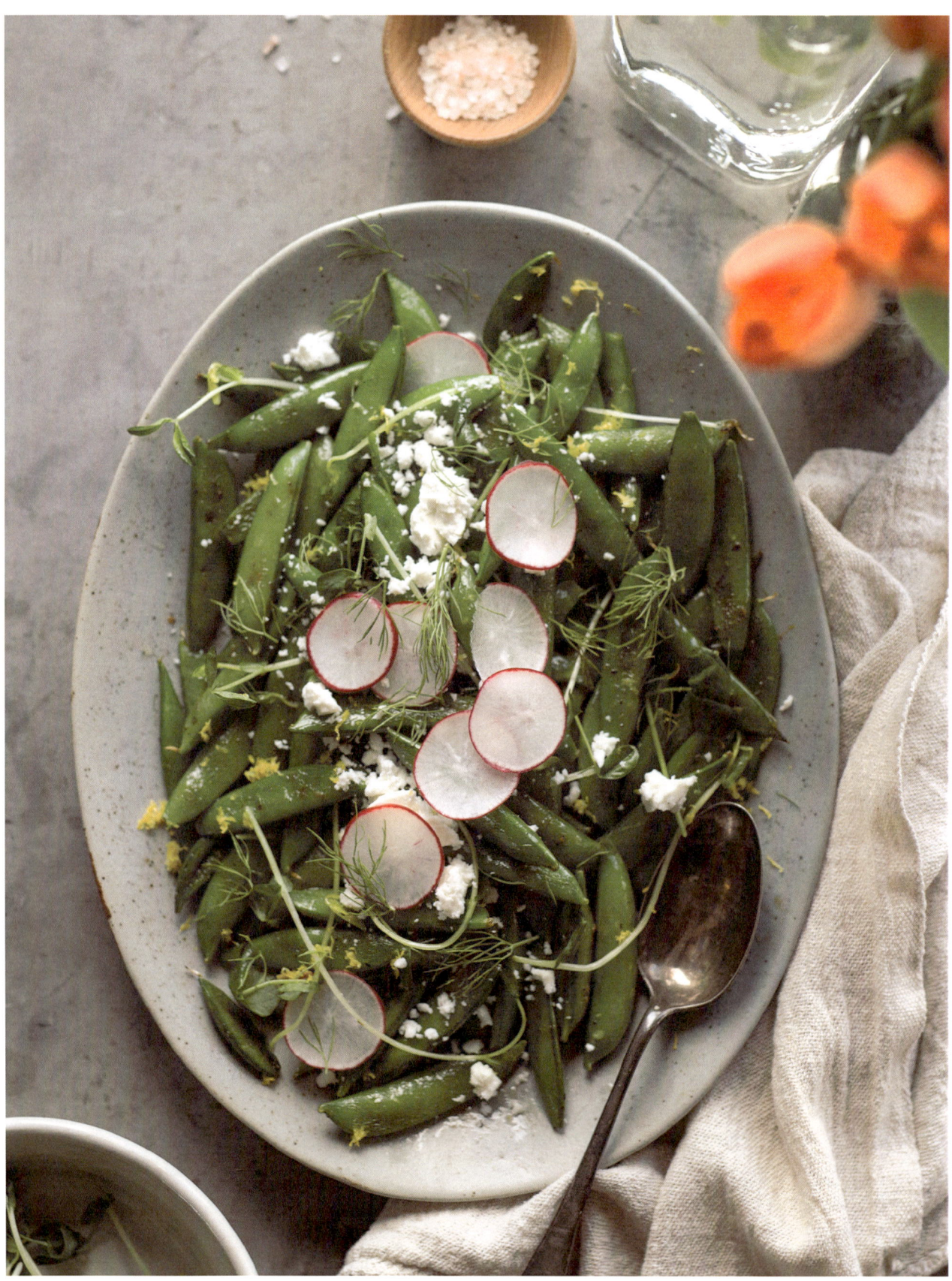

TABLE OF CONTENTS

THE NOURISHED SPROUT

How to Use This Cookbook 1
Stocking a Whole Foods Pantry 3
Weekly Grocery List 9

FIRST TRIMESTER
Introduction 13
Steel-Cut Oats with Coconut Cream and Poached Plums 17
Avocado Toast Four Ways 19
Ginger Granola with Coconut and Sliced Almonds 21
Brussels Sprout Hash with Sweet Potatoes and Poached Eggs 23
Salmon and Kimchi Tacos with Citrus Avocado Crema 25
Spring Quinoa Salad with Mint and Swiss Chard Pesto 27
Vermicelli Noodle Salad with Lemongrass Shrimp 29
Lentil and Spinach Dal with Cauliflower "Rice" 31
Cauliflower Carbonara with Peas and Pancetta 33
Veggie Crust Pizza with Bison, Figs, and Arugula 35
Hazelnut-Crusted Chicken with Miso Lemon Collard Greens 37
Salmon Niçoise Salad with Poached Salmon and Tarragon Vinaigrette 39
Watermelon Limeade: The Happy Tummy Tonic 41
Carrot Dip with Walnuts, Orange, and Red Pepper Flakes 43
Banana Carrot Bread with Cinnamon Pecans 45
Chocolate Sesame Truffles, Two Ways 47
Chocolate Hazelnut Chia Pudding with Smashed Raspberries and Nut Crunch 49
Super Digestive Smoothie with Cucumber, Pineapple, Mint, and Lime 51

SECOND TRIMESTER
Introduction 53
Muesli Cookies with Apricot, Walnuts, and Coconut 57
Fruit Crisp with Blueberries and Pear 59
Salmon & Egg Toast with Roasted Broccoli and Tarragon Chimichurri 61
Butternut Squash Breakfast Buns with Tomato Jam and Arugula 63
Lemon Broccoli Soup with Miso and French Lentils 67
Pumpkin Truffle Pasta with Chanterelles and Parmesan 69

Kimchi Quesadilla with Shiitakes and Greens 71
Ginger Soy Sushi Bowl with Edamame, Avocado, and Mango 73
Grilled Lemon Halibut with Miso-corn, Shiitakes, and Swiss Chard 75
Chicken Souvlaki Salad with Olives, Dates, and Parsley 77
Seared Elk Steak with Ginger Carrot Sauce and Greens 79
Spicy Pineapple Miso Shrimp with Grilled Avocado and Kohlrabi Slaw 81
Vegan Kimchi "Cheez" Dip with Carrots and Potatoes 83
Spanikopita with Spelt Phyllo and Dandelion Greens 85
Smooth Skin Smoothie Bowl, Two Ways 87
Chocolate Avocado Brownies with Date and Cacao Frosting 89
Guava Kombucha Freezies with Raspberries and Chia Seeds 91
Mint Chocolate Nice Cream with Cacao Nibs 93

THIRD TRIMESTER

Introduction 95
Labour Prep by Dr. Carrie 96
Shakshuka with Beans and Greens 101
Tropical Bircher Muesli with Quinoa, Papaya, and Kiwi 103
Superhero Pancakes with Vanilla Coconut Sauce 105
Pumpkin Caramel Smoothie with Coconut and Dates 107
Beet, Citrus, and Lentil Salad with Citrus Gremolata 109
Sesame Ginger Soba Noodles with Mango and Avocado 111
Mediterranean Quinoa Salad: with Feta, Artichokes, and Mint 113
Cauliflower Fried Rice with Shredded Chicken and Veggies 115
Mulligatawny with Apples, Lentils, and Rice 117
Bison Borscht with Beets, Cabbage, and Potatoes 119
Dairy-Free Salmon Chowder with Celery Root and Tarragon 121
Shepherd's Pie with Elk and Eggplant 123
Red Raspberry Leaf Mojito with Kombucha, Strawberries, and Mint 125
Avocado and Corn Salsa with Swiss Chard Stems 127
Hot Cacao: Relaxing and Magnesium-Rich 129
Beet Dip with Mint and Lemon 131
Red Raspberry Bites: Dr. Carrie's Ripe and Ready Snacks 133
Bliss Balls with Banana, Walnut, and Figs 135
Labour Prep Chocolate Pudding with Dates, Avocado, and Chia Seeds 137
Chocolate Brittle with Peanut Butter and Cinnamon 139

FOURTH TRIMESTER

Introduction 141
Post-Birth Healing Broth 145
Coconut Cardamon Millet Pudding with Spiced Pears and Pomegranate Molasses 147
Mini Frittatas with Asparagus and Roasted Tomatoes 149
Ayurvedic Kitchari Stew with Mung Beans, Cauliflower, and Spices 151
Blueberry Lemon Doughnuts with Citrus Glaze 153
Postpartum Nourish Bowl with Root Vegetables and Tahini Dressing 155
Creamy Wild Rice Soup with Cremini Mushrooms and Kale.. 157
Soothing Miso Ramen with Bone Broth and a Jammy Egg 159
Yam and Ginger Soup with Lentils and Greens... 161
Roasted Salmon & Bok Choy with Coconut Lemongrass Broth 163
Root Vegetable Soup with Tomato, Mirin, and Roasted Garlic.................................... 165
Venison Meatballs with Ancestral Blend, Garlic, and Parsley 167
Ginger Turmeric Chicken Soup with Apricots and Chickpeas 169
Elk Larb Gai with Mango Avocado Salad 171
Peanut Butter Cookies with Chocolate, Oats, and Fenugreek...................................... 173
Vanilla Coconut Custard with Honey-Stewed Rhubarb and Pistachios........................ 175
No-Bake Granola Bars with Goji Berries, Dates, and Cranberries................................ 177
Lactation & Immunity Smoothie with Berries, Moringa, and Camu-Camu 179
Beet & Apple Bundt Cakes with Cinnamon-Sugar Glaze... 181
Spiced Muffins with Parsnips and Carrots 183
Postpartum Healing Tea 185
Relaxing Reishi Rose Elixir 187
Energizing Matcha Latte 189
Grounding Coconut Chai 191

Acknowlegements 192
About the Authors... 193
Index.. 194

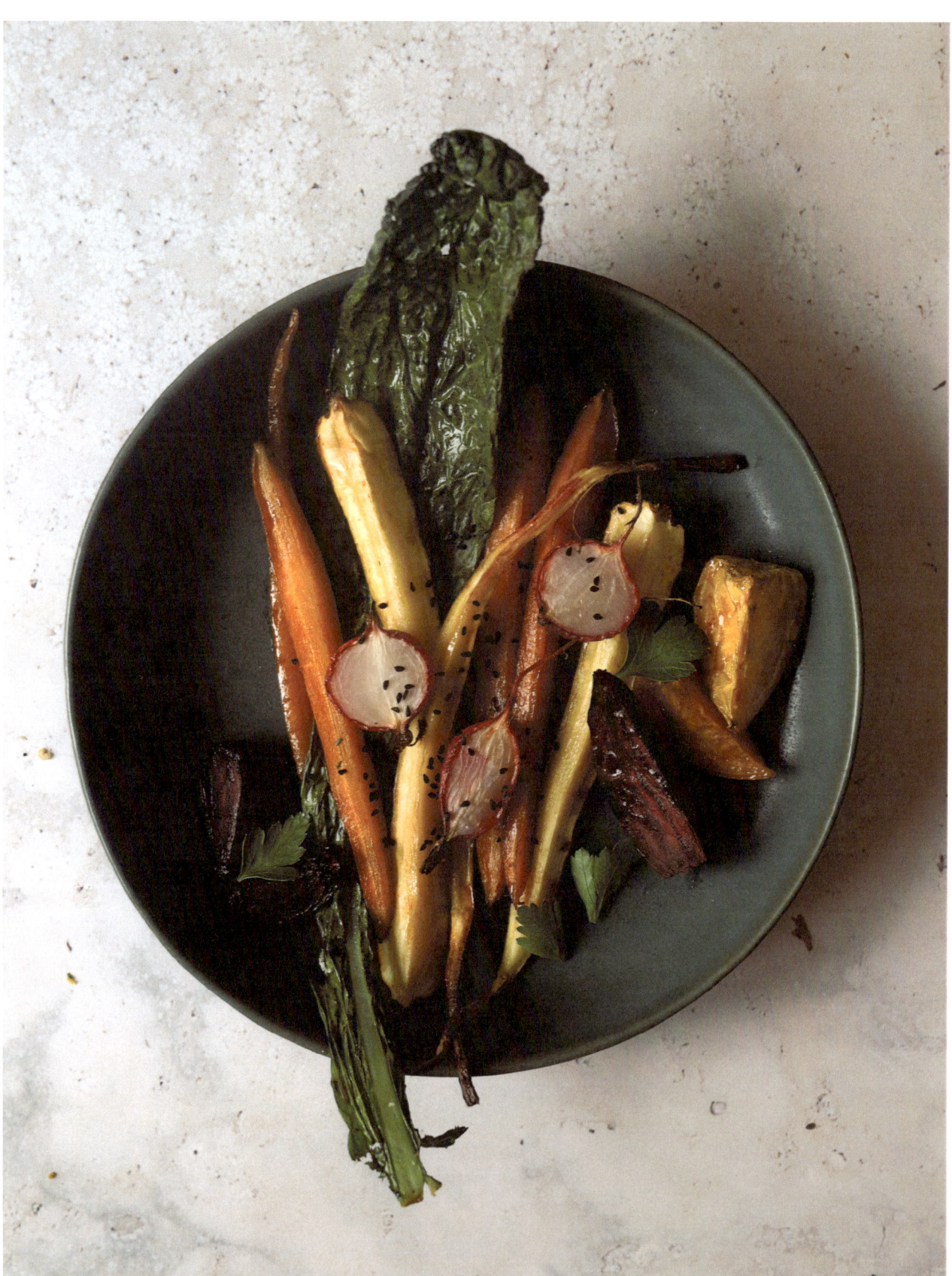

HOW TO USE THIS COOKBOOK

This cookbook is divided into four parts: the traditional three trimesters of pregnancy plus the postpartum stage or "fourth" trimester. Pregnancy brings about a massive increase in your body's caloric and nutritional demands. Keeping the baby's growth and development-specific nutritional requirements in mind, this book gives you ideas on how to incorporate specific nutrients at the perfect time, in fun and inventive ways.

We also want you to have a vibrant and healthy pregnancy with fewer pregnancy symptoms. We often see that a mother who is deficient in certain vitamins, minerals, or vital nutrients feels worse symptoms throughout her pregnancy and postpartum period. That is why we have included therapeutic recommendations for certain pregnancy symptoms, such as in our recipes for the Super Digestive Smoothie, which combats constipation, and the Happy Tummy Tonic and Ginger Coconut Granola, which address nausea. We even have a smoothie bowl for stretch marks and a hot cacao for leg cramps. We are especially proud of the "Prepping for Labour" section, which features everything from how to tone and strengthen the uterus to Dr. Carrie's famous Labour Aid.

Though we tailored the recipes in this book to week-by-week developmental considerations, you can use them interchangeably, especially as you find your favourites—you can snack on the amazing Carrot Walnut Dip any time your appetite knocks!

After delivery, during the first three months postpartum, the bundled babe is fully dependent on Mom as they adjust to the world outside the womb. Mama's body is a hormone roller coaster as it deals with sleep deprivation and other physical and emotional changes.

There is no better time to let others help take care of *you*. Anise developed most of the recipes in the third and fourth trimesters to be freezable—and easy enough for a family member or friend to make for you. Don't be afraid to pass along a screenshot of these pages so visitors don't come empty-handed when they arrive to meet your new little one.

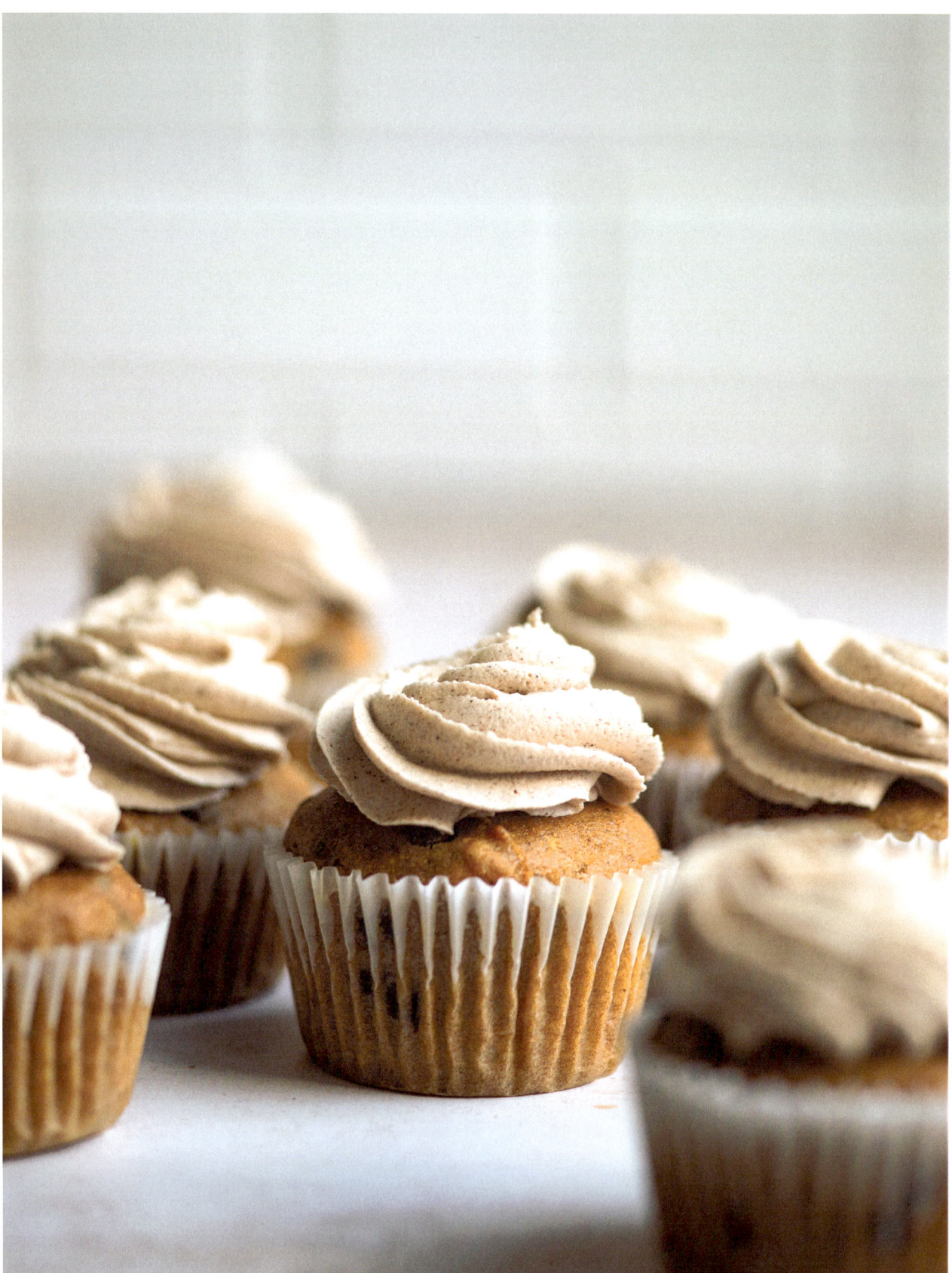

STOCKING A WHOLE-FOODS PANTRY

Otherwise known as Pregnancy Whole Foods 101, this section is your resource to build a powerhouse pantry and learn the foundations of whole-food eating. Building a pantry allows for easy and functional meal planning, and it will put great options at your fingertips, no matter your cravings or preferences in pregnancy.

WHAT IS A WHOLE FOOD?

A whole food is a natural food in its purest form, with all its nutrients intact. It is a food to which nothing has been added, from salt and sugar to chemicals and preservatives. An apple straight off the tree is a whole food; applesauce is a modified or processed food.

An amazing synergy happens when we consume whole foods: our bodies more effectively absorb and use vitamins and minerals, which are more "bioavailable" in whole foods. By eating how nature intended, the vitamins, minerals, antioxidants, enzymes, and phytonutrients in whole foods work together harmoniously to give our body the nutrition it requires for optimum health.

Although most women are proactive about taking prenatal vitamins, there is no substitute for the health benefits of a nourishing whole-foods diet.

WHAT ARE FOOD SENSITIVITIES?

Food sensitivities are non-allergic inflammatory responses to food-specific proteins that cause unwanted symptoms in the body.

The most common food sensitivities are in response to dairy, gluten, egg, soy, and peanuts, but there can be others. In The Nourished Sprout, we strive to offer options that are free of these foods. However, one of the great changes we see in pregnancy is that some women can actually eat more of the foods that previously caused them discomfort, perhaps because the immune system is slightly subdued in pregnancy.

A WHOLE-FOODS PANTRY

A well-stocked pantry makes whole-food recipes easily accessible at home. Having a supply of the quality ingredients listed below allows for effortless meal prep and the creation of last-minute meals that are still nourishing.

WHOLE GRAINS

- *Quinoa.* Technically a seed, quinoa is a great option when you crave "carby" foods but want the added nutrition and amino acid content of this protein-rich superfood.
- *Brown rice.* An easy switch from white rice that retains the nutrition of the grain's outer bran and B vitamins.
- *Steel-cut oats.* An easy, gluten-free breakfast option—and a great whole food for breast milk production.
- *Millet.* A great source of phosphorus and magnesium that helps build a strong skeletal system in the developing babe.
- *Barley.* A protein-dense carbohydrate that keeps your blood glucose stable, it's perfect for combating pregnancy nausea.
- *Buckwheat groats.* These flavourful, nutty, triangular "fruit seeds" are packed with manganese and copper, essential for the production of red blood cells.

NUTS AND SEEDS

- *Almonds.* Along with tons of other minerals and vitamins, almonds are packed with biotin, which gives you energy and strengthens hair and nails for both you and babe.
- *Cashews.* Cashews are perfect for adding smoothness to snacks and sauces, and they are rich in protein, fat, and copper. Our need for copper increases in pregnancy because it is essential for organ growth and development.
- *Walnuts.* Walnuts are a rich source of heart-healthy monounsaturated fats and an excellent vegetarian source of "brain fat": omega-3 fatty acids.
- *Pistachios.* With high B6 content and packed with protein and fibre, pistachios are a great snack or meal ingredient to calm nausea.
- *Pumpkin seeds.* A great source of zinc and magnesium, they are perfect eaten fresh as a snack or as toppers for salads and soups.
- *Sunflower seeds.* Rich in magnesium and fibre, which helps maintain the digestive tract and keep bowel movements moving, sunflower seeds are also a valuable source of folic acid.
- *Chia seeds.* A superfood containing proteins, essential fatty acids, and dense mineral and vitamin content, these seeds can be added to a maternal diet to increase energy and prevent deficiencies. They're also a great source of soluble fibre to maintain a healthy digestive tract.

- *Hemp hearts.* Hemp hearts are 33 percent protein, and they offer the growing babe tons of essential fatty acids—omega-3, 6, 9, and gamma linolenic acid (GLA)—for skin health and postpartum mental health.
- *Flaxseeds.* The fibre content of this gluten-free seed bulks stools and allows for more regular bowel movements, preventing constipation during pregnancy. It's better to eat them ground because the body doesn't always fully digest them.

BEANS AND LEGUMES

- *Lentils.* Small but mighty, lentils are rich in folic acid and a fantastic vegetarian protein. Lentils blend smoothly into sauces and soups for added nutrition.
- *Chickpeas.* Rich in fibre and low on the glycemic index, this protein and carbohydrate source improves energy and digestion in pregnancy.
- *Black beans.* The dark skin of black beans is packed with the phytonutrient anthocyanin, which can help manage the increased oxidative stress that occurs with pregnancy.
- *Green peas.* These provide a protein with low allergenic properties—perfect for moms experiencing tummy troubles from other dairy-based proteins.
- *Kidney beans.* Kidney beans are nourished with iron, folic acid, and copper to aid blood building and increase energy.

FLOURS

- *Cassava flour.* A relatively new flour on the market, cassava is a great grain-free and nut-free option for baking. Be careful, as you can't substitute this in a one-to-one ratio for all-purpose flour.
- *Coconut flour.* With ample fibre and healthy fats, and measuring low on the glycemic index, coconut flour is perfect for maintaining healthy blood sugar levels. This flour absorbs quite a bit of liquid so cannot be substituted one-to-one in other recipes. A good rule of thumb: for every ¼ cup of coconut flour, add an extra egg.
- *Oat flour.* Higher in fibre than any other grain, it also packs in manganese, selenium, phosphorus, magnesium, and zinc.
- *Almond flour.* Dense with nutrients and calories, almond flour adds substance to baking. It's a great gluten-free option with a great fat-to-carbohydrate-to-protein ratio that will keep you feeling full longer.
- *Brown rice flour.* Rich in B vitamins and manganese, it helps in the proper development of bones and cartilage.
- *Spelt flour.* While spelt flour is not gluten free, it's a great whole-foods option. Spelt substitutes easily for all-purpose flour while keeping its bran and germ—and all of its nutrients—intact.

- *Starches for gluten-free baking*. Pick a light starch like arrowroot powder, potato starch, or tapioca flour. These can be added to gluten-free baking to provide the structure and binding properties that gluten typically provides.

NATURAL SWEETENERS

- *Honey.* A natural sugar with B vitamins and minerals, honey is lower on the glycemic index than refined sugars. It helps you avoid the "cookie crash" that other sweeteners can trigger. Please ensure that you consume only pasteurized honey while pregnant!

- *Maple syrup.* High in manganese and zinc, this sap-based sweetener also has calcium to strengthen babe's growing connective tissues like hair, nails, and bones.

- *Coconut sugar.* This has a lower glycemic index than white sugar thanks to inulin, a fibre that slows the sugar's absorption into the body. With a natural sweetness and the added benefits of a few minor nutrients, it is a great choice for baking.

- *Dates.* A pre-birth superfood said to soften the cervix and reduce time in labour, these naturally sweet fruits are like candy. You can blend them easily into puddings, smoothies, or baked goods. You can also find date sugar at whole-food stores.

OTHER SUPERFOODS

- *Seaweed.* This is a nutrient-dense food full of iodine, iron, and trace minerals for strong maternal health and fetal development.

- *Goji berries.* This protein-rich berry is high in antioxidants and vitamin C, both essential to the bone, cartilage, and connective tissue development of a growing babe.

- *Apple cider vinegar.* Apple cider vinegar is fruitier and sweeter than white vinegar. It is made from crushed apples, which give it added nutrients and antioxidants. This vinegar has an alkaline pH effect in the body. When the body is in an acidic state, inflammation and disease are more prevalent. Despite their acidic taste, things like apple cider vinegar and lemon water actually bring our body closer to an alkaline state.

- *Chlorella and spirulina.* Nature's super algae are full of chlorophyll, iron, beta carotene, and essential fatty acids as well as a source of protein. It's a green booster to maternal energy and fetal growth and development.

OILS AND FATS

- *Grass-fed butter or ghee.* Nothing beats grass-fed butter—a whole food in its purest form! It's perfect for high heat points like the oven. Butter has a high cholesterol and lecithin content and a high ratio of vitamins A, D, E, and K. It also contains DHA for brain development and function. Don't underestimate this nutrient-dense food during pregnancy, despite its bad rap! Ghee is butter that has been clarified to remove the milk protein, casein, and whey, leaving only the pure fat behind. Due to its lower lactose content, ghee is an ideal option for individuals with dairy intolerances.

- *Coconut oil.* With a high stability point, coconut oil is great for frying and cooking on high heat. It's also amazing for our pregnancy skin: the perfect oil for belly rubs.
- *Avocado oil.* Another oil great for high-heat cooking, although not as stable as butter or coconut oil, avocado oil is rich in monosaturated fats.
- *Extra-virgin olive oil.* The quality of olive oil makes a difference to the health benefits that result. Choose an extra-virgin olive oil—oil from the first pressing of the olive fruit—to ensure you and the babe get the anti-inflammatory benefits.
- *Flaxseed or hemp oil.* These polyunsaturated fats are essential to cellular development in the growing fetus and can also have beneficial effects on maternal hair, skin, and nails. These oils are highly sensitive and should be kept in the fridge in dark bottles. They should never be heated and should be used only in salad dressings and in smoothies where they will be kept cold. Never heat an omega-3 oil because it destroys all the nutrients and becomes rancid, creating free radicals in the body.

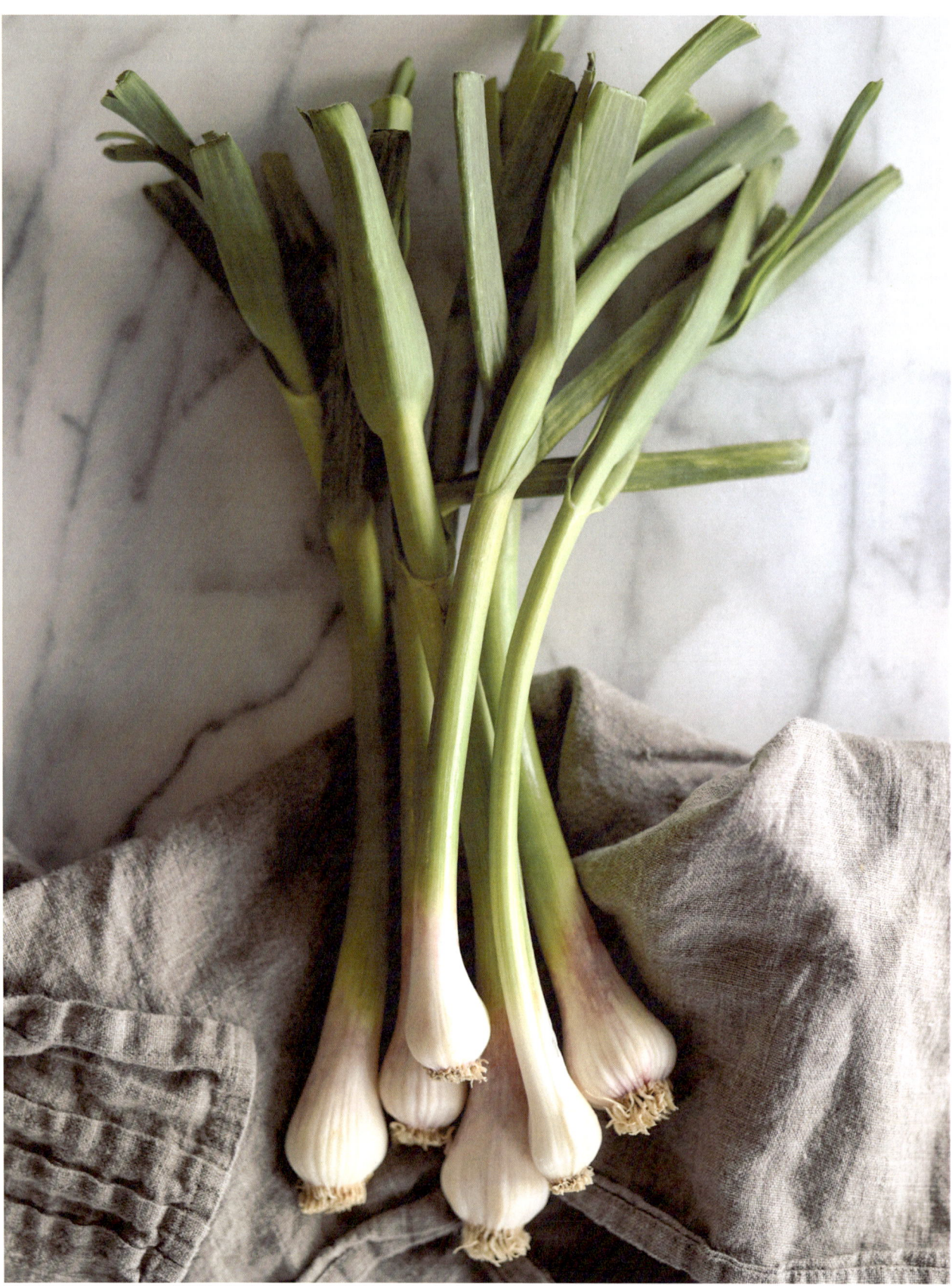

WEEKLY GROCERY LIST

What you eat during pregnancy can have dramatic effects on your baby's development and health. It can also affect your experience and symptoms of pregnancy and even your postpartum health. There really isn't a better time to focus on a vibrant diet!

Below we discuss the types of food to gravitate towards at the grocery store each week, their key nutrients, and the importance of increasing food quality and quantity during this magical time.

PROTEIN

Protein is a fundamental engine of tissue growth in both the baby and the placenta. It supports hormonal changes in the body and builds digestive enzymes that properly break down food. Quality protein sources from meat, fish, and eggs also improve progesterone secretion, which creates a supportive environment in your uterus.

- *2 fish, like salmon, anchovies, sole, or tilapia.* Fish is high in omega-3, which is important for brain and nervous system development. Salmon has the highest levels of docosahexaenoic (DHA) and eicosapentaenoic (EPA) fatty acids. Insufficient levels of DHA have been linked to low birth weight in babies and premature births. Look for fish with low mercury ratings, like salmon, anchovies, tilapia, haddock, and trout. Avoid large game fish like swordfish, marlin, mackerel, and tuna.

- *At least 2 pieces of red game meat.* Game meat has a higher omega-3 content and lower saturated fat than traditional red meat. Some great sources are bison, elk, and venison. Red meat is also high in B vitamins and the minerals zinc and iron. If you choose farmed game, look for meat that does not contain added hormones or antibiotics. Using an "ancestral blend" of organ meat and ground meat is an amazing way to incorporate extra iron and minerals.

- *Lentils and other legumes.* Legumes are great for soups, or you can prepare them in advance for salads. They are high in fibre as well as folic acid, which helps your baby's DNA production and combats neural tube defects. Dried beans should be soaked the night before to remove phytate, a naturally-occurring plant compound that can inhibit the absorption of nutrients.

- *Organic, free-range eggs.* Egg yolks are a great source of good cholesterol—yes, there is good and bad cholesterol! Cholesterol often gets a bad reputation, but it is essential for our hormone production, whether that's progesterone or cortisol or estrogen. It is also vital to the healthy development of the baby's brain, nervous system, and intestinal tract. Eggs are also high in choline, which is necessary for the formation of neurons and their connections.

- *Poultry.* Try to use both white and dark meat in chicken and turkey. The dark meat has more minerals—hence the darker colour!

- *Organic dairy.* Sheep and goat dairy are more easily digested than cow, so opt for those when possible. Consume plain, full-fat yogourt (avoid the extra-sugar varieties!), milk, and cheese in moderation.

CARBOHYDRATES

Carbohydrates provide energy and minerals to support a healthy metabolism, as well as folic acid and B vitamins such as B12, which are important in pregnancy. Choosing complex carbohydrates such as whole grains—quinoa, brown rice, millet, rye, buckwheat—instead of simple, refined carbs—white rice, white bread, white pasta—will keep your blood sugar level stable, which is extremely important during pregnancy. Stable blood sugar levels improve energy, reduce nausea, help control hormone imbalance, and reduce your likelihood of developing gestational diabetes.

Vegetables

- *In-season produce.* You can never have too many vegetables and their amazing phytochemicals—think varied, colourful, seasonal, organic, and local if possible. The fall harvest yields root vegetables with amazing grounding properties, while spring and summer bring peas, radishes, and asparagus. Farmers markets are a great place to see what is in season!
- *At least 2 green, leafy vegetables.* Switch up your produce! Instead of picking up spinach every time you go to the store, try something new like beet greens, dandelion greens, or arugula. I feel as though greens are in a category of their own: they are high in most vitamins and minerals, high in antioxidants and fibre, anti-inflammatory, and high in phytochemicals that can reduce the risk of cancer, heart disease, and diabetes. But be careful eating too much raw spinach and kale: they contain oxalates that can disrupt kidney function and cause inflammation and bone pain.

Fruit

- *Berries.* These are high in antioxidants and easy to add to smoothies, oatmeal, and more.
- *Apples and pears.* Low in sugar, these are great as on-the-go snacks and served with nut butter.
- *Bananas.* High in potassium, bananas are an ideal ingredient for smoothies and baking.
- *Citrus.* Lemons add zing to soups, salad dressings, and drinks—including water. Oranges are a high source of vitamin C.
- *In-season wild cards.* Try something new, like a pomegranate or figs! Peaches and nectarines are a blessing in late summer, and watermelon was made for hot climates.

Whole Grains

By swapping your white rice, white bread, and white pasta for whole grains, you are reaching an entirely different nutritional profile that includes bran, germ, and endosperm. Soak your grains before cooking to remove phytic acid thus making them easier to digest.

- *2–3 whole grains for salads, soups, and "power bowls."* Examples are brown rice, quinoa, wheatberries, and black rice.
- *1 whole grain for breakfasts.* Try steel-cut oats, buckwheat, and millet.
- *1 dry good.* Whole-food dry goods include quinoa or cassava pasta, organic sourdough bread, and seed crackers.

Whole-grain flours for baking. My favourites are coconut flour, oat flour, brown rice flour, and almond flour. I find they work best in combination and make lovely muffins and cakes. See "Flours" in our "Stocking a Whole-Foods Pantry" section for more info.

HEALTHY FATS

Although fats can have a bad reputation, they are actually essential for our general health and a healthy pregnancy and baby. Fats surround every cell in the body and make up over 60 percent of your baby's brain. Fats are also needed for the absorption of vitamins such as A, D, E, and K.

- *4–5 avocados*. This well-known fruit is high in healthy fats like a-Linolenic acid (omega-3) and oleic acid, a monounsaturated fat.

- *Nuts and seeds*. These are also high in omega-3s and omega-6s. Soak your raw nuts to break down the phytic acid and make them easier to digest. Vary your nuts each time you go to the store, as each one has a different nutritional profile. Keep a few on hand at all times for quick, on-the-go snacks.

- *Oils*. You can consume healthy fats in the form of oils from coconut, hemp seed, flaxseed, pumpkin seed, and others. See our "Oils and Fats" entry in the "Stocking a Whole-Foods Pantry" section for more info. Try to switch it up, and always have an omega-3 option, like hemp or flaxseed, handy in the fridge.

- *Flaxseed or chia seed*. These contain the perfect balance of soluble and insoluble fibre. They're easy to add to smoothies, too.

- *Grass-fed butter or ghee*. These fats are saturated, so they're stable at high temperatures. For people with a low tolerance for dairy protein, ghee is a great alternative because the milk proteins have been removed. See our "Oils and Fats" entry in the "Stocking a Whole-Foods Pantry" section for more info.

WHAT TO AVOID

Alcohol	Deli meats and cured meats
Cigarettes	Raw sprouts
Caffeine—reduce coffee to 1 cup a day	Green tea
Soft, unpasteurized cheese	Chamomile tea
Uncooked or undercooked meats	Medicinal herbs like ginseng, black or blue cohosh, and goldenseal, unless otherwise stated by your health-care provider. (Cooking herbs are safe.)
High-mercury fish	
Sushi	

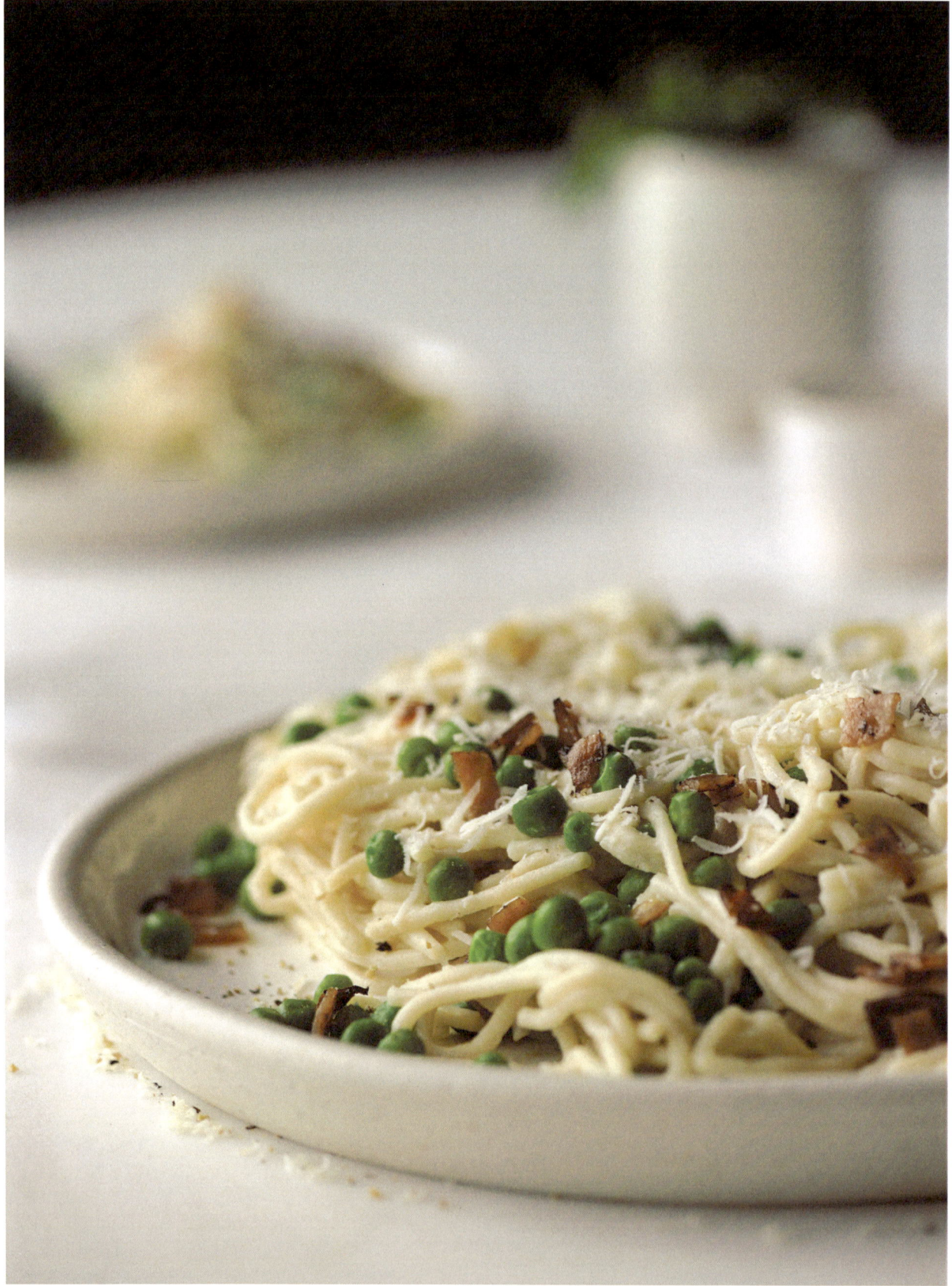

FIRST TRIMESTER

AN EARLY CONGRATULATIONS!

Everything is so new, exciting, intense, and dynamic. Your newly pregnant body is changing every day, matching the rapid growth and development of your little sprout. The first trimester is a time of caution, sometimes secret elation—and the majority of intense pregnancy symptoms. Food aversions and cravings, appetite ups and downs, and extreme fatigue are just some of the new challenges. All the while, you are more focused than ever on prioritizing a healthy diet.

This first trimester is uniquely important because baby is developing rapidly, building all the major cells and systems of its body. During these foundational 12 weeks, the neurological system, cardiovascular system, skeletal system, and organs are all being created. No wonder most mamas are exhausted!

During this roller-coaster first trimester, many women need to be delicate with their eating habits. So don't worry too much about getting extra calories. Instead, add nutrients when you can and eat what you tolerate the best. Listen to your body—you may need to eat much more frequently than you did pre-pregnancy. Some people find they need to eat every 2 hours! Lots of expectant mamas gravitate to carbohydrates and more easily digestible foods.

The key nutrients we focus on in our first-trimester recipes are folic acid, omega-3 fatty acids, vitamins B6 and B12, zinc, magnesium, and fibre. These crucial building blocks, combined with carb- and protein-rich meals and snacks, will help ease the nausea, unsettled stomach, and constipation of the first trimester.

These delicious recipes are gentle on the stomach and pleasing to the palate, while giving your baby and body all the nutrient-rich ingredients they need to grow and thrive.

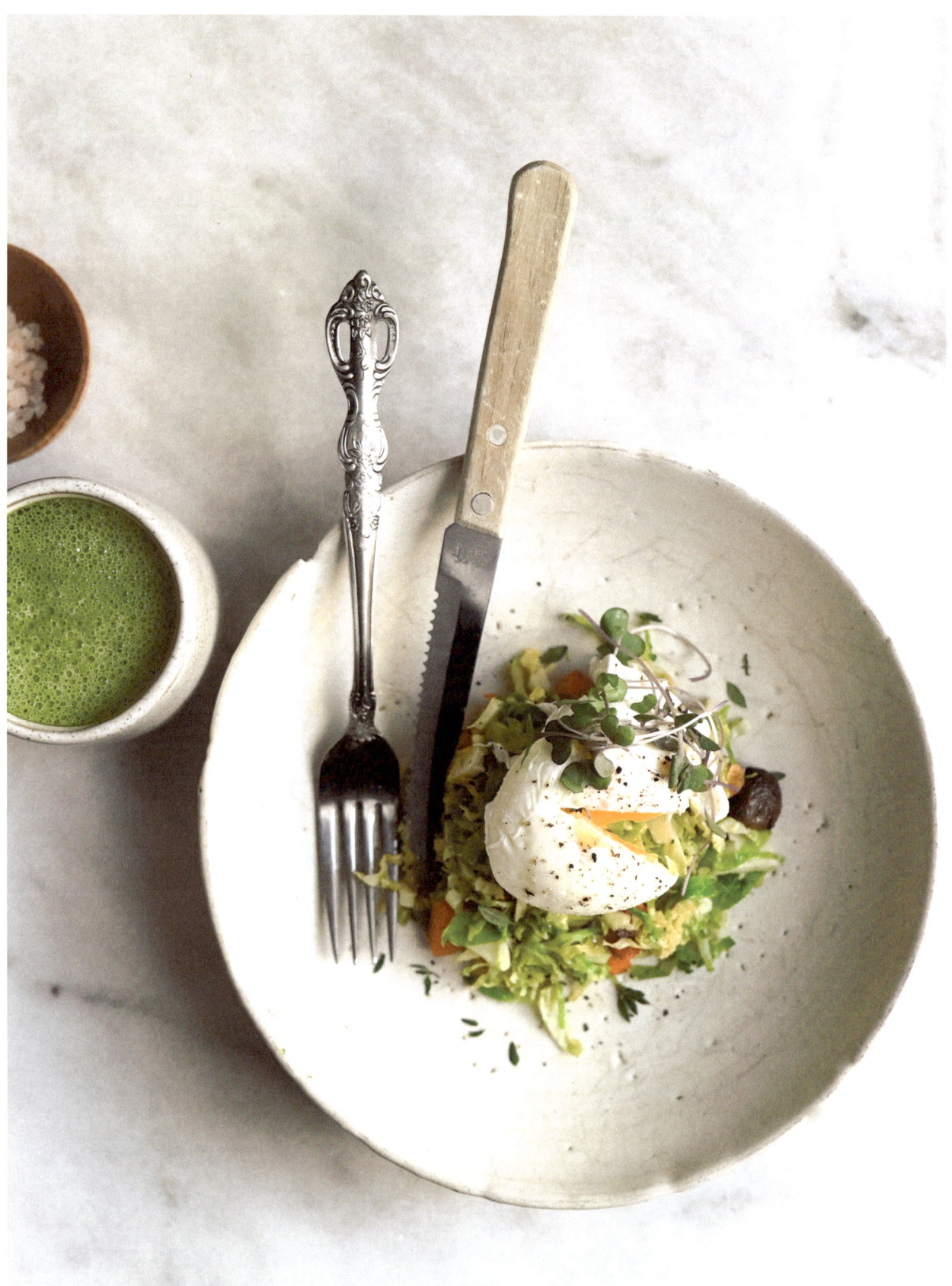

FIRST TRIMESTER

TABLE OF CONTENTS

BREAKFAST
Steel-Cut Oats with Coconut Cream and Poached Plums 17
Avocado Toast Four Ways 19
Ginger Granola with Coconut and Sliced Almonds 21
Brussels Sprout Hash with Sweet Potatoes and Poached Eggs 23

LUNCH
Salmon and Kimchi Tacos with Citrus Avocado Crema 25
Spring Quinoa Salad with Mint and Swiss Chard Pesto 27
Vermicelli Noodle Salad with Lemongrass Shrimp 29
Lentil and Spinach Dal with Cauliflower "Rice" 31

DINNER
Cauliflower Carbonara with Peas and Pancetta 33
Veggie Crust Pizza with Bison, Figs, and Arugula 35
Hazelnut-Crusted Chicken with Miso Lemon Collard Greens 37
Salmon Niçoise Salad with Poached Salmon and Tarragon Vinaigrette 39

SNACKS AND SWEETS
Watermelon Limeade: The Happy Tummy Tonic 41
Carrot Dip with Walnuts, Orange and Red Pepper Flakes 43
Banana Carrot Bread with Cinnamon Pecans 45
Chocolate Sesame Truffles, Two Ways 47
Chocolate Hazelnut Chia Pudding with Smashed Raspberries and Nut Crunch 49
Super Digestive Smoothie with Cucumber, Pineapple, Mint, and Lime 51

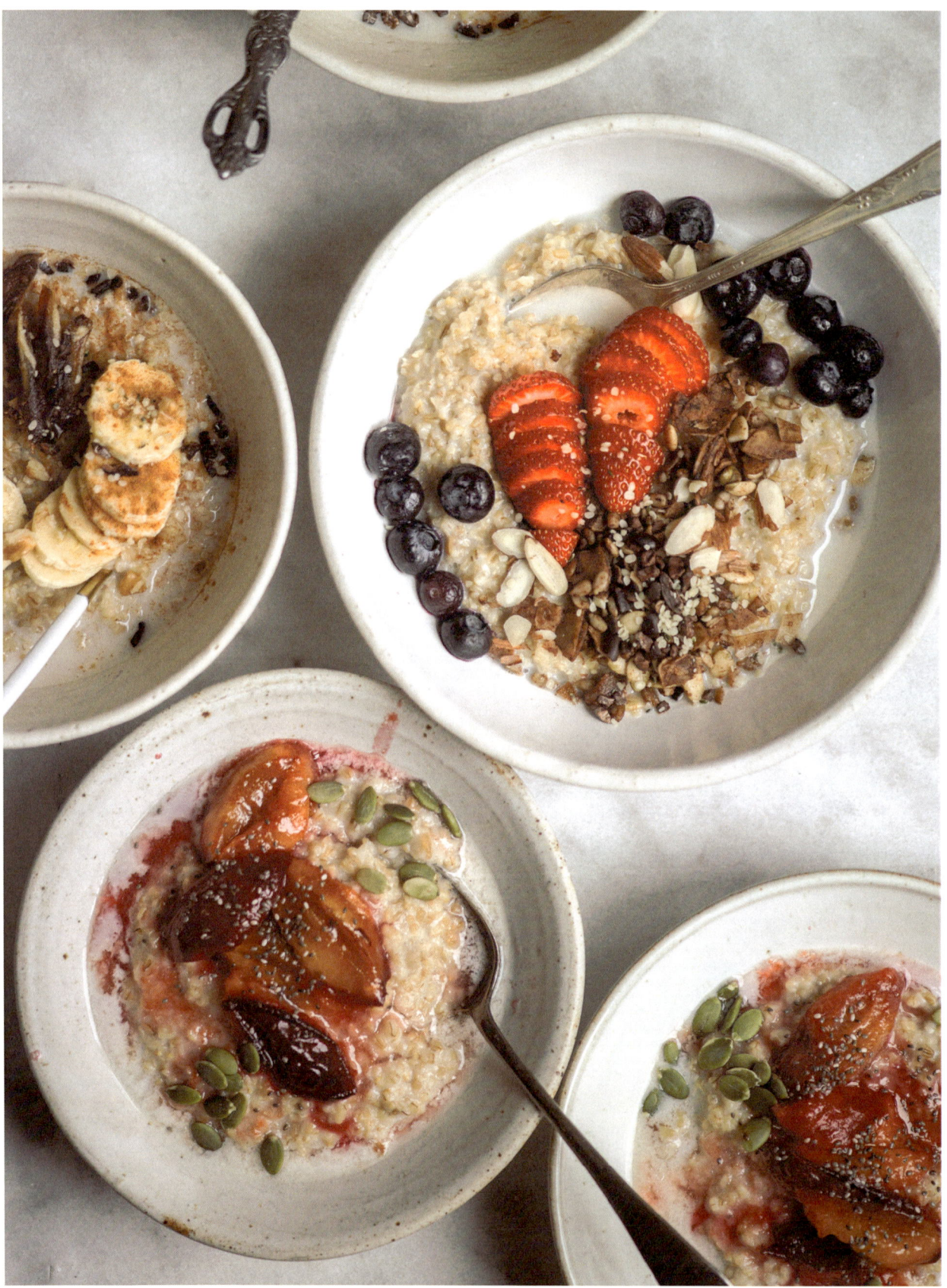

STEEL-CUT OATS

WITH COCONUT CREAM AND POACHED PLUMS

This is a warm and nourishing foundation for the first-trimester stomach, and it is easy to prepare at the beginning of the week and use for future breakfasts. Steel-cut oats are less refined than traditional oats and full of texture and flavour. They are also a great source of fibre and magnesium for an easy, fast, and gentle start to your day. Digestion often slows during pregnancy, but this fibre-packed breakfast can keep you regular and set you up for a day of success!

INGREDIENTS | SERVES 4

1 tablespoon grass-fed butter or ghee
1 cup steel-cut oats
⅛ teaspoon sea salt
2 small plums (or any in-season stone fruit)
½ tablespoon coconut oil
2 tablespoons plus ¼ tablespoon maple syrup
½ teaspoon vanilla extract
¼ teaspoon cardamom or spice of your choice (e.g., cinnamon, ginger, lavender)
3 tablespoons coconut cream
Pumpkin seeds to garnish

DIRECTIONS

1. In a medium Dutch oven or saucepan, heat the butter or ghee over medium heat. Once it is melted, add the steel-cut oats. Stir for a few minutes until a toasty aroma begins to develop.
2. Pour in 3 cups of filtered water and add the salt; bring to a boil.
3. Cover, remove from heat, and leave overnight. (If you aren't preparing this the night before, continue cooking for 20–25 minutes, stirring occasionally.)
4. In the morning, prepare the fruit: Slice the fruit and sauté in a medium frying pan with the coconut oil, 2 tablespoons maple syrup, vanilla, and cardamom. Continue sautéing for a few minutes until the mixture is soft and fragrant. Set aside.
5. If you prepared the oats overnight, bring the oats back to a simmer and add the remaining ¼ tablespoon maple syrup and coconut cream. Stir thoroughly. Once warmed through, serve with the fruit and top with pumpkin seeds.

Other combinations to try: banana, almond butter, cacao nibs, and dates or berries, cinnamon, coconut granola, and hemp hearts.

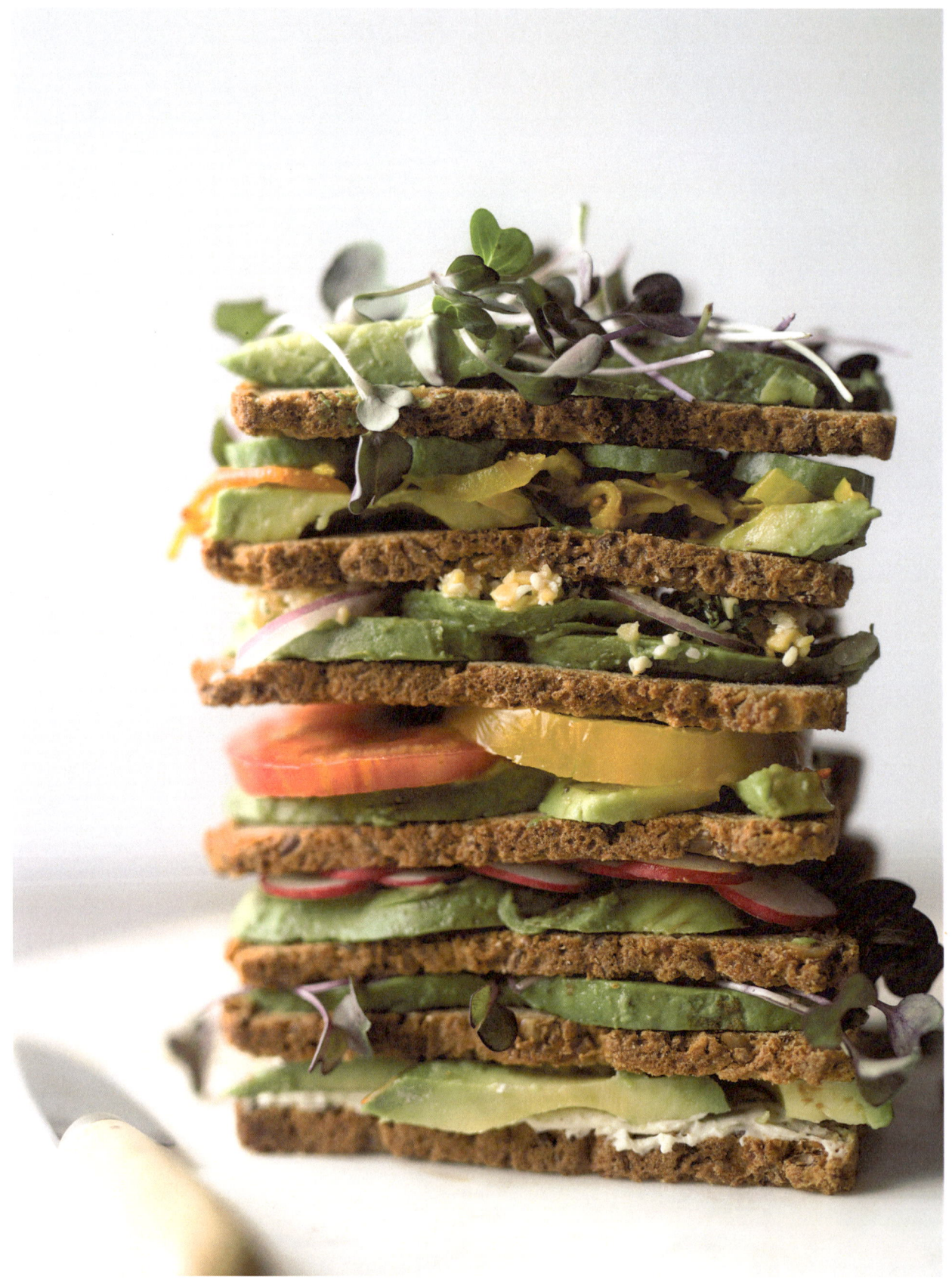

AVOCADO TOAST

FOUR WAYS

Trendy yet humble, this breakfast caters perfectly to early-pregnancy cravings and needs. Protein, whole-grain complex carbs, and healthy fats are the ideal ingredients for a happy tummy and growing baby. Avocado is an amazing source of monounsaturated fats that supports good heart health and blood glucose levels. Avocado also provides a great dose of vitamin B6, which helps with morning sickness.

The possibilities are endless! Rather than a true "recipe," what follows is more an inspiration for various combinations. Here are some of our favourite combos—just serve them on two toasted slices of sourdough or whole rye bread such as Mestemacher.

INGREDIENTS

The Cali:
1 avocado
1 free range, organic egg, poached or boiled
microgreens
2 radishes, thinly sliced
hemp hearts

The Gut Buster:
1 avocado
kimchi or beet kraut
pea shoots
crushed nuts and seeds

The Vegan:
1 avocado
cashew cheese to spread on bread
tomatoes, sliced and sprinkled with salt
everything bagel spice or za'atar seasoning
fresh basil or other fresh herbs

The Inferno:
1 avocado
1 free range, organic egg, poached or boiled
pickled onions
sesame seeds
gochujang or samba oelek to drizzle over the avocado or egg

DIRECTIONS

1. Prepare the flesh of the avocados by slicing, chopping, or mashing. Season with salt, fresh cracked pepper and lemon juice. Set aside.
2. Toast your bread and spread with grass-fed butter or vegan soy-free butter.
3. Place the avocados and remaining toppings on your toast, and enjoy!

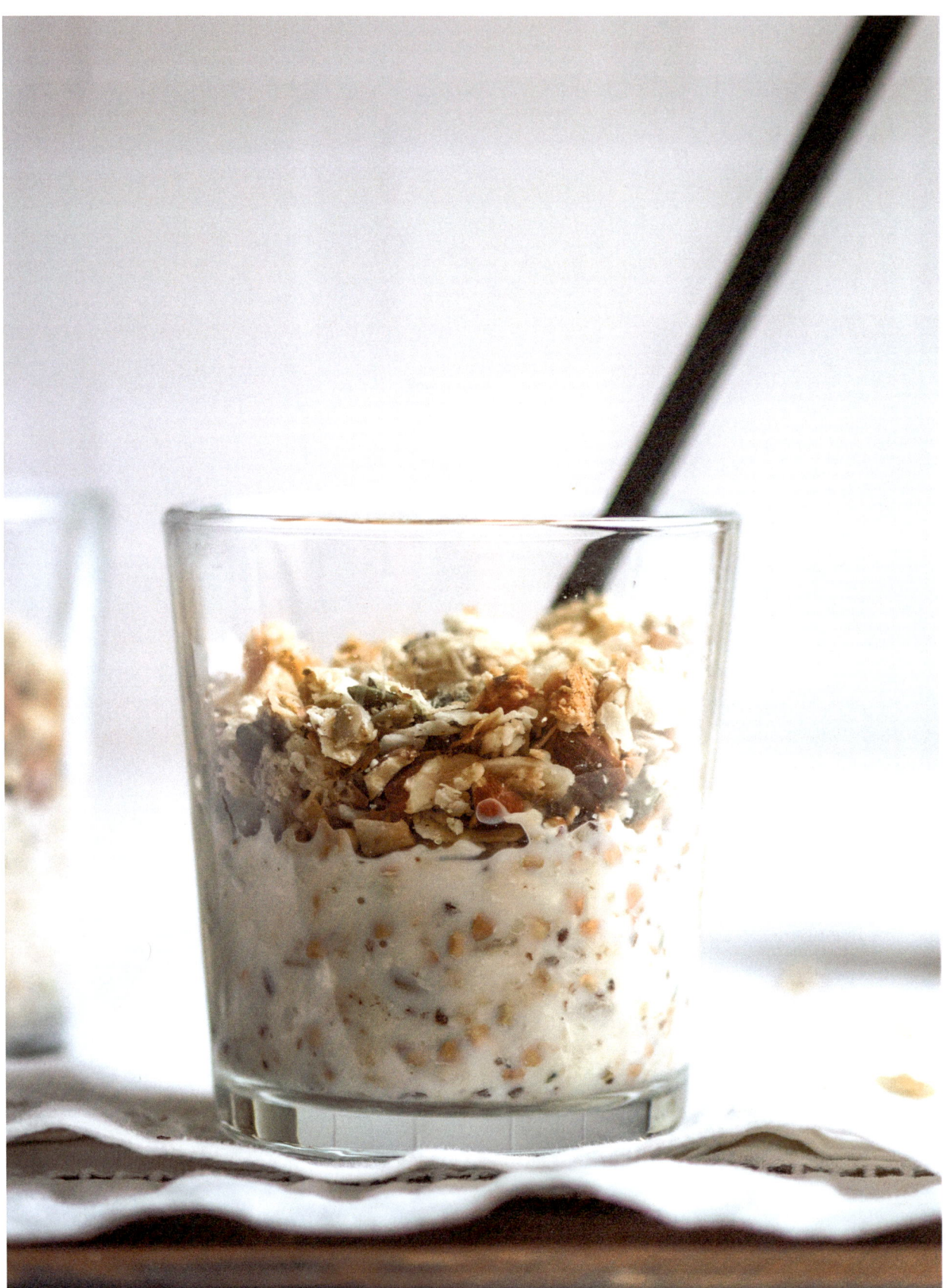

GINGER GRANOLA

WITH COCONUT AND SLICED ALMONDS

"Morning" sickness can actually strike anytime of the day. The nausea of early pregnancy is often due to pregnancy hormones, low blood glucose, slowed digestion, and other physiological changes. If you struggle with nausea in the morning, try popping a bowl of this granola on your bedside table and eating a bit right upon waking. It will help calm your stomach and balance blood glucose levels before you even get out of bed.

INGREDIENTS | SERVES 4

- 1 ½ cups rolled oats
- 1 ½ cups large-flake, unsweetened coconut
- ½ cup walnuts
- ½ cup sliced almonds
- ½ cup pumpkin seeds
- ⅔ cup coconut oil
- ⅓ cup maple syrup
- 1 teaspoon vanilla extract
- 2–4 teaspoons ginger powder (depending on how spicy you like it)
- ½ teaspoon sea salt
- ½–1 cup candied ginger, chopped (optional—for a real anti-nausea bang!)

DIRECTIONS | PREHEAT THE OVEN TO 350° F

1. Line a baking sheet with parchment paper.
2. In a bowl, mix together the rolled oats, unsweetened coconut, walnuts, almonds, and pumpkin seeds. Set aside.
3. Place the coconut oil in a small oven-safe dish and melt in the oven. Carefully remove and add maple syrup, vanilla, ginger powder, and salt. Stir to combine.
4. Add the wet ingredients to the bowl of dry ingredients and mix thoroughly.
5. Spread the mixture over the parchment paper.
6. Bake at 350° for 20 minutes, stirring every 4–5 minutes for the first 15 minutes. Let it bake untouched for the last 5 minutes.
7. Remove from the oven and let cool. Add in the chopped candied ginger, if using. Can be stored in an airtight container at room temperature for up to 1 week.

QUICK TIP: Can't stomach making breakfast in the morning? Prepare breakfast foods and other meals at a time of the day when you are feeling the best.

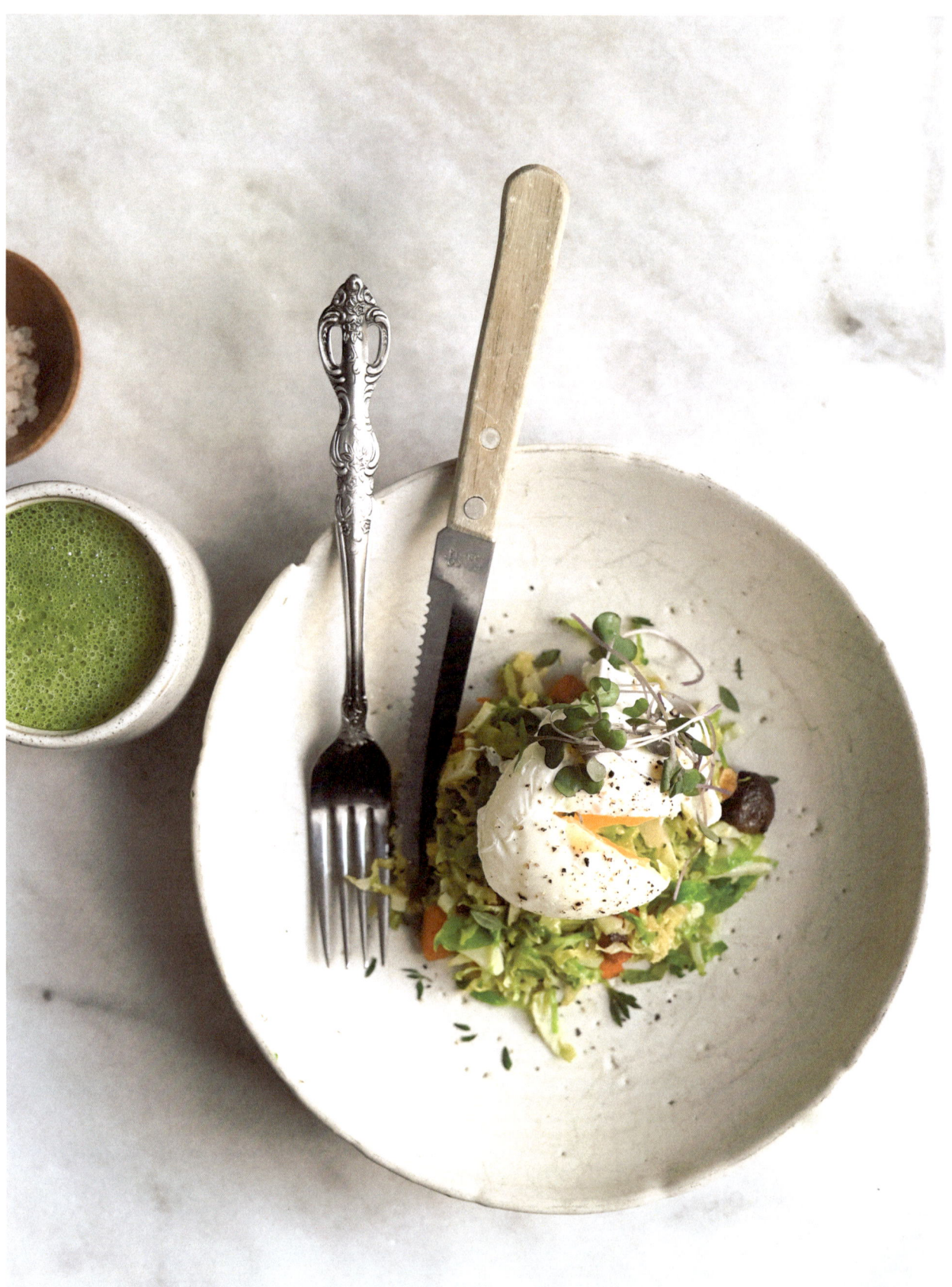

BRUSSELS SPROUT HASH

WITH SWEET POTATOES AND POACHED EGGS

Eggs are a great natural source of choline and biotin, essential vitamins for your diet in the first trimester. Choline, like folic acid and other B vitamins, plays a role in a healthy neural-tube and the neurological system in the fetus. Maternal intake during pregnancy can also have a positive effect on baby's cognition, memory, and neurological development into childhood.

INGREDIENTS | SERVES 2

Hash:
2 tablespoons coconut oil, divided
½ cup chopped cremini mushrooms
¼ cup diced onions
4 sprigs of thyme
3 sage leaves, minced
½ teaspoon sea salt, divided
1 ½ cups cubed sweet potatoes (½ inch chunks)
1 ½ cups Brussels sprouts, ends trimmed off, outer leaves removed, thinly sliced

Poached eggs:
2 free range, organic eggs
1 tablespoon white vinegar
½ teaspoon sea salt

DIRECTIONS

1. In a large cast-iron skillet or frying pan, heat 1 tablespoon of coconut oil over medium-low heat and add mushrooms, onions, thyme, sage, and ¼ teaspoon of salt. Sauté for 3–4 minutes or until mushrooms have softened, adding additional oil if they begin to stick.

2. Add the sweet potatoes, the other ¼ teaspoon of salt, and the last tablespoon of coconut oil. Sauté for another 8–10 minutes until the sweet potatoes are cooked through.

3. While the sweet potatoes are cooking, prepare the eggs: fill a large saucepan with water to about 4 inches. Add the vinegar and salt and bring to a low boil. Crack an egg in a very small bowl and set aside. If the water is at a rapid boil, turn down so there are few or no bubbles. With a spoon, swirl the water in the saucepan to create a whirlpool. Place the bowl close to the water and gently pour your egg into the middle of the whirlpool. Let the egg cook for 6–7 minutes. Remove with a slotted spoon and place on a paper towel. Repeat with the other egg.

4. Once the sweet potatoes have softened in the skillet, add the sliced Brussels sprouts and sauté for another 2–3 minutes, or until the sprouts have softened.

5. Remove the thyme sprigs and divide the hash between 2 plates and top with poached eggs. Season with salt and pepper.

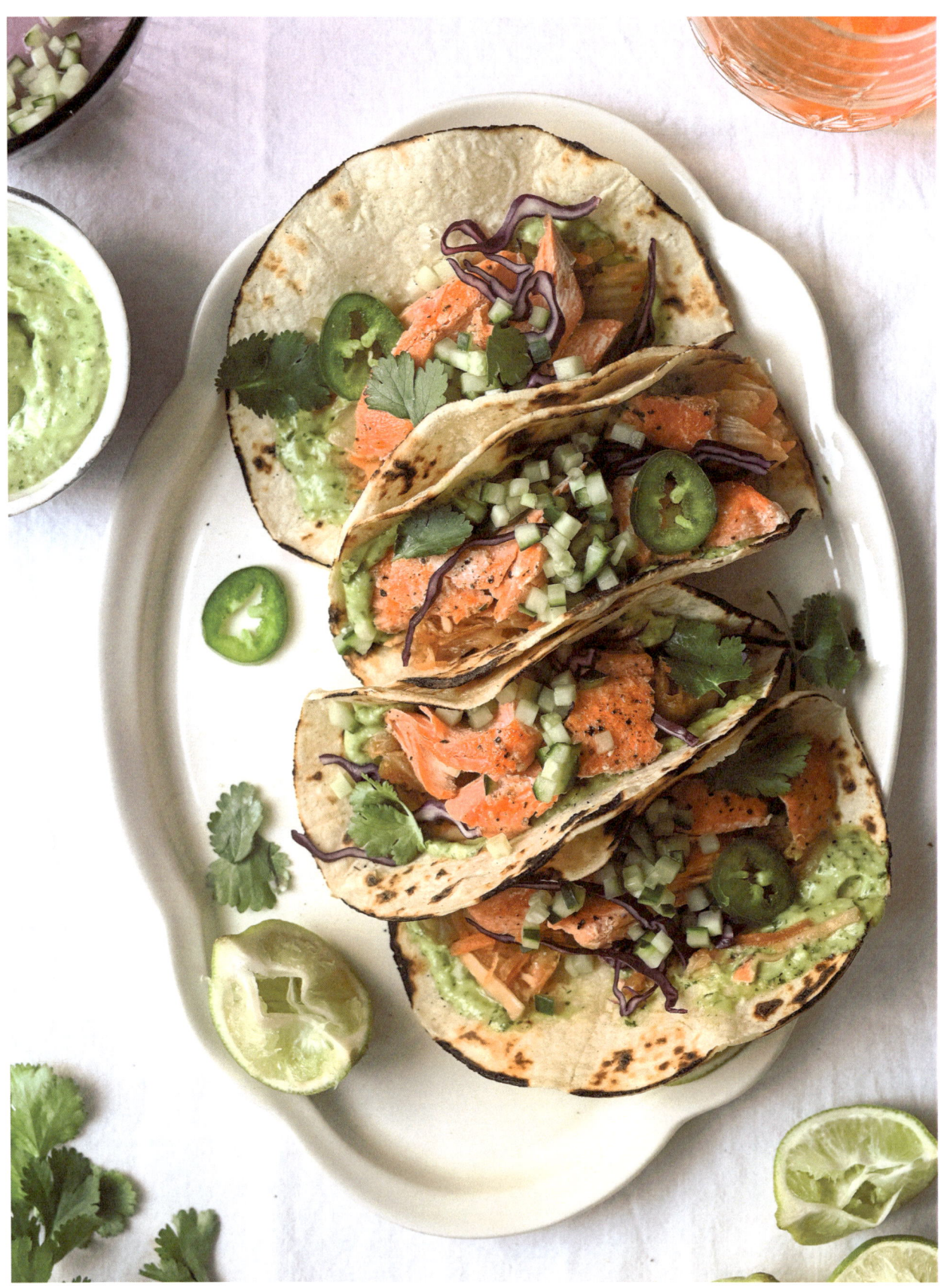

SALMON AND KIMCHI TACOS

WITH CITRUS AVOCADO CREMA

Salmon and other fatty fish are rich sources of omega-3 essential fatty acids, which are critical for early brain and eye development. Opt for wild salmon when possible, as studies show that farmed salmon has higher levels of toxins than wild salmon. Fermented foods, such as yogourt, kimchi, sauerkraut, kombucha, and kefir, are tasty ways to increase your probiotic intake. Probiotics are the commensal or "good" bacteria that live in our guts and contribute to healthy digestive and immune systems. These yummy tacos blend abundant nutrition and varying flavour profiles, making them a family favourite for the first trimester.

INGREDIENTS | SERVES 2

Citrus avocado crema:
1 medium avocado
¼ cup basil, tightly packed
2 tablespoons fresh orange juice
2 tablespoons fresh lemon juice
½ teaspoon freshly minced garlic
2 tablespoons extra-virgin olive oil

Tacos:
340 grams wild sockeye salmon fillets (12 ounces)
¼ teaspoon sea salt
freshly cracked pepper
½ fresh lemon
1 tablespoon coconut oil
4 corn, cassava, or whole grain tortillas
1 cup kimchi or kraut of your choice, drained of juice
½ cup shaved red cabbage
¼ cup finely diced cucumber
Fresh cilantro and sliced jalapeños to garnish (optional)

DIRECTIONS | PREHEAT OVEN TO 450° F

1. In a food processor, combine all crema ingredients and purée until smooth. Set aside.
2. Arrange the salmon fillets on a plate and season with ¼ teaspoon salt, freshly cracked pepper and the juice from the half lemon.
3. In a large cast-iron skillet or ovenproof frying pan, heat the coconut oil over medium heat. When the pan is hot, add the salmon, skin side down, and cover. Cook for 4 minutes until the skin is nice and crispy. Move the salmon around the pan to ensure it isn't sticking. (Please be careful of the hot oil! I held a lid between the pan and myself and wore an oven mitt.)
4. Transfer the skillet with the salmon to the oven and bake at 450° for another 4–5 minutes for medium-moist, or until the salmon is opaque in the centre. Cooking time will depend on the thickness of the fish and the desired level of doneness, so please check after approximately 4 minutes.
5. Remove from the oven and set aside.
6. Warm your corn tortillas in the oven, or heat them on top of a stove grate until lightly charred. Transfer to a plate.
7. Assemble the tacos: Place shaved red cabbage and kimchi on the tacos, then add chunks of salmon. Drizzle over the crema and top with the cucumber, cilantro, and jalapeños.

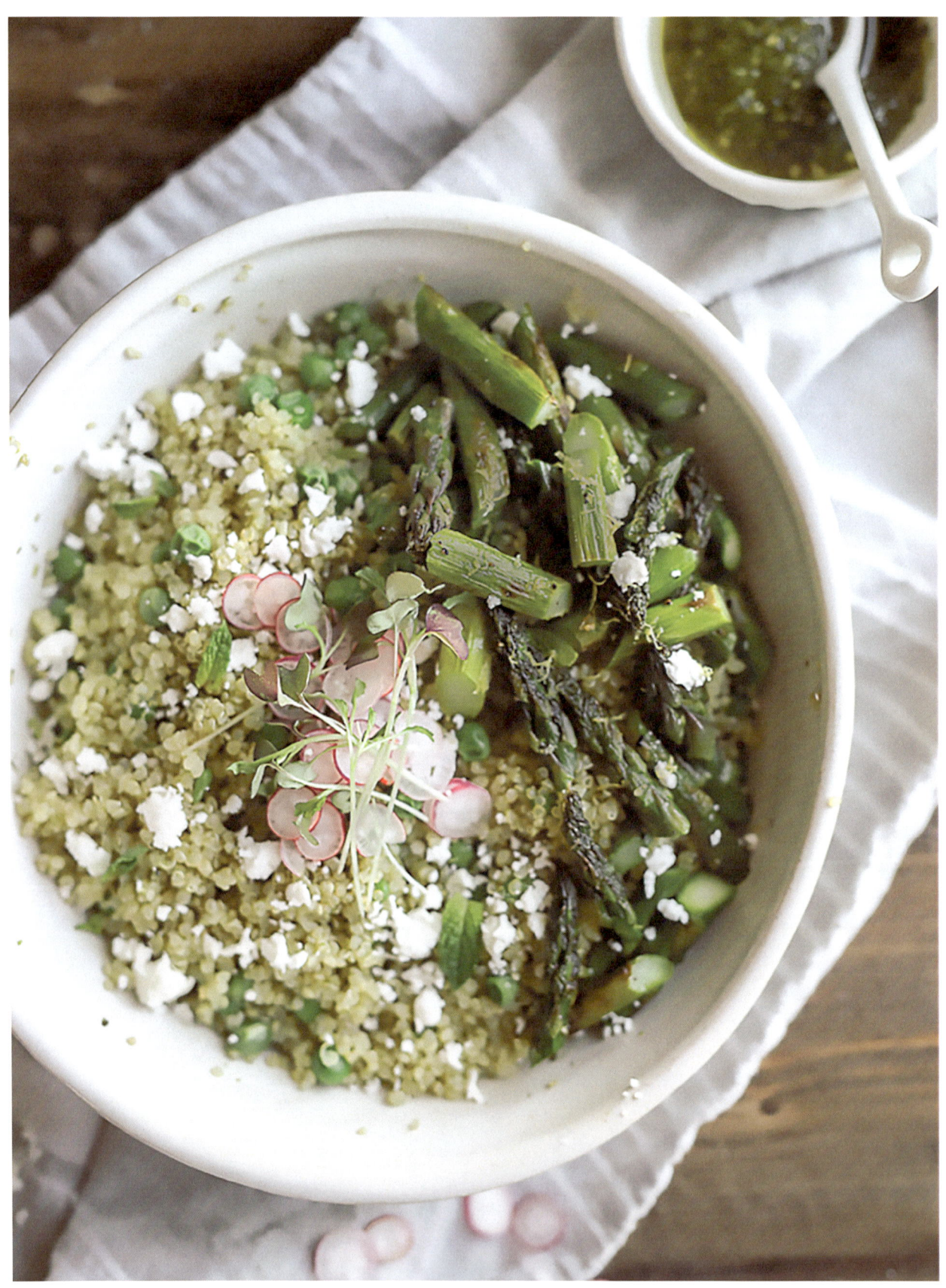

SPRING QUINOA SALAD

WITH MINT AND SWISS CHARD PESTO

Quinoa is a beautiful balance of protein, carbohydrates, and fat, with micronutrients that rival a good multivitamin. Although it can look and feel like a fluffy starch, quinoa is technically a seed and a "complete" protein, providing all nine essential protein building blocks, so it's an ideal option for vegans or expectant mamas who are turned off of meat. Our need for protein increases dramatically during pregnancy, so finding ways to boost our intake is important. This quinoa bowl is the perfect lunch for busy workdays or days spent chasing around a toddler. Prep the pesto a day or two in advance, and you are one step closer!

INGREDIENTS | SERVES 2 AS MAIN COURSE

Quinoa Salad:

1 pint cherry tomatoes, halved
1 teaspoon sea salt, divided
1 cup quinoa, thoroughly rinsed
½ cup spring peas
1 tablespoon coconut oil
1 bunch asparagus, woody ends trimmed
Pepper to taste
Zest of ½ lemon, lemon reserved
½ cup crumbled sheep feta cheese
1 ½ tablespoons chopped fresh mint
2 small radishes, very thinly sliced, for garnish (optional)
Microgreens for garnish (optional)

Pesto:

¼ cup + 2 tablespoons pumpkin seeds
2 small garlic cloves
½ cup fresh mint leaves
½ cup tightly packed fresh basil
2 large Swiss chard leaves, ribs and stems removed, chopped
3 tablespoons lemon juice
1 teaspoon sea salt
2 teaspoon good quality spirulina, optional
½ cup extra-virgin olive oil, hempseed oil, or flaxseed oil

DIRECTIONS

1. Place the cherry tomatoes in a large bowl. Sprinkle with ¼ teaspoon sea salt and stir to coat.

2. In a medium saucepan, bring 2 cups of water plus ¼ teaspoon sea salt to a boil. Add the quinoa. Cover, reduce heat to low, and simmer for 15 minutes. Remove from the heat and let stand for 5 minutes, covered. Fluff with a fork and transfer to the tomato bowl.

3. While the quinoa cooks, make the pesto: In a food processor, pulse pumpkin seeds until they resemble bits. Add garlic and pulse again. Add mint, basil, Swiss chard, lemon juice, salt, and spirulina if using. Pulse until all ingredients are smooth and well combined. Stir in the oil. Add half the pesto to the quinoa and tomato mixture and stir gently.

4. Place the peas in the same saucepan you used to cook the quinoa, then add water to cover and ¼ teaspoon salt. Bring to a boil, cover, reduce heat to low, and simmer for 3 minutes. Strain the peas and add to the quinoa.

5. Heat a grill pan over medium-high heat. Add the coconut oil and asparagus and sprinkle with ¼ teaspoon salt and freshly cracked pepper. Toss to combine, and grill the asparagus for 5 minutes, turning it to avoid burning. (Reduce the heat or add more oil if they start to burn.) Remove from the grill pan, and cut the asparagus on the bias into 1-inch pieces. Sprinkle with the lemon zest, stir to coat, and add to the quinoa mixture.

6. Toss the quinoa and vegetable mixture with the feta cheese and mint. Mix in the remaining pesto and squeeze the reserved fresh lemon over the salad. Top with sliced radishes and microgreens.

Have leftover pesto?! Mix with cashew cream cheese to make a creamy pasta sauce!

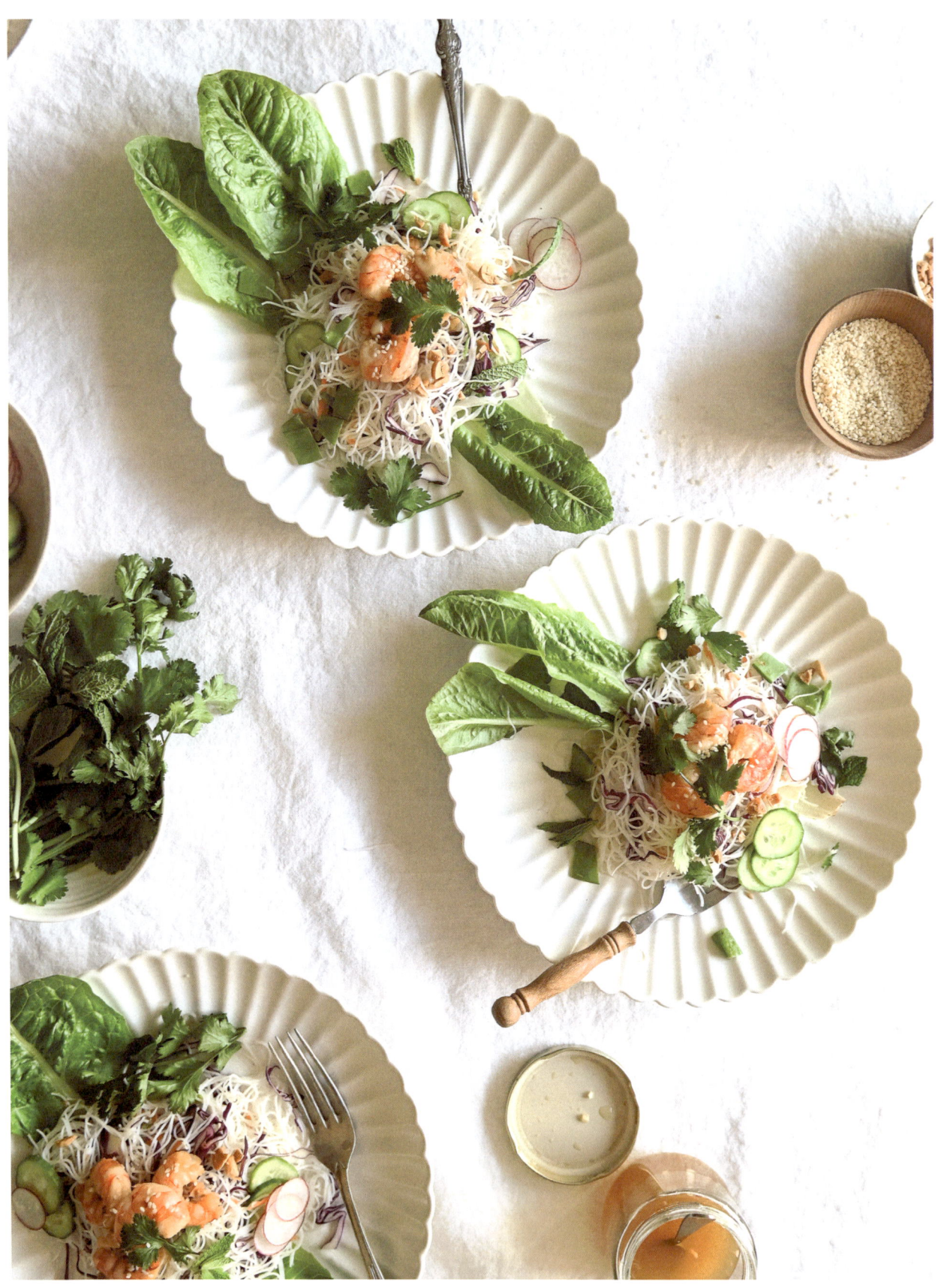

VERMICELLI NOODLE SALAD

WITH LEMONGRASS SHRIMP

This gorgeous salad will please the senses as well as the taste buds. It is fresh, delicious, and super versatile. You can switch up the vegetables with what you have on hand or pop the ingredients into rice wraps for an easy, grab-and-go lunch or snack. Light but nourishing, it's perfect for the first-trimester appetite—especially on hot summer days.

INGREDIENTS | SERVES 4

Lemongrass shrimp:
2 teaspoons lemongrass paste
2 teaspoons lime juice
1 tablespoon extra-virgin olive oil
1 teaspoon freshly minced garlic
¾ tablespoon organic cane sugar
¾ tablespoon fish sauce
2 pinches red pepper flakes
330 grams organic, raw, large shrimp, peeled, deveined, tails removed (12 ounces)

Salad:
220 grams snap peas, sliced thin on the bias (8 ounces)
½ English cucumber, chopped or cut julienne
¼ head red cabbage, shaved thin
2–3 radishes, sliced thin
½ cup each chopped fresh mint and basil
200 grams brown-rice vermicelli noodles (7 ounces)
½ a head of romaine lettuce

Dressing:
¼ cup water
¼ cup lime juice
4 ½ teaspoons freshly minced garlic
3 tablespoons fish sauce
3 tablespoons pasteurized honey warmed until thin and easily pourable
2 tablespoons rice vinegar
1–2 pinches red chili flakes (optional)

DIRECTIONS

1. In a jar with a tight-fitting lid, combine all the dressing ingredients and shake vigorously. Set aside.
2. In a large baking dish or bowl, combine all the lemongrass shrimp ingredients except the shrimp and whisk thoroughly to combine. Add the raw shrimp and let the combination sit while you prepare the rest of the salad.
3. Cook noodles per package instructions. Drain, set aside, and let cool slightly.
4. Heat a frying pan over low-medium heat. Add the shrimp and all the marinade. Poach the shrimp in the marinade until they are cooked through, about 3–4 minutes, stirring occasionally. Remove from the heat, drain the liquid, and set aside.
5. Assemble your bowls! Place a few romaine lettuce leaves in a bowl, add your desired amount of noodles, drizzle a bit of dressing on top, pile on your veg and a few shrimp, and finish with more dressing and fresh herbs.

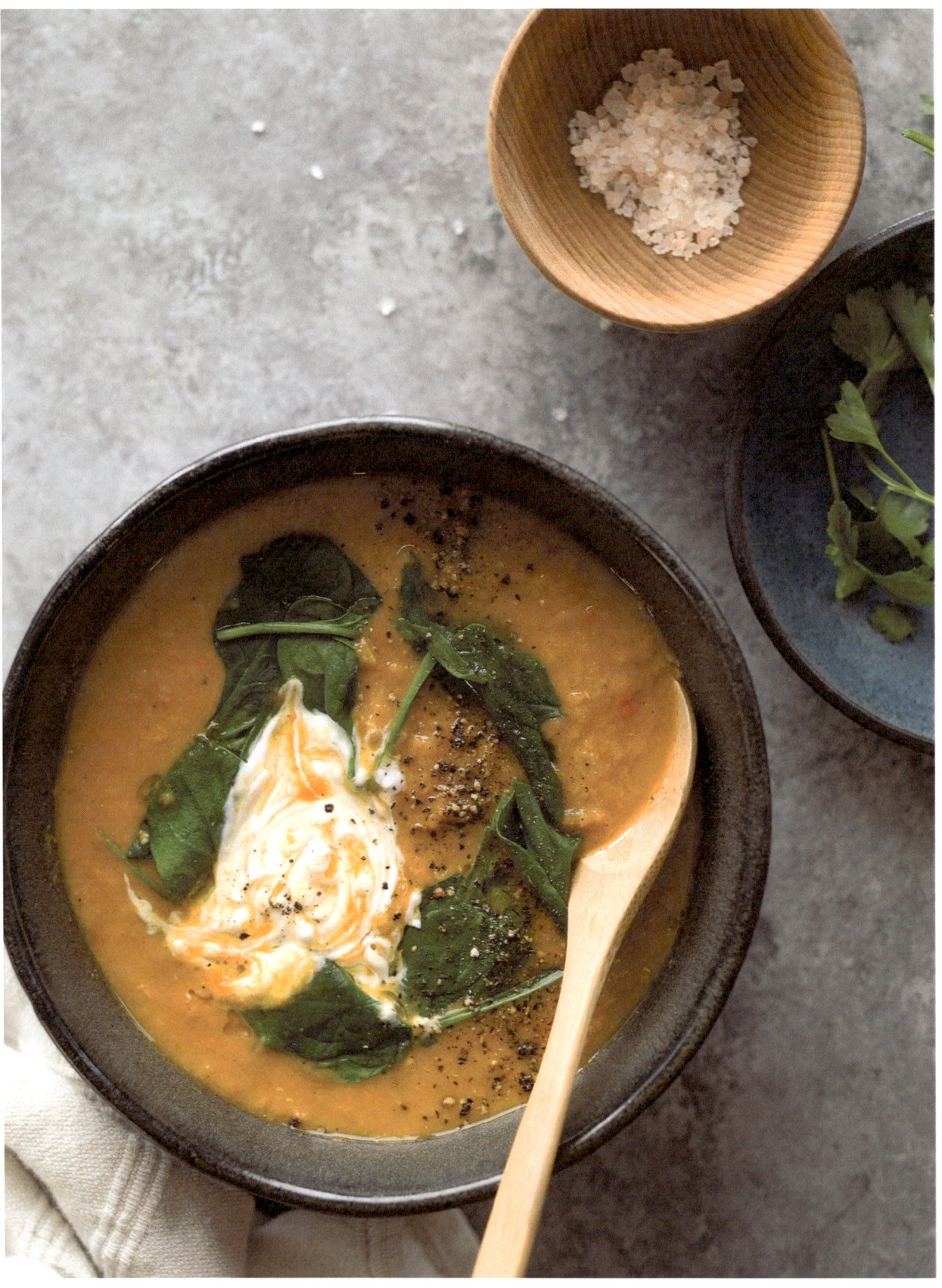

LENTIL AND SPINACH DAL

WITH CAULIFLOWER "RICE"

Lentils and spinach: the folic acid dynamic duo! Folic acid is essential not only for baby's neural tube development but also for a pregnant mama's mental health, energy, and digestion. Go over and above your daily prenatal vitamin by adding spinach and other leafy greens to soups, stews, eggs, and smoothies.

INGREDIENTS | SERVES 4

1 small yellow onion, diced
5 cloves garlic, minced
4 teaspoons freshly grated ginger
1 ½ tablespoons coconut oil
2 Roma tomatoes, cut into chunks (about 1 ½ cups)
3/4 cup canned, full-fat coconut milk
2–3 cups vegetable stock or bone broth
1 cup red lentils
1 ½ teaspoons cumin
¾ teaspoon turmeric
1 teaspoon garam masala
½ teaspoon sea salt
3 cups fresh spinach leaves

Cauliflower rice:
1 ½ cups chopped cauliflower
½ teaspoon sea salt
Freshly cracked pepper
½ tablespoon extra-virgin olive oil

Honey mint yogourt:
½ cup plain or coconut yogourt
2 tablespoons chopped mint
1 tablespoon pasteurized honey

DIRECTIONS

1. In a large skillet with a lid, sauté the onions, garlic, and ginger with the coconut oil over medium heat for 6–7 minutes until onions are soft but not brown and aromatics are fragrant. Stir frequently to avoid it sticking to the bottom. Add more coconut oil if needed.
2. Add tomatoes and let them reduce for 3–4 minutes.
3. Add coconut milk, 2 cups of stock, lentils, cumin, turmeric, garam masala, and salt. Reduce heat to low and simmer, covered, for 25 minutes. You may need to add more stock if it becomes dry before the lentils are cooked through.
4. While the lentils are simmering, make the cauliflower rice: In a food processor, pulse 1 ½ cups of chopped cauliflower until it is about the consistency of rice. (Pulse, please. Do not hold the button down or you will have cauliflower purée!) Place the cauliflower rice in a large frying pan on the stove over medium heat. Sprinkle with ½ teaspoon of salt, freshly cracked pepper, and ½ tablespoon of extra-virgin olive oil. Stir to combine and cook over medium heat for 7–8 minutes, stirring frequently. Taste and add more salt and pepper if needed. Remove from the heat and set aside.
5. To make the honey-mint yogourt, stir together all yogourt ingredients. Set aside.
6. Once the lentils are soft, add 3 cups of fresh spinach and cover the skillet again. Let the spinach steam until wilted, then stir.
7. Serve dal over cauliflower rice and top with honey-mint yogourt.

A root with amazing first-trimester benefits, ginger (Zingiber officinale) is an anti-nauseant, anti-emetic (prevents vomiting), and antioxidant. It also has a calming effect on the entire gastrointestinal system.

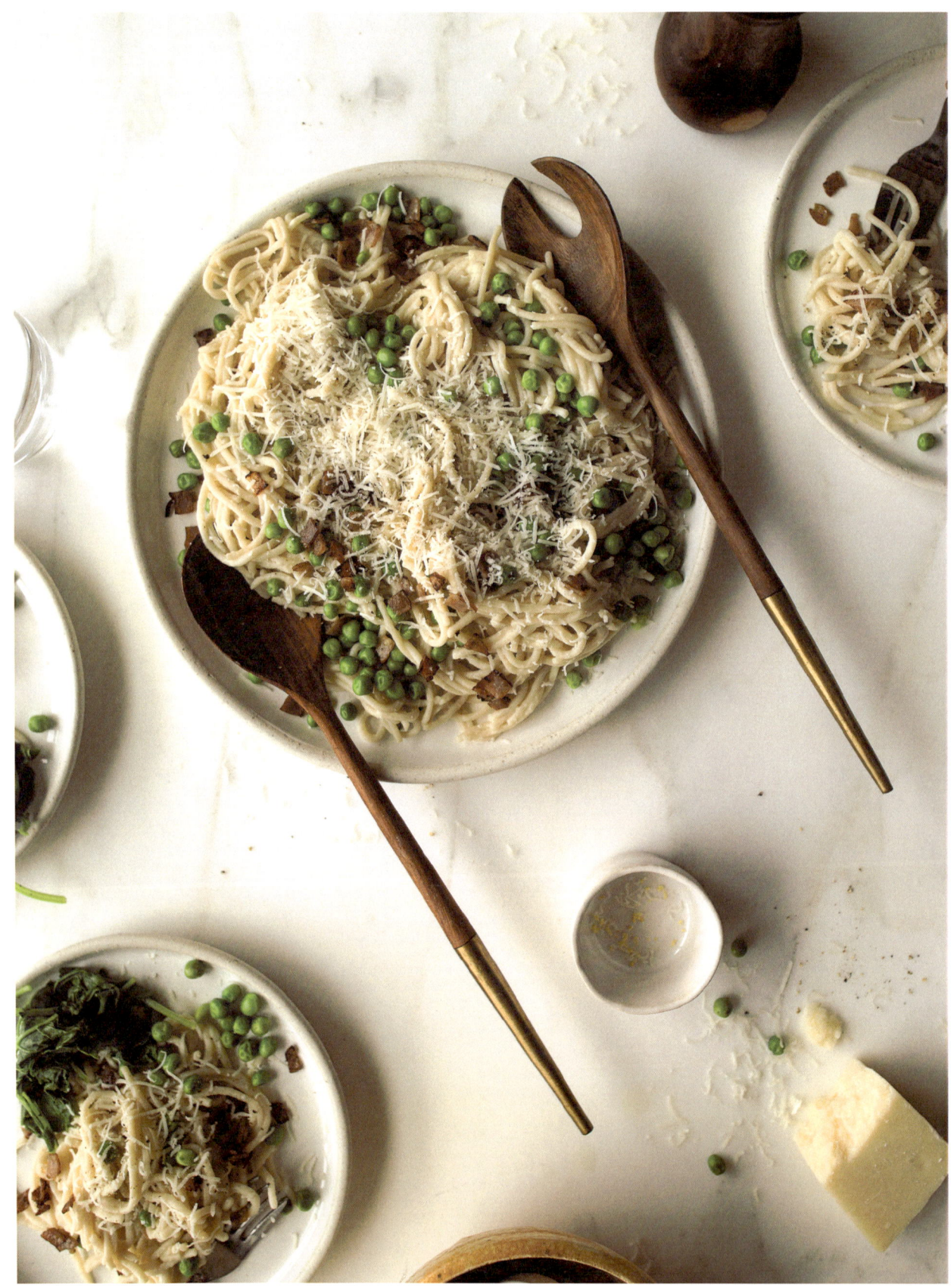

CAULIFLOWER CARBONARA

WITH PEAS AND PANCETTA

The trick of hiding vegetables is an open secret among all seasoned mamas, especially with our volatile toddlers. It comes in handy on the days when you can't stomach the thought of eating vegetables and are getting those oh-so-familiar carb cravings. Provide key nutrients like fibre, vitamin B6, vitamin C, and magnesium with this creamy carbonara—while even the pickiest eaters are none the wiser!

INGREDIENTS | SERVES 4

1 medium head of cauliflower (or ½ a large head), cut into small chunks—approximately 6 cups chopped

5 cups chicken or vegetable stock

2 tablespoons coconut oil, ghee, or butter

2 tablespoons freshly minced garlic

2 shallots, minced

1 ½ tablespoons lemon juice

1 ¼ tablespoons nutritional yeast

1 tablespoon extra-virgin olive oil

1 teaspoon sea salt

Pepper to taste

Whole-grain or brown-rice spaghetti or linguine

4 strips turkey bacon, pancetta, or tempeh, cut into cubes or small squares

1 cup peas

Shredded Parmesan, to taste (optional)

DIRECTIONS

1. Place cauliflower chunks in a large saucepan. Add stock, ensuring it coveres the cauliflower. If not, add more until the cauliflower is fully submerged. Simmer over medium-low heat for about 15 minutes or until cauliflower is tender. Reserve a few tablespoons of the cooking liquid.

2. While the cauliflower is cooking, sauté the garlic and shallots in 2 tablespoons of oil or butter in a frying pan over low heat for approximately 5 minutes, stirring frequently, until shallots are translucent but not brown. Set aside.

3. Once the cauliflower is cooked through and soft, used a slotted spoon to transfer to a blender, being careful not to get too much liquid in the blender.

4. Add the cooked onions and garlic, lemon juice, nutritional yeast, 1 tablespoon of extra-virgin olive oil, salt, and pepper to the blender. Blend until creamy. If it is too thick, add the cauliflower cooking liquid a spoonful at a time until the sauce reaches your desired consistency. Taste, and season with more salt if needed. Set aside.

5. Cook pasta in heavily salted water according to package directions. Add peas to the pasta water during the last 3 minutes of cooking time.

6. While the pasta is cooking, fry up the turkey bacon, pancetta, or tempeh in the same pan you used for the onions and garlic. Set aside.

7. When the pasta and peas are done, drain and return them to the empty saucepan. Toss the pasta and peas with the sauce: start with ⅔ of the sauce and add more according to your preference. Add turkey bacon, pancetta, or tempeh. Garnish with shredded Parmesan if you like.

This sauce also works great with salmon and asparagus instead of bacon!

Sunchokes can be hard to find, but they a great source of prebiotics for the gut. If you can find them, substitute half the cauliflower with peeled and chopped sunchokes.

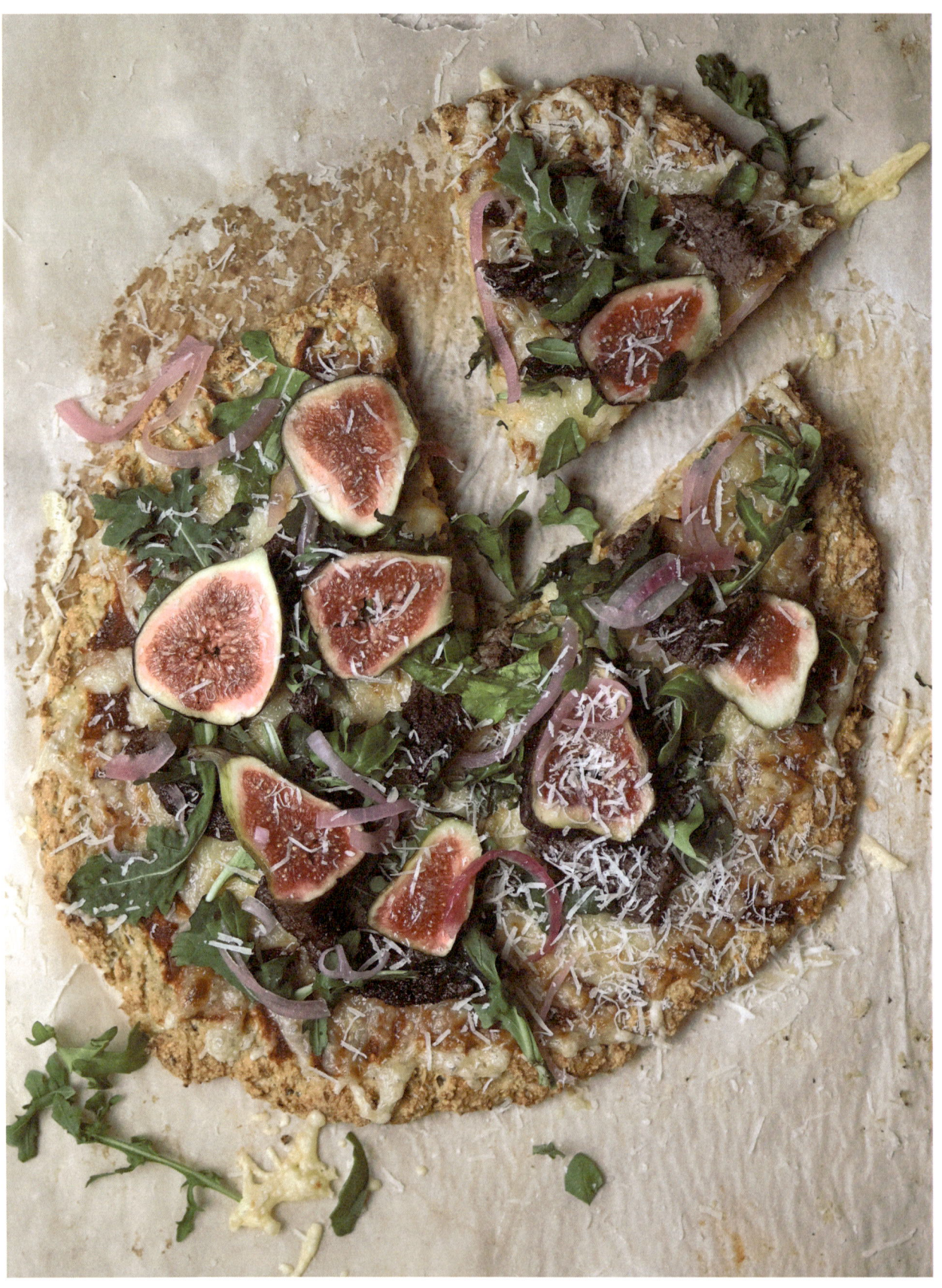

VEGGIE CRUST PIZZA

WITH BISON, FIGS, AND ARUGULA

A sweet and tangy twist on your typical pizza night. Figs are rich in vitamin A, which is necessary for baby's organ development, as well as fibre and antioxidants. Adding a wild game meat to this recipe ups the mineral content and nutritional profile. A tangy or spicy barbecue sauce is a great option for this pizza; it goes well with the peppery arugula and sweet figs! But always watch the sugar content in condiments like barbecue sauce.

INGREDIENTS | YIELDS 2 SMALL PIZZAS

Cauliflower crust:

5 cups grated or riced cauliflower

1 cup grated Parmesan, plus more for garnish

1 small free range, organic egg

2 teaspoons Italian seasoning

1 teaspoon onion powder

1 teaspoon garlic powder

¼ teaspoon sea salt

¼ teaspoon pepper

Pizza toppings:

1–2 tablespoons coconut oil

170 grams bison cut into stir-fry pieces or thin strips (6 ounces)

½ teaspoon sea salt

Organic, all-natural barbecue sauce

1–1 ½ cups shredded mozzarella or vegan mozzarella

¼ cup thinly sliced red onions or pickled red onions

8 fresh figs, halved, or dried figs softened in hot water with hard stems removed

½ cup arugula

DIRECTIONS | PREHEAT OVEN TO 400° F

1. Line a baking sheet with parchment paper.
2. In a small saucepan, combine cauliflower rice, a large pinch of salt, and just enough water to steam (about ½ inch of water in the bottom of the saucepan). Bring to a simmer and let the cauliflower steam, covered, for 4 minutes. Strain in a mesh sieve.
3. Transfer the strained cauliflower rice to a cheesecloth or nut-milk bag, and squeeze out all the liquid. You will be amazed at all the liquid that comes out! Keep squeezing gently until the cauliflower is almost dry. Transfer to a medium bowl and add Parmesan, 2 tablespoons beaten egg, Italian seasoning, onion powder, garlic powder, salt, and pepper. Mix well with your hands until fully combined.
4. Transfer the mixture to the parchment-lined baking sheet and mould into two circles or rectangles. You can make the crust thin or thick—a thick crust will obviously result in a smaller pizza. Bake at 400° for 30 minutes or until pizza crust is browned. If you don't cook it long enough, it will be rubbery instead of crisp.
5. While the pizzas are baking, cook the bison: In a cast-iron skillet, heat the coconut oil over medium heat. Add the sirloin pieces and sprinkle with ½ teaspoon of salt. Cook until the outside is browned, about 3 minutes.
6. When the crusts are done, remove from the oven and top with the barbecue sauce, mozzarella, and raw red onions (if using). Bake at 400° until the cheese is melted, brown, and bubbly, about 10 minutes. (Vegan mozzarella will not brown.)
7. Remove the pizzas from the oven and top with bison, arugula, pickled onions (if using), figs, and more fresh Parmesan.

Cooking food in a cast-iron skillet actually fortifies the food with iron. It is a great chemical-free alternative to non-stick cookware. So, when possible, opt for cast iron!

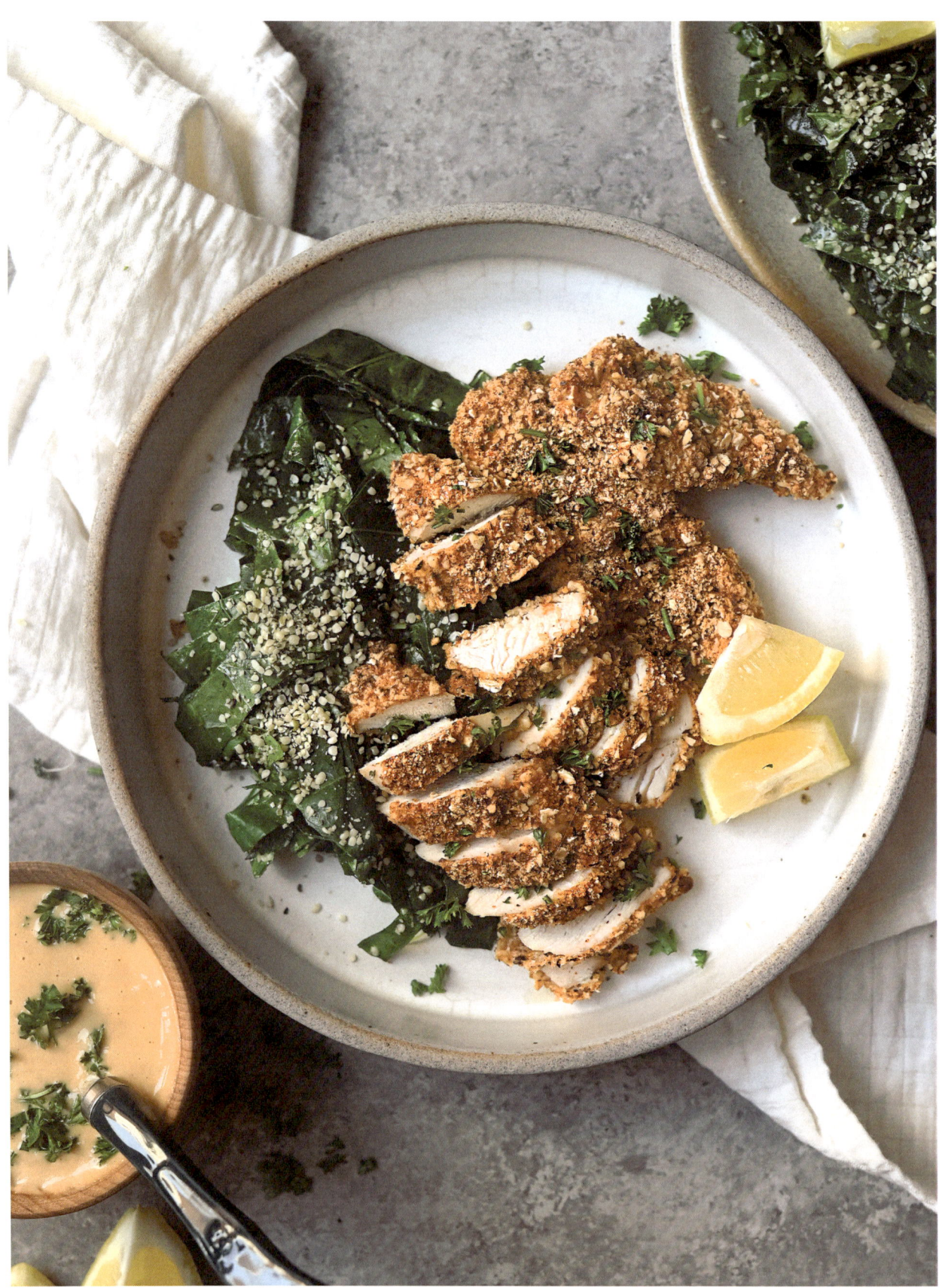

HAZELNUT-CRUSTED CHICKEN

WITH MISO LEMON COLLARD GREENS

This recipe is crispy and satisfying for parents and small fingers alike. Dark meat contains more zinc, iron, and vitamins B6 and B12 than white meat, so rotate more chicken thighs into your routine. Vitamin B12 deficiency is common during pregnancy, but B12 is essential to neurological development, red blood cell production, and energy for Mama. All the more reason to keep up with your B12!

INGREDIENTS | SERVES 4

Hazelnut-Crusted chicken:

450 grams boneless, skinless chicken thighs, excess fat removed, sliced into strips (1 pound)

¾ cup nuts, such as hazelnuts, cashews, or almonds

½ cup plus 1 tablespoon rolled oats

3 teaspoons onion powder

1 ½ teaspoons paprika

1 ½ teaspoons garlic powder

¼ plus ⅛ teaspoon cayenne pepper

1 ½ teaspoons sea salt

¾ teaspoon pepper

3 free range, organic eggs

Miso lemon collard greens:

3 tablespoons fresh lemon juice

3 tablespoons white miso paste

3 tablespoons flaxseed oil

2 bunches of collard greens

2 tablespoons of coconut oil

2 garlic cloves, minced

¼ teaspoon sea salt

3 tablespoons hemp hearts

2 tablespoons coconut flakes

This is a great recipe to use for "fish sticks" as well! Try tilapia, cod, halibut, or any wild white fish.

DIRECTIONS | PREHEAT OVEN TO 475° F

1. In a food processor, pulse nuts until crumbly and small. Add oats, and pulse again until oats are breadcrumb size.

2. Add onion powder, paprika, garlic powder, cayenne, sea salt, and pepper. Pulse to combine. Transfer the nut-and-oat mixture to a bowl and set aside.

3. In a separate bowl, beat the eggs and set aside.

4. Line a baking sheet with parchment paper. Arrange the baking sheet, breadcrumb mixture, egg mixture, and raw chicken in a row. Using a fork, dip one chicken finger into the egg mixture. Let the excess egg drip off the chicken, then transfer the chicken finger to the nut-and-oat mixture.

5. Using a separate fork, roll and toss the chicken finger in the nut-and-oat mixture, shaking off the excess before laying it on the baking sheet. Continue with remaining chicken fingers.

6. Place the baking sheet with chicken in the oven and bake at 475° for 15 minutes. Turn the chicken over then bake for another 5 minutes. Check the middle of the largest chicken finger before serving—there should be no pink!

7. While the chicken bakes, prepare the collard green dressing: In a jar with a tight-fitting lid, combine the lemon juice, miso paste, and flaxseed oil. Shake vigorously to combine, then set aside.

8. Make the collard greens: Wash and trim the greens, removing the stalks. Arrange the greens in a pile, roll them up, cut the roll into thin strips, and then cut once through the middle. Set aside.

9. In a cast-iron skillet over medium-low heat, warm the coconut oil and garlic for 30 seconds. Once the garlic becomes fragrant (but not burned), stir in the greens and sea salt. Turn the heat to medium and sauté the greens for 3–4 minutes, stirring frequently until they are soft and bright green. Remove from the heat and season with more sea salt and pepper if desired.

10. Drizzle with dressing and toss to combine. Sprinkle hemp hearts and coconut flakes on top and serve immediately with chicken fingers.

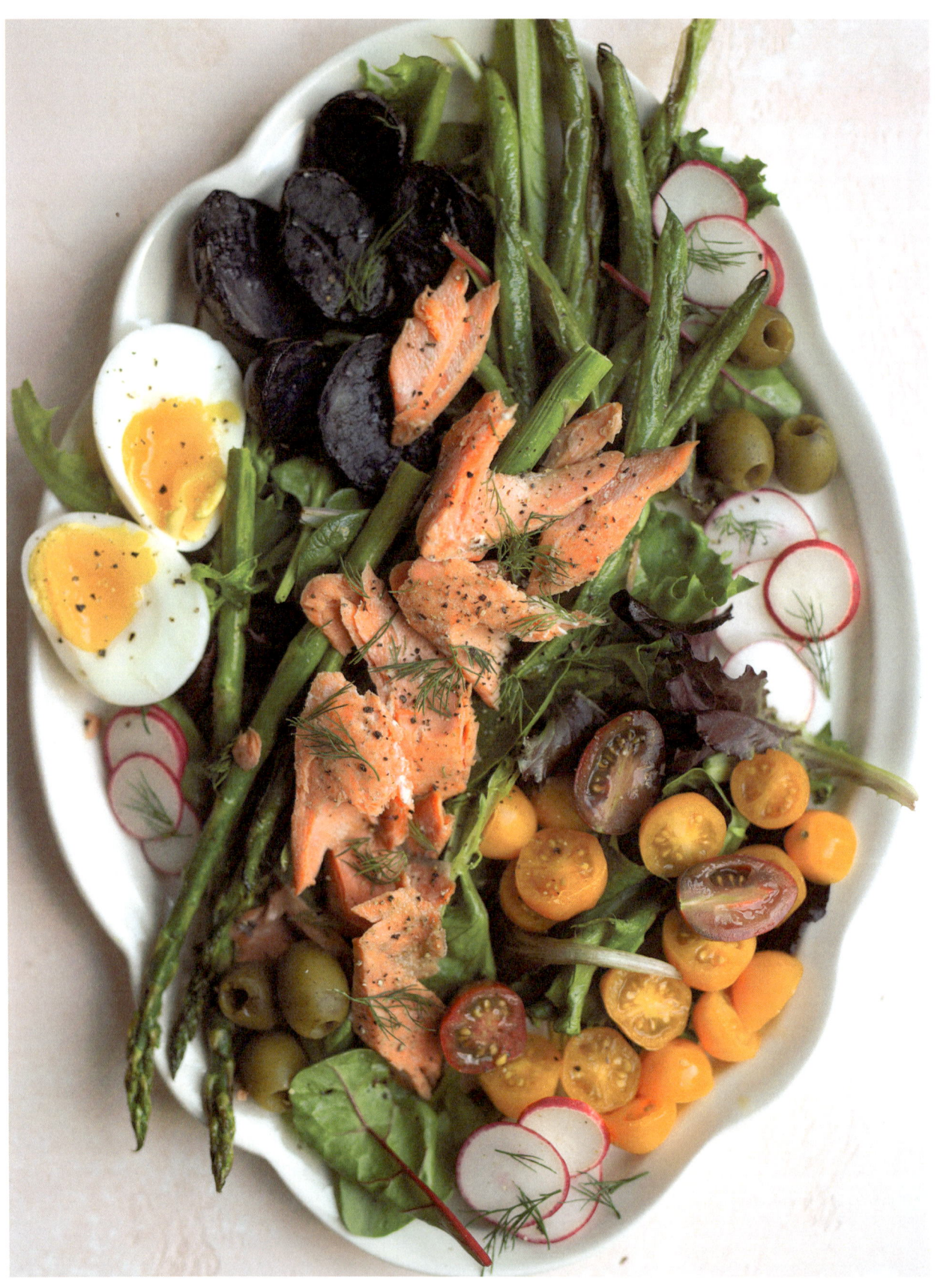

SALMON NIÇOISE SALAD

WITH POACHED SALMON AND TARRAGON VINAIGRETTE

This power-packed salad combines all the essential fatty acids your growing baby could need as well as protein from the eggs and salmon. Asparagus is a lesser-known pregnancy superfood that provides prebiotics and serves your daily need for folic acid, potassium, and vitamins A, C, and K.

Feel free to customize this low-maintenance meal. For example, in the summer, Anise likes to boil the potatoes and beans. In the winter, she likes to roast them. Anise also adds pickled onions and avocado if she has them handy. This gorgeous salad will surely satisfy on those low-energy evenings early in your pregnancy.

INGREDIENTS | SERVES 4

Dressing:

¼ cup extra-virgin olive, hemp, or flaxseed oil
3 tablespoons lemon juice
1 ½ teaspoons Dijon mustard
½ tablespoon apple cider vinegar
¾ teaspoon freshly minced garlic
1 teaspoon minced shallot
⅛ teaspoon sea salt
Freshly cracked pepper
2 teaspoons chopped fresh tarragon

Salmon:

1 whole wild sockeye salmon fillet, 450-680 grams (1-1 ½ pounds)
½ cup white wine
1 lemon, sliced
1 fennel bulb, sliced
1 leek, sliced
2 teaspoons sea salt, divided

Niçoise salad:

1 pint cherry tomatoes, halved
12 mini red or purple potatoes, halved or quartered
¾ teaspoon salt, divided
1 bunch asparagus, ends removed
220 grams haricots verts, ends trimmed (8 ounces)
4 free range, organic eggs
1 head butter lettuce
¼–½ cup castelvetrano olives
2 radishes, quartered or sliced
Salt and pepper, to taste

DIRECTIONS

1. Combine all dressing ingredients in a jar with a tight-fitting lid. Shake vigorously then set aside.

2. Place the tomatoes in a bowl and sprinkle with ¼ teaspoon salt and freshly cracked pepper. Toss to combine and set aside.

3. In a large deep skillet or even a high-sided baking tray that is safe for stovetop use, combine the wine, lemon, fennel, leek, 1 ½ teaspoons salt, and 6 cups water. Bring to a boil, reduce to a simmer, cover, and cook 8 minutes.

4. Season the salmon fillet with ½ teaspoon salt and slowly lower into the poaching liquid. Reduce to a gentle simmer, cover, and cook until the salmon flakes easily when pushed—about 5–7 minutes, depending on the thickness of the salmon. Carefully remove and set aside.

5. Put potatoes in a medium saucepan, cover them with water, and season with ½ teaspoon salt. Bring to a simmer over medium-high heat and cook until fork-tender, about 8–12 minutes, depending on the size of your potatoes. During the last 3 minutes of cooking, add the haricots verts and asparagus and cook until slightly tender and bright green. Drain all vegetables and set potatoes aside. Rinse asparagus and haricots verts in a colander under cold water. Set aside.

6. Fill the same saucepan with water and bring to a simmer. Place the eggs in the boiling water and simmer over medium-low heat for 7 ½–8 minutes. The cooking time for the eggs depends on your tolerance for runny yolks. Boil 7 minutes for a runny yolk, 7 ½ minutes for a "gummy" yolk, and 8 minutes for hard-boiled. Research has shown that runny yolks are safe to consume during pregnancy. Leaving the yolk a tad runny also makes the choline—a key nutrient for baby's brain health—more bio-available. However, you should cook based on your comfort level. Fill a bowl with ice water and set aside. Drain and transfer the eggs to the ice water.

7. Assemble the salad! Arrange the lettuce on a large platter and place the potatoes, haricots verts, and asparagus on top. Drizzle with half the dressing. Place tomatoes, olives, and radishes on top. Peel and halve the cooled eggs and place on the salad. Top with flaked salmon and more dressing. Enjoy!

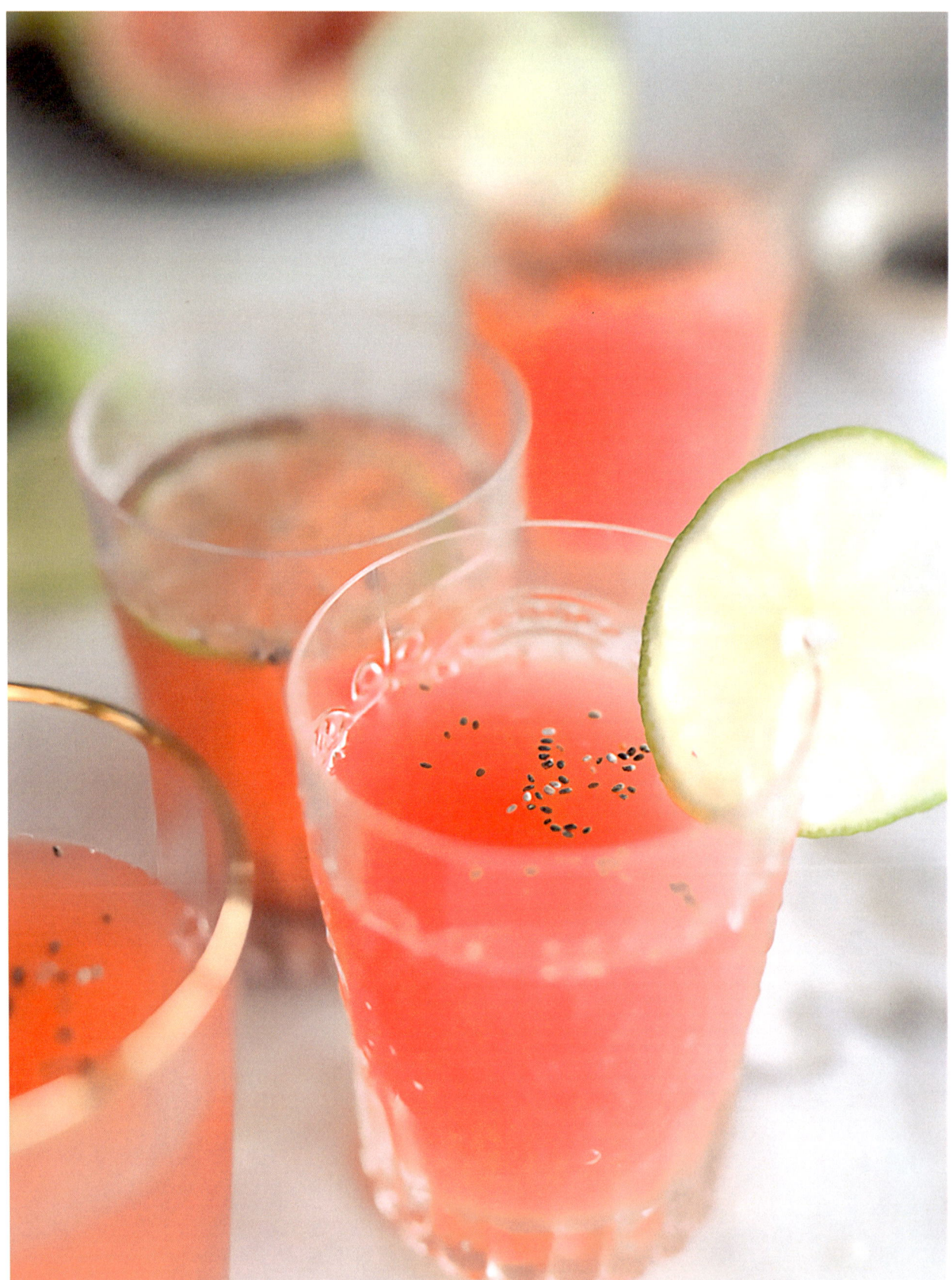

WATERMELON LIMEADE

"THE HAPPY TUMMY TONIC"

Constipation is one of the most common complaints in the first trimester. Drink this hydrating, nourishing, and calming tonic to help keep your digestion moving and grooving throughout pregnancy. Aloe vera has natural laxative properties, and the chia seeds, with their soluble fibre, act as little bubbles of hydration for your clogged pipes. Ginger is also a game changer for a queasy stomach!

INGREDIENTS | SERVES 2

1 ½ cups fresh pressed watermelon juice, or a combination of watermelon, grapefruit, pear, or other fresh fruit juices
¼–½ teaspoon freshly grated ginger (to your taste)
1 tablespoon fresh lime juice
½ tablespoon pasteurized honey
2 tablespoons aloe vera juice*
2 tablespoons chia seeds

DIRECTIONS

1. If you are making your own juice, blend the watermelon in a high-speed blender then strain through a cheesecloth. Otherwise, you can purchase store-bought fresh pressed juice.

2. Place all ingredients except chia seeds in a large jar with a tight-fitting lid. Shake vigorously until ingredients are combined. This can be kept in the fridge until ready to drink. Stir in the chia seeds 5 minutes before serving.

*Aloe vera juice can be found at your local health food or whole foods store.

Keeping your fluids up will help ward off early pregnancy symptoms such as headaches, fatigue, constipation, nausea, and vomiting. Try a homemade flavoured water, coconut water (no sugar added), or herbal tea to mix it up.

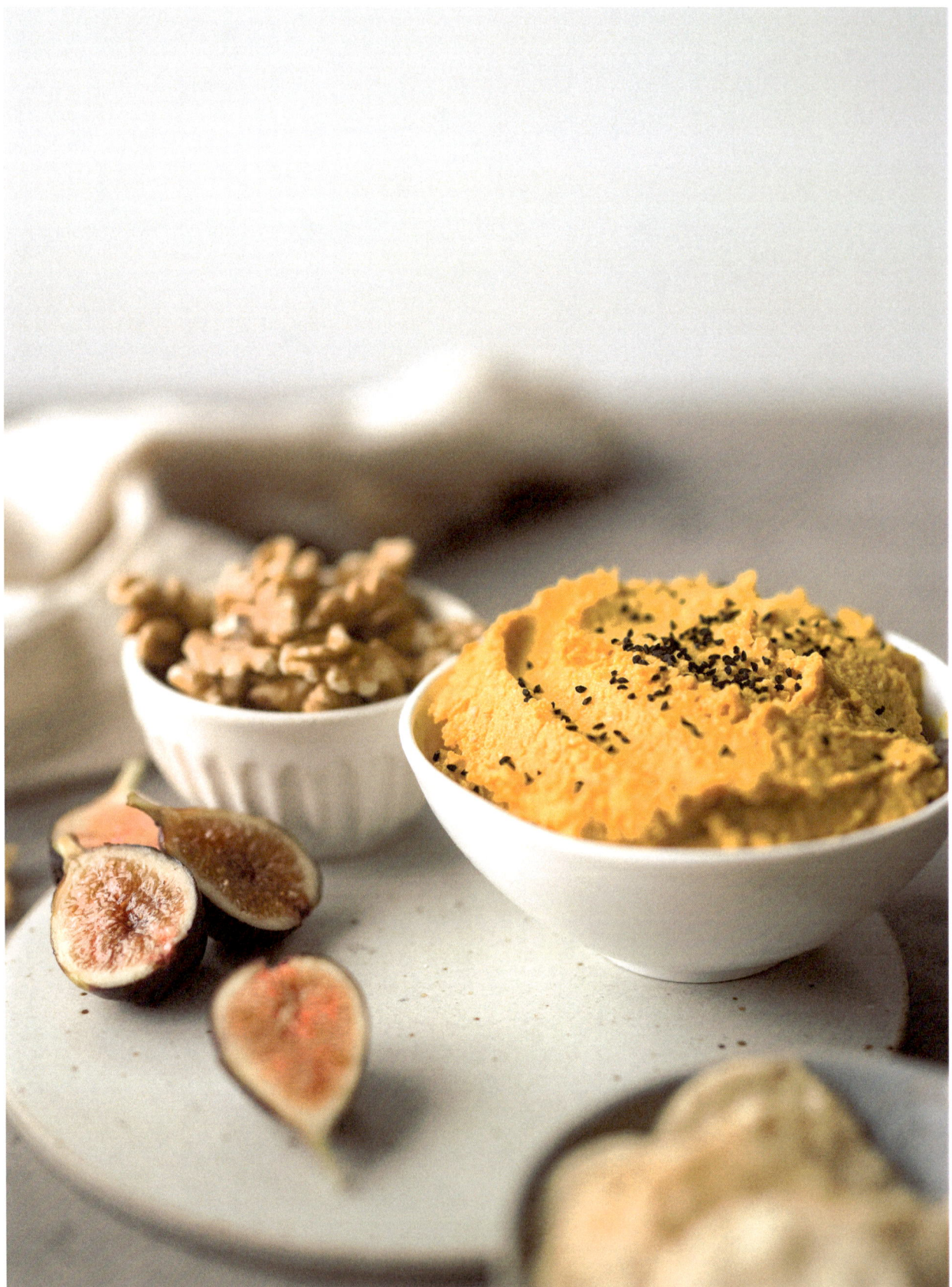

CARROT DIP

WITH WALNUTS, ORANGE, AND RED PEPPER FLAKES

Incorporating nutrition in everyday snacks is a great way to boost nutrient and caloric intake since many women aren't able to go as long between meals as they did pre-pregnancy. Carrots are a whole-food source of beta carotene (vitamin A) for eye development; biotin for hair, skin, and nail growth; vitamin K; and potassium. The complex sugars from the carrots combine with the protein and fat from the nuts for a satisfying, blood-stabilizing snack that will keep you going until dinner.

INGREDIENTS | YIELDS 1 1/2 CUPS

1 ½ cups chopped carrots
¼ teaspoon sea salt
½ cup walnuts
3 tablespoons fresh orange juice
1 garlic clove
3 pinches red pepper flakes
1 teaspoon cumin
1 teaspoon sea salt
1 green onion, chopped
½ sheet nori seaweed, torn into pieces
Crackers or cucumber slices to serve

DIRECTIONS

1. Place carrots and salt in a small saucepan and add enough water to cover. Steam the carrots until soft, approximately 5 minutes.
2. Transfer the carrots and 2 tablespoons of the carrot water to a food processor. Add walnuts, orange juice, garlic, red pepper flakes, cumin, and salt. Purée until smooth. Add the green onions and nori and pulse to combine.
3. Serve with crackers or cucumber slices.

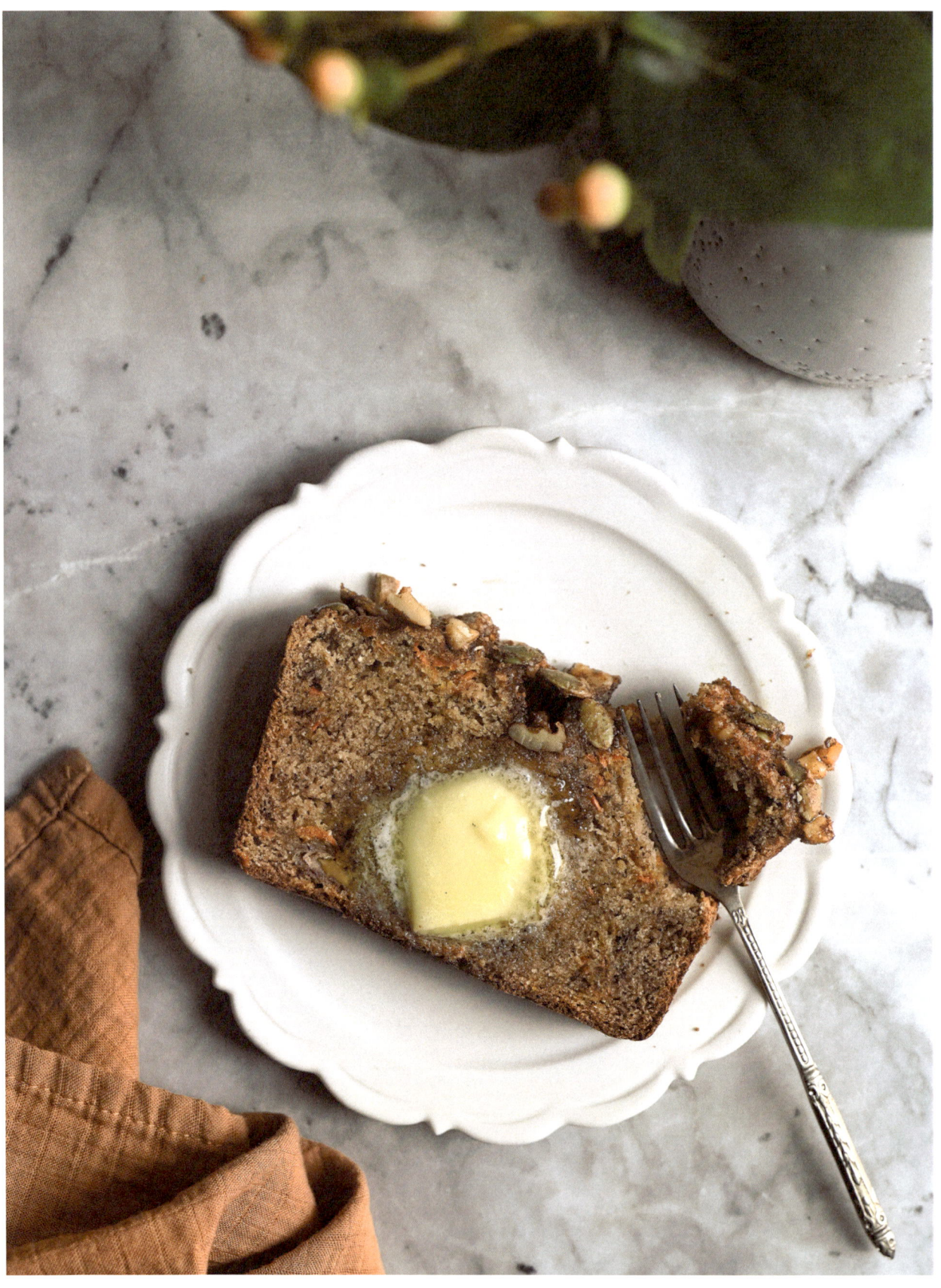

BANANA CARROT BREAD

WITH CINNAMON PECANS

This simple recipe is open to endless flavour possibilities: switch up the nuts, or substitute the carrots for another vegetable such as parsnips, beets, or zucchini. This carb-rich food is great when our first-trimester appetite can't stomach veggies or protein—it hides vegetables, healthy fats, and protein in a crave-worthy loaf. The key to the most amazing banana bread? Using bananas that are ripe with brown spots, then frozen, then thawed! They become a sweet, ooey, gooey dream and create a strong banana flavour in the bread!

INGREDIENTS | YIELDS 1 LOAF

Dry ingredients:

1 cup oat flour or spelt flour
½ cup cassava flour
½ cup coconut flour
½ cup coconut sugar
1 teaspoon baking powder
½ teaspoon baking soda
½ teaspoon sea salt
1 teaspoon cinnamon
½ teaspoon ginger
½ teaspoon nutmeg or cardamom

Wet ingredients:

1 ½ cups very ripe, pre-frozen bananas, thawed and mashed (5–6 bananas)
3 free range, organic eggs
1 teaspoon vanilla
½ cup melted coconut oil or grass-fed butter
1 ¼ cup grated carrots

Topping:

⅓ cup crushed pecans or walnuts
1 ½ tablespoons pumpkin seeds
2 tablespoons maple syrup
1 tablespoon coconut sugar
½ teaspoon cinnamon or cardamom
¼ teaspoon vanilla extract

DIRECTIONS | PREHEAT OVEN TO 350° F

1. Line a loaf pan with parchment paper.
2. In a small bowl, mix together all topping ingredients and set aside.
3. In a medium bowl, stir together the dry ingredients. Set aside.
4. In a large bowl, stir together all the wet ingredients except the carrots.
5. Stir the dry ingredients into the wet mixture until combined. Gently fold in the grated carrots.
6. Pour the mixture into the loaf pan and top with nut topping. Bake at 350° for 55–60 minutes or until a toothpick inserted into the centre of the loaf comes out clean.
7. Remove from the oven, and let the bread cool completely in the loaf pan before removing.

Karma cooking is a heartwarming way to nourish your body and soul, and to share good health with others. Doubling a batch of bread, muffins, or other baking, and gifting one batch to a local women's centre, charity, or another expectant mama, spreads good karma all around

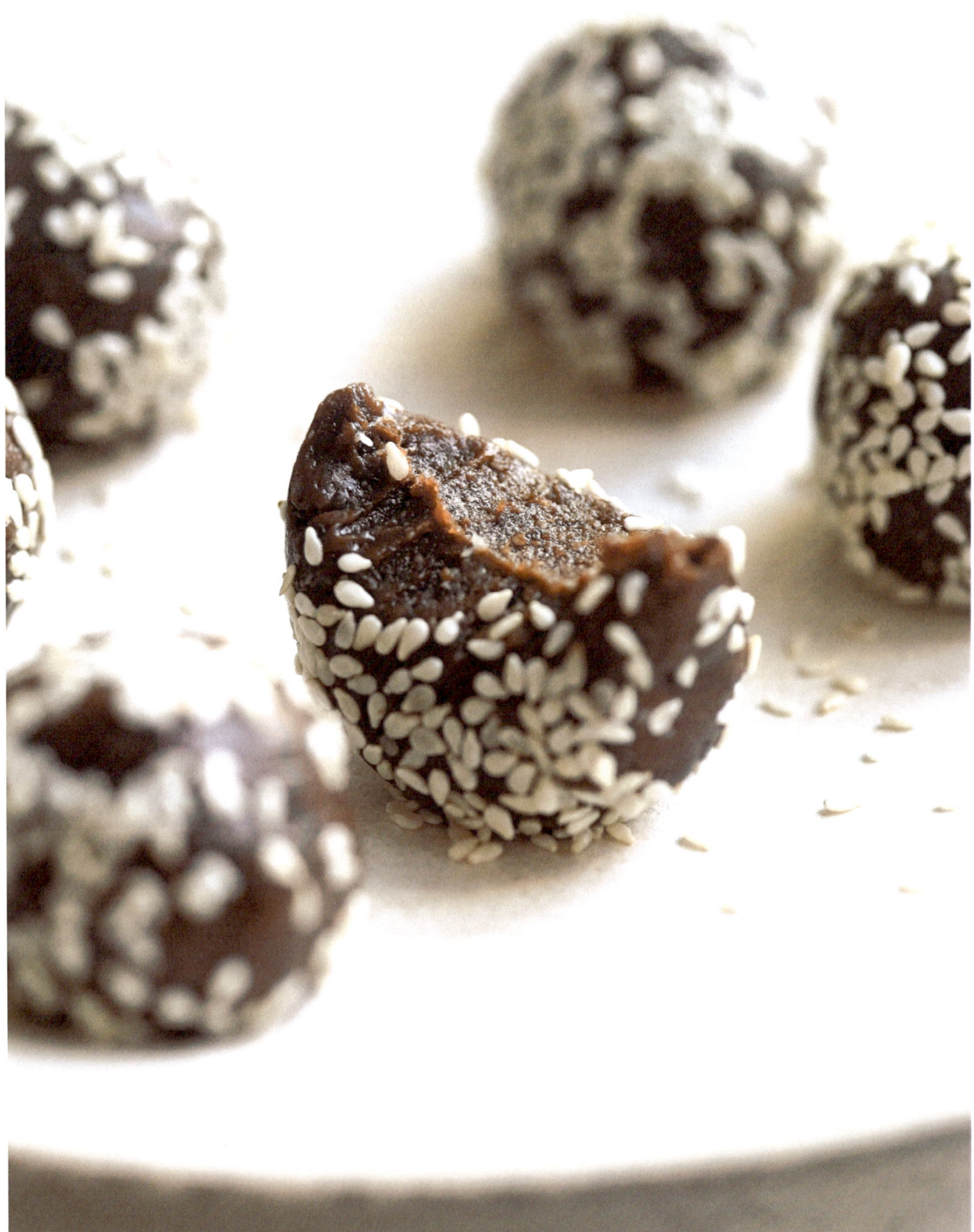

CHOCOLATE SESAME TRUFFLES

TWO WAYS

The huge shift in maternal metabolism that takes place during pregnancy makes it important to prioritize eating every few hours in order to stabilize blood glucose levels. Because of the healthy fats in the nuts and seeds, these handy snacks provide protein and sustained energy. Figs are also high in calcium and other minerals, which we can't get enough of during pregnancy! These are the perfect snack for hungry kids on the go, or even to share with the other mamas at your next prenatal yoga class.

INGREDIENTS | YIELDS 10 TO 12 TRUFFLES

½ cup dried figs, stems removed (approximately 14 figs)
½ cup nut butter
2 tablespoons chocolate green superfood mix* or vegan chocolate protein powder or cacao powder
2 tablespoons pumpkin seeds
2 tablespoons maple syrup
3 tablespoons sesame seeds
1 tablespoon cacao powder
2 tablespoons hemp hearts

Nut-free option:
15 soft dates
3 tablespoons pumpkin seed butter
½ cup sunflower seed butter
¼ cup chia seeds
1 cup rolled oats
2 tablespoons chocolate green superfood mix* or vegan chocolate protein powder or cacao powder
½ cup maple syrup
2 tablespoons hemp hearts

Anise likes "Botanica Perfect Greens- Chocolate" which can be found online or at your local health food store

DIRECTIONS

1. Reconstitute the figs or dates by putting them in a bowl of hot water for a few minutes. Remove from the water, pat dry, and cut into small pieces. (I find that if you put them straight in to the food processor without cutting, they get "stuck").
2. Add the remaining ingredients to the food processor, except the hemp seeds. Pulse until well combined.
3. Add the figs or dates and pulse again until mixed thoroughly.
4. Take about 1 tablespoon of the mixture, roll it into a ball, and roll the ball in hemp hearts. Repeat with the rest of the truffle mixture. Store truffles in the fridge for up to 2 weeks.

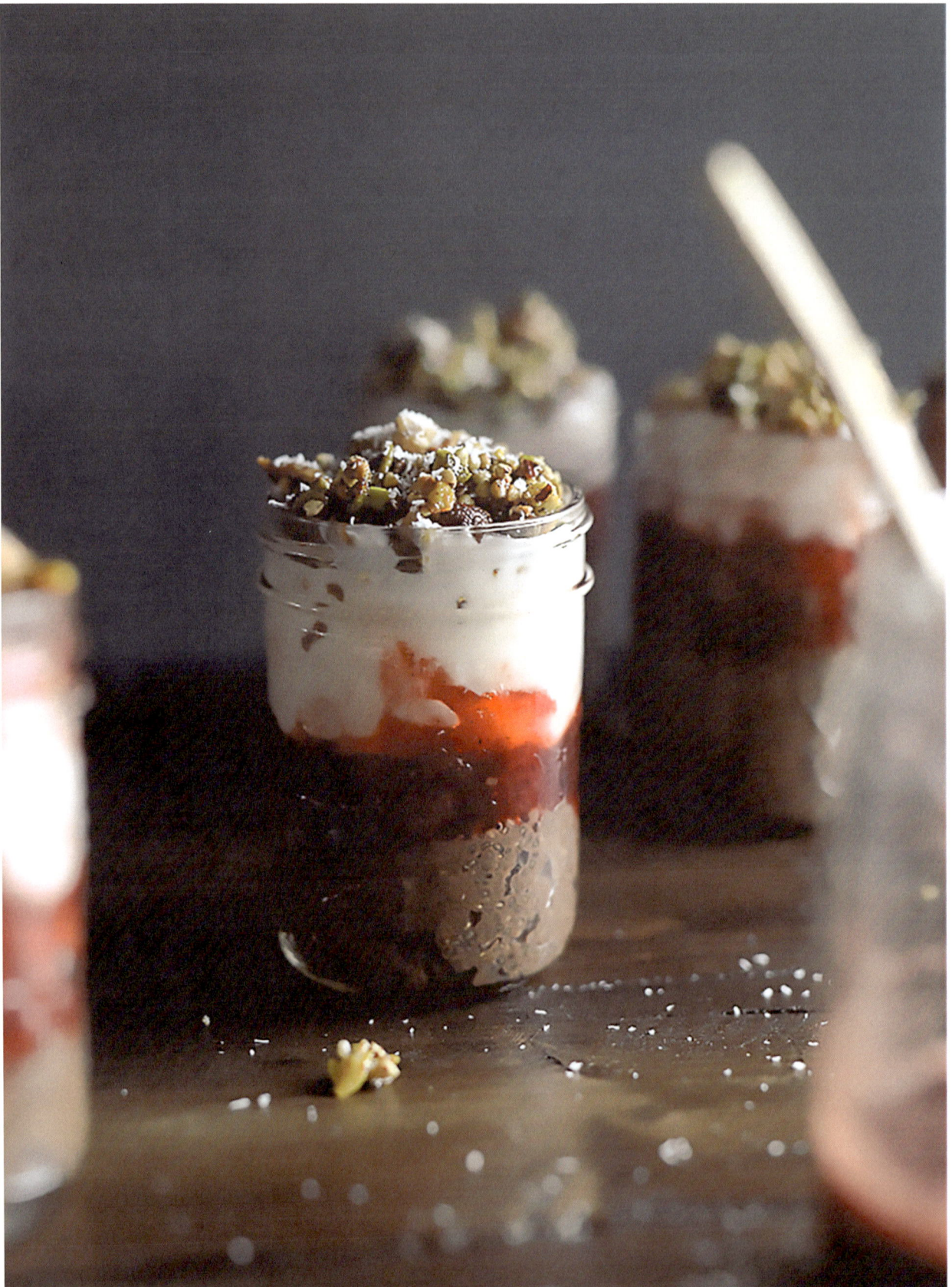

CHOCOLATE HAZELNUT CHIA PUDDING

WITH SMASHED RASPBERRIES AND NUT CRUNCH

This is one of Anise's staple recipes! This chia parfait is a satisfying way to stabilize blood sugar and gain extra fibre from the chia seeds. Cacao powder is also a great source of iron and protein—perfect for the growing mama and babe. And who doesn't love a little chocolate in the afternoon?!

INGREDIENTS | SERVES 4

Chia pudding:
1 cup light coconut milk
2 tablespoons hazelnut butter (or almond-hazelnut butter)
¼ cup maple syrup
2 tablespoons cacao powder
¼ teaspoon vanilla extract
¼ cup chia seeds

Skillet nut crunch:
2 tablespoons coconut oil
3 tablespoons maple syrup
¼ cup assorted nuts, roughly chopped
¼ cup pumpkin seeds
½ cup buckwheat groats
1 teaspoon ground cardamom

Parfaits:
1 cup raspberries, smashed with the back of a spoon
Coconut yogourt or plain Greek yogourt

DIRECTIONS

1. Make the chia pudding: In a glass container with a lid, combine the coconut milk, hazelnut butter, maple syrup, cacao powder, and vanilla. Whisk or stir until well combined. Add the chia seeds, stir, and let the mixture sit for 30 minutes.

2. Make the nut crunch: In a cast-iron skillet over medium-low heat, warm the coconut oil and maple syrup. Add the nuts, seeds, buckwheat, and cardamom and cook for 8 minutes, stirring occasionally so it doesn't stick. If the mixture gets too dry, add more coconut oil. Remove from heat and transfer to a plate to cool and harden. After about 15 minutes, crumble it with your hands.

3. Assemble: Layer the chia pudding, smashed raspberries, and yogourt in a small jar; top with the nut crunch.

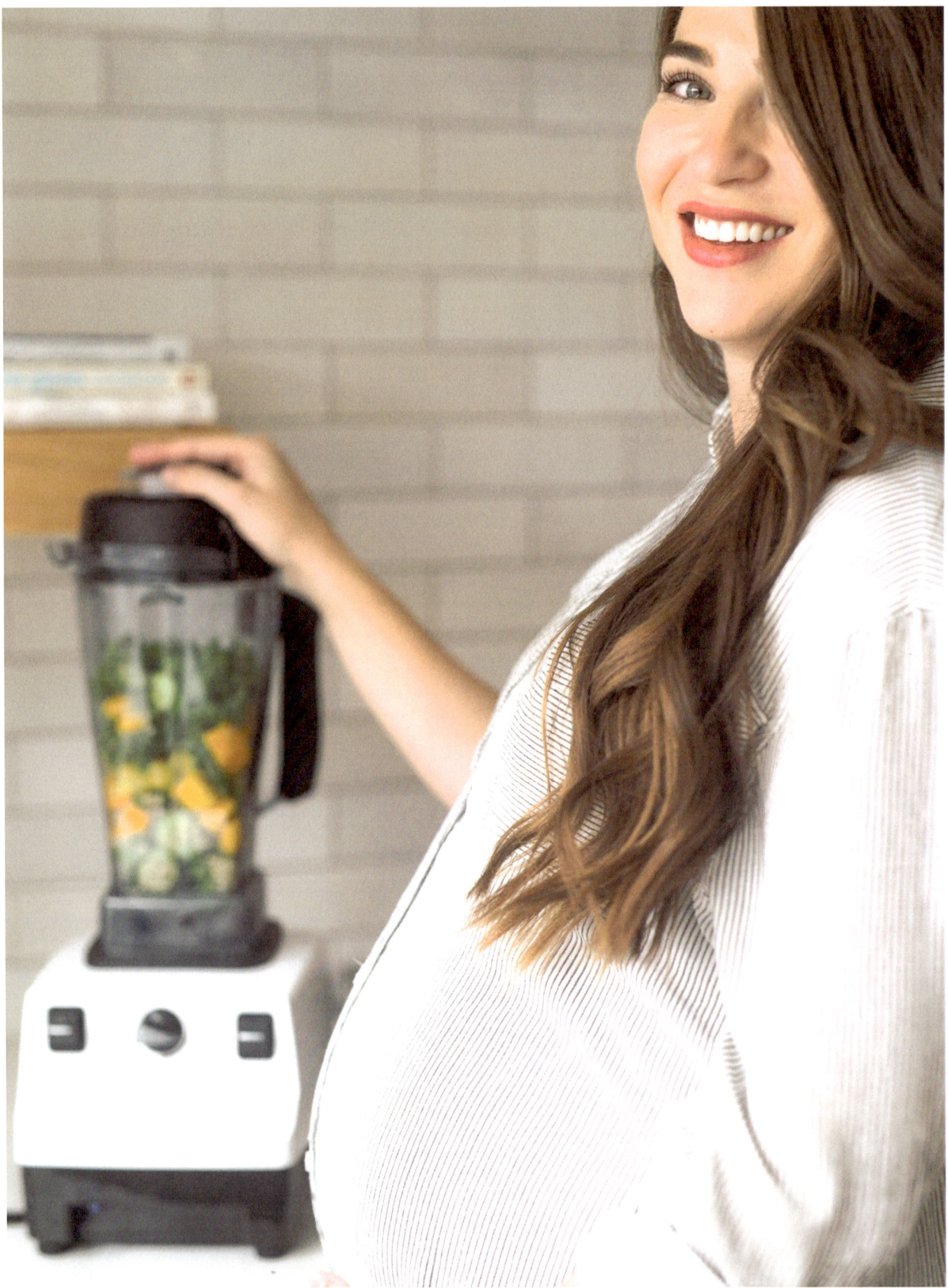

SUPER DIGESTIVE SMOOTHIE

WITH CUCUMBER, PINEAPPLE, MINT, AND LIME

The gastrointestinal tract is often where we first notice changes after becoming pregnant. A slower overall digestion, coupled with the diversion of blood flow to the growing fetus, causes constipation. Nausea, shifts in appetite, and novel food cravings and aversions can make constipation worse.

Coconut water is a great source of hydration. By keeping the body and bowels hydrated, food will move more smoothly through your gastrointestinal tract, and toxins will be cleared from the body more easily. Staying hydrated will also help keep your blood pressure down, which is especially important during pregnancy, when your blood volume increases by 50 percent! The pineapple in this smoothie also provides bromelain, a bonus digestive enzyme!

This hydrating, fibre-rich smoothie will help keep your digestive tract balanced and regular, any time of the day.

INGREDIENTS | SERVES 1

1 ¼ cup coconut water, no sugar added
¾ cup frozen pineapple chunks
2 ribs of kale, stems removed and discarded
¼ cup chopped cucumber
¼ cup avocado (approximately ½ small avocado)
2 tablespoons tightly packed mint
2 tablespoons chia seeds
2 tablespoons hemp hearts
2 ½ tablespoons lime juice
Handful of ice

DIRECTIONS

1. Blend all ingredients in a blender and enjoy!

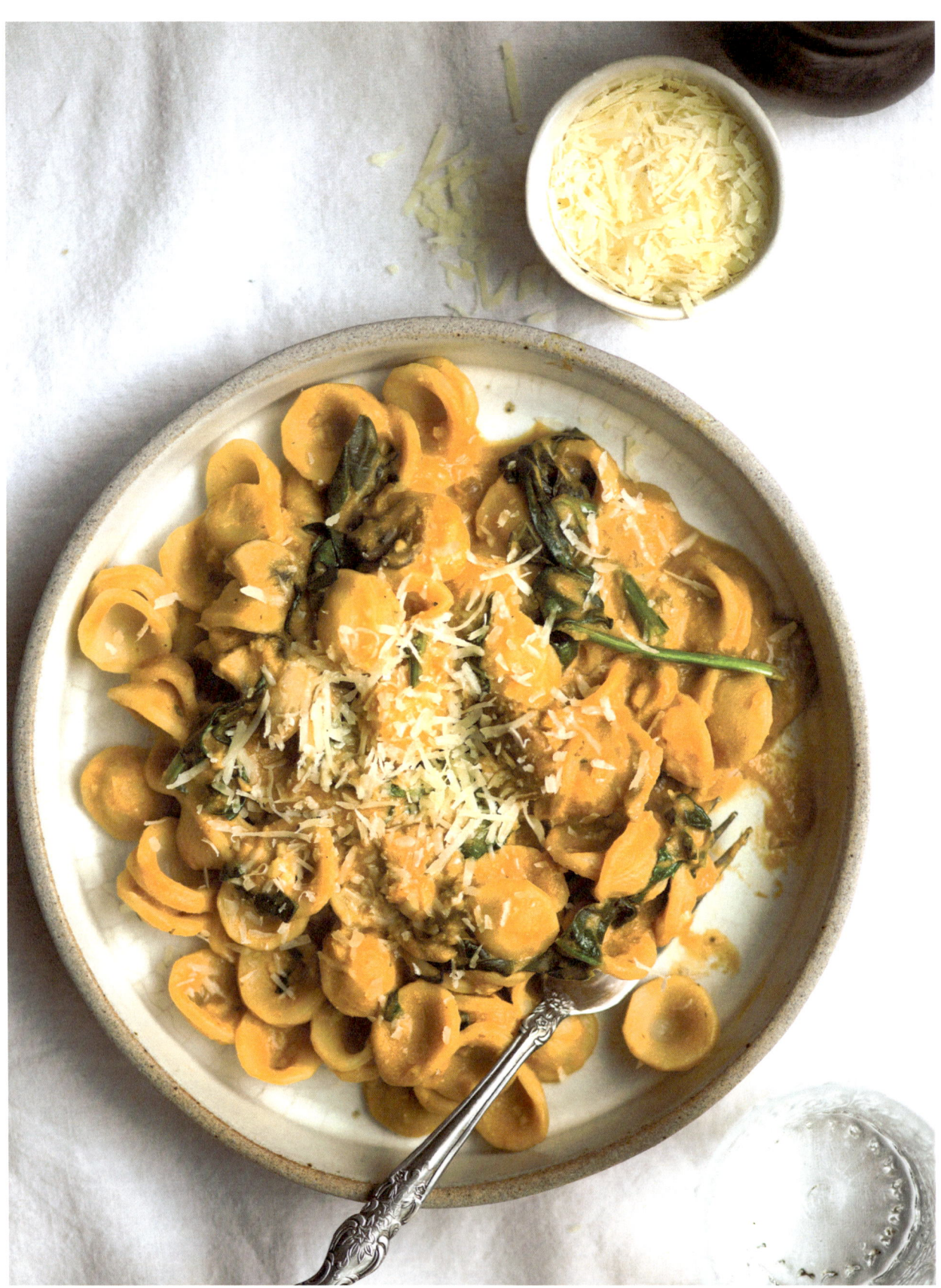

SECOND TRIMESTER

THE HONEYMOON PHASE

The time of the emerging goddess. Most women catch their stride in the second trimester: they regain vibrant energy, their nausea and vomiting often subside, their bellies start to pop, and the baby sprouts rapidly, finishing the development of their cells and organs. Excellent nutrition is still key during this time and can keep second-trimester symptoms at bay. Iron, B vitamins, magnesium, and amino acids remain important for maternal bone, brain, and bone health, and a whole variety of micro-minerals and vitamins support babies' continued growth.

Many mamas see their appetites ramp up and their food aversions disappear in the second trimester. It's time to give yourself a lift with an extra 300 to 400 calories daily. For some, this means an extra snack—but a well-balanced one. Others will choose to eat slightly larger meals. These extra calories are especially important for working or busy parents who experience a late-afternoon energy crash.

Moms-to-be often have the most energy for cooking and meal prep in the second trimester, so put on your chef's hat, pull out the superfoods, and get creative in the kitchen. Wee babe is putting on weight and has greatly increased nutrient needs, so now is the time for vibrant eating. Stretch your wings this trimester and connect with the precious babe growing inside of you by nourishing yourself with these delicious snacks and meals.

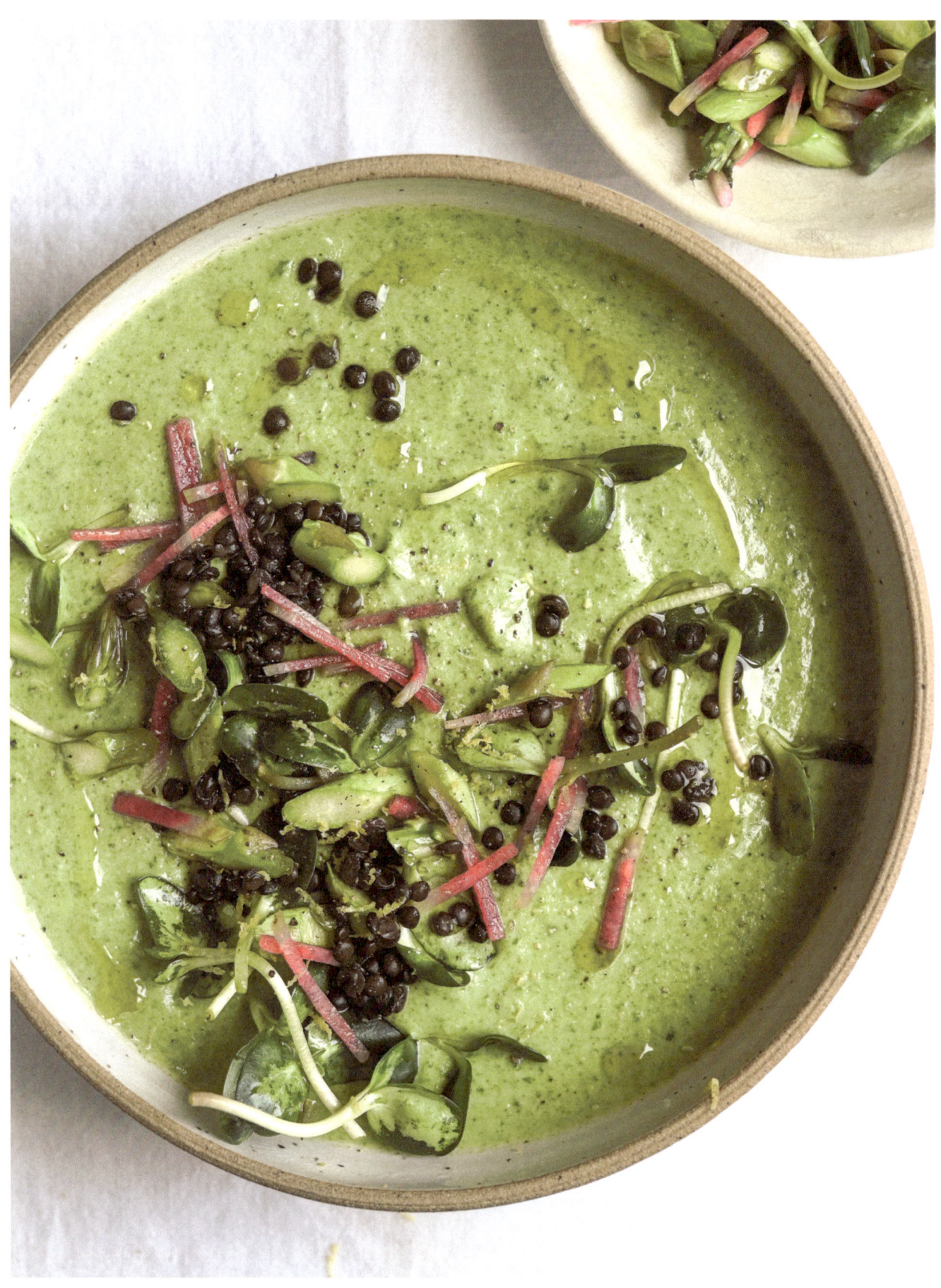

SECOND TRIMESTER

TABLE OF CONTENTS

BREAKFAST
Muesli Cookies with Apricot, Walnuts, and Coconut 57

Fruit Crisp with Blueberries and Pear 59

Salmon & Egg Toast with Roasted Broccoli and Tarragon Chimichurri 61

Butternut Squash Breakfast Buns with Tomato Jam and Arugula 63

LUNCH
Lemon Broccoli Soup with Miso and French Lentils 67

Pumpkin Truffle Pasta with Chanterelles and Parmesan 69

Kimchi Quesadilla with Shiitakes and Greens 71

Ginger Soy Sushi Bowl with Edamame, Avocado, and Mango 73

DINNER
Grilled Lemon Halibut with Miso-corn, Shiitakes, and Swiss Chard 75

Chicken Souvlaki Salad with Olives, Dates, and Parsley 77

Seared Elk Steak with Ginger Carrot Sauce and Greens 79

Spicy Pineapple Miso Shrimp with Grilled Avocado and Kohlrabi Slaw 81

SNACKS AND SWEETS
Vegan Kimchi "Cheez" Dip with Carrots and Potatoes 83

Spanikopita with Spelt Phyllo and Dandelion Greens 85

Smooth Skin Smoothie Bowl, Two Ways 87

Chocolate Avocado Brownies with Date and Cacao Frosting 89

Guava Kombucha Freezies with Raspberries and Chia Seeds 91

Mint Chocolate Nice Cream with Cacao Nibs 93

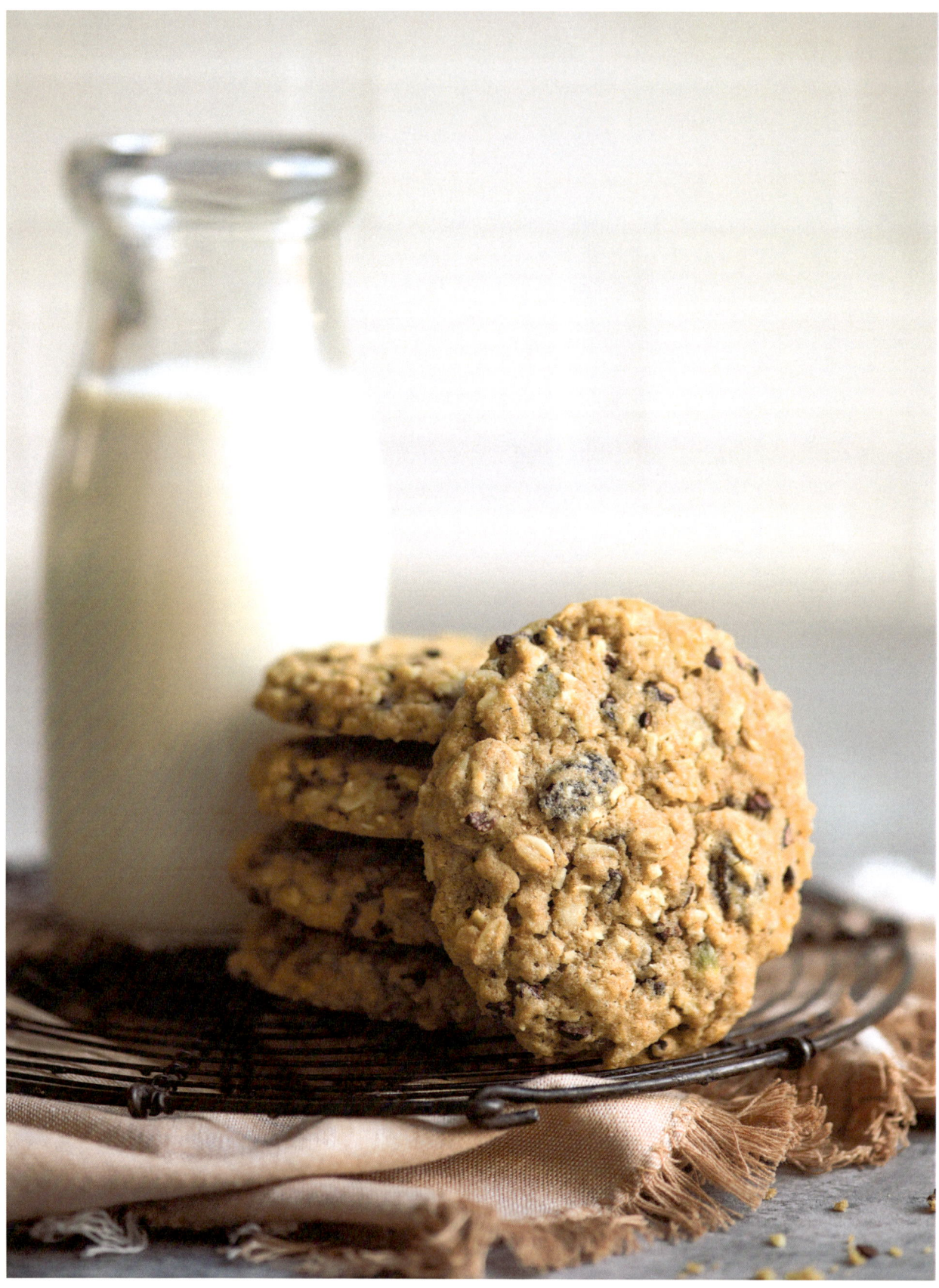

MUESLI COOKIES

WITH APRICOT, WALNUTS, AND COCONUT

Cookies for breakfast?! When they are basically oatmeal in cookie form and jam-packed with healthy fats, protein, vitamins, and minerals, they make for a deliciously fun morning meal. Prep these early in the week so you can take them on the run. Moms with toddlers will also appreciate the convenience for little hands!

INGREDIENTS | YIELDS 12 COOKIES

¼ cup coconut oil, melted and cooled

3 tablespoons drippy tahini or smooth almond butter

3–4 tablespoons maple syrup

¼ teaspoon vanilla extract

½ cup mashed banana

1 cup rolled oats

2 tablespoons pumpkin seeds

¼ cup chopped walnuts

¼ cup shredded, unsweetened coconut

8 dried Turkish apricots, chopped

½ teaspoon cinnamon

⅛ teaspoon sea salt

DIRECTIONS | PREHEAT OVEN TO 350° F

1. In a medium bowl, combine the melted coconut oil, tahini or almond butter, maple syrup, and vanilla. Mash the banana into the wet ingredients until the mixture is smooth.

2. Add the oats, pumpkin seeds, chopped walnuts, coconut, apricots, cinnamon, and salt. Stir well to combine.

3. Line a baking sheet with parchment paper and drop heaping tablespoons of the mixture onto the paper with a bit of space in between each mound. Flatten with your fingers. (These won't rise or get bigger because there is no baking soda or baking powder.)

4. Bake at 350° for 18 minutes. Remove from the oven and let cool. Keep these cookies in an airtight container, and they will remain soft and chewy!

If you prefer chocolate-flavoured cookies, swap the apricots and cinnamon for 2 tablespoons of cacao powder.

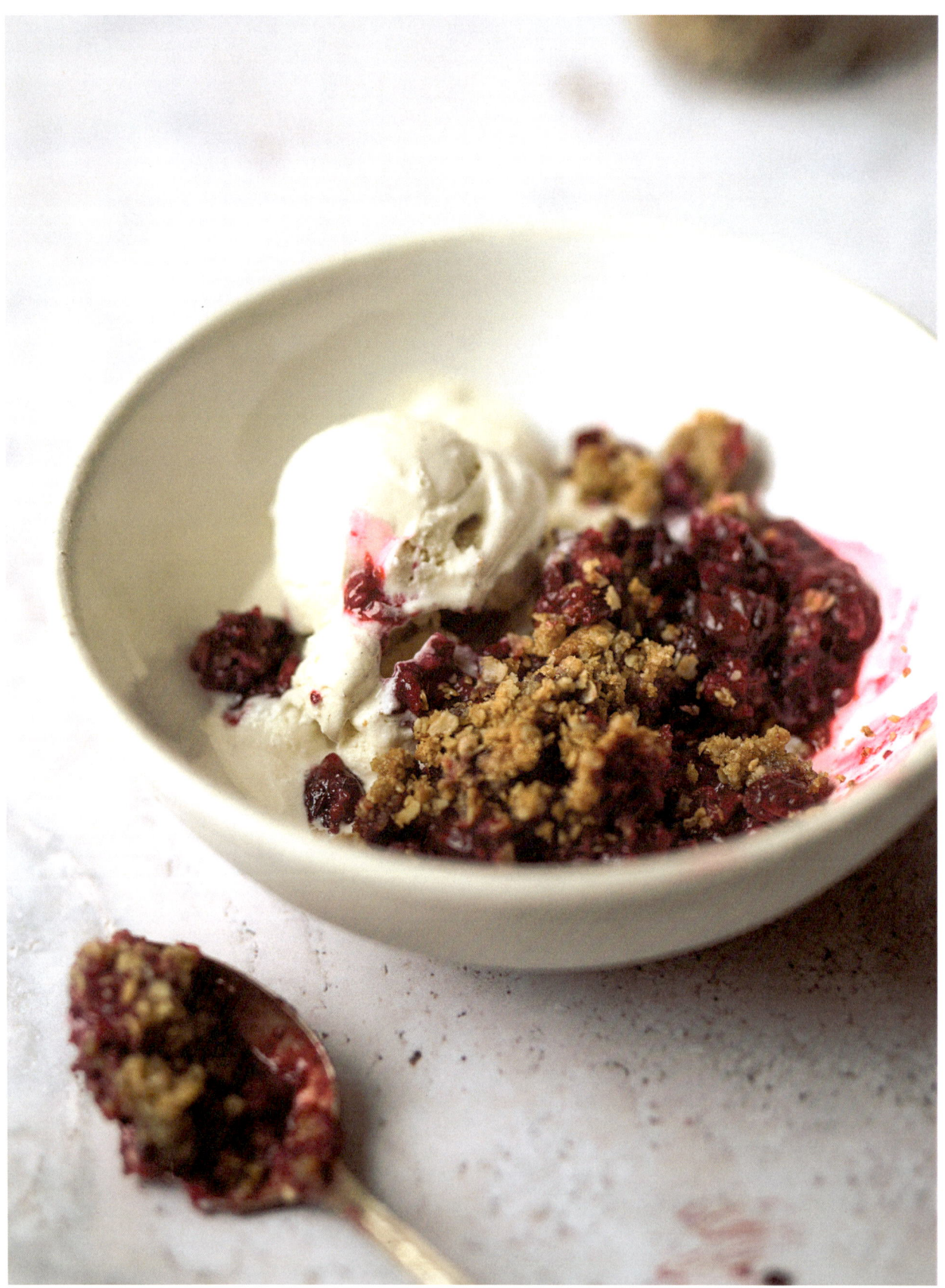

FRUIT CRISP

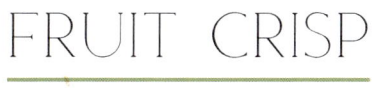

WITH BLUEBERRIES AND PEAR

In their second trimester, pregnant mamas are screened for healthy blood glucose regulation via the glucose tolerance test. And, contrary to appearances, this dessert-like breakfast is a blood glucose winner. Chia seeds and oats are perfect for balancing blood glucose levels. Combining higher-sugar foods with fibre, fat, and protein is a great way to regulate blood sugar levels and set you up for success throughout your pregnancy.

INGREDIENTS | YIELDS 1 CRUMBLE PIE

Filling:
2 cups chopped pears
2 cups fresh blueberries
¼ teaspoon freshly grated ginger
3 tablespoons maple syrup
2 tablespoons orange juice
Zest from ½ an orange
1 ½ tablespoons chia seeds
½ teaspoon vanilla powder

Topping:
2 cups rolled oats
1 ⅓ cups buckwheat groats
3 tablespoons pumpkin seeds
⅓ cup maple syrup
¼ cup coconut oil, melted
¼ cup almond butter
1 teaspoon vanilla extract or powder

Coconut cream, organic yogourt, or coconut ice cream to serve

DIRECTIONS | PREHEAT OVEN TO 375° F

1. Mix together the filling ingredients in a deep pie dish.
2. Make the topping: In a separate bowl, combine the oats, buckwheat groats, and pumpkin seeds. Add maple syrup, coconut oil, almond butter, and vanilla and mix thoroughly with your hands.
3. Evenly spread the topping over the filling.
4. Bake at 375° for 30–40 minutes, or until the fruit begins to bubble along the sides and the top is lightly brown and firm.
5. Enjoy with a dollop of organic yogourt or coconut ice cream.

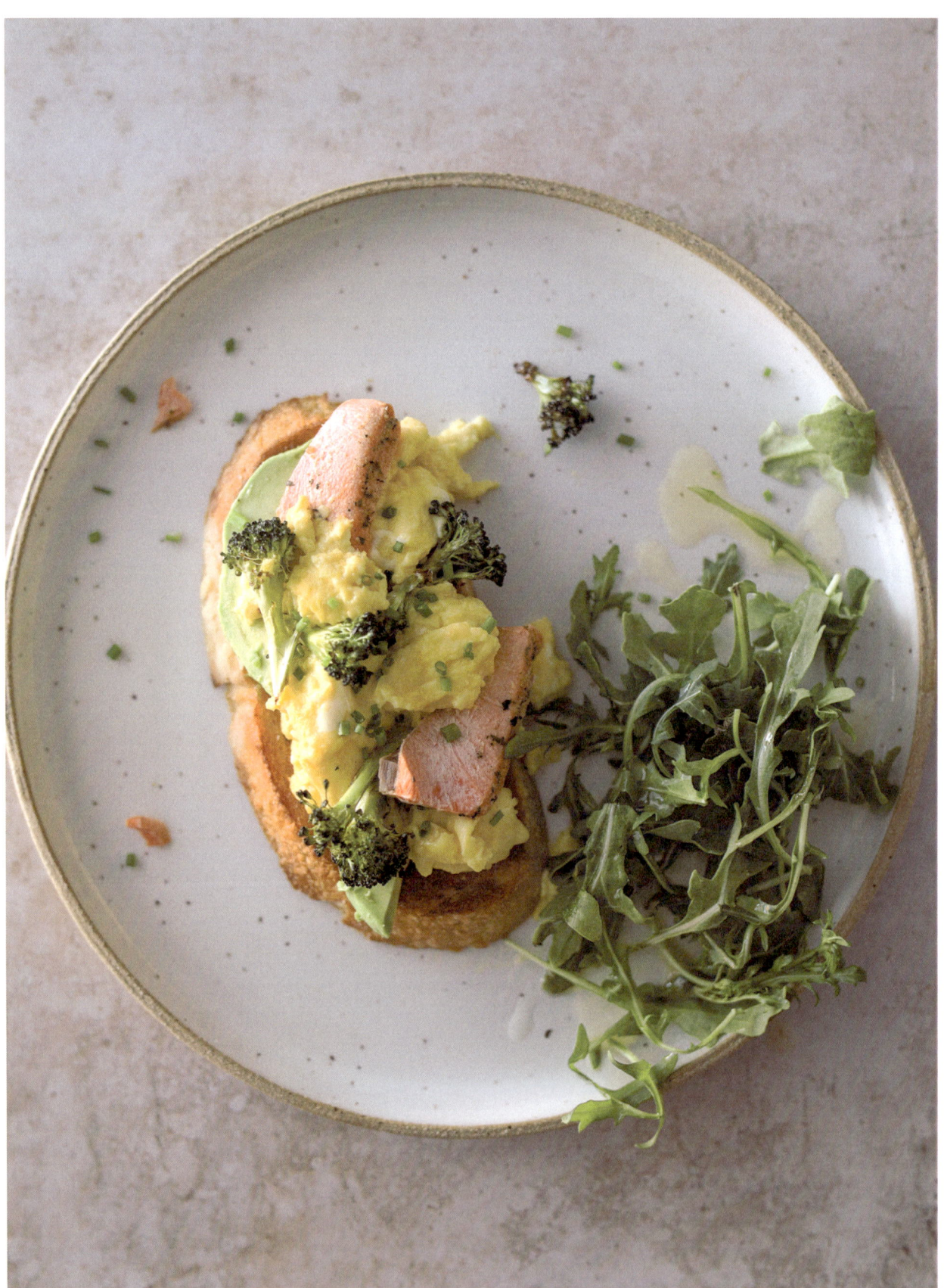

SALMON & EGG TOAST

WITH ROASTED BROCCOLI AND TARRAGON CHIMICHURRI

Perfect for Sunday brunch, this dish uses up leftover salmon from the night before. Your little sprout is starting to put on fat stores, which helps them balance their temperature and metabolism. Organic, free-range eggs offer cell-building protein, cholesterol, and essential fatty acids. They have more brightly coloured yolks compared to their factory farm counterparts due to higher amounts of carotenoids and vitamins A, E, and D. Many people also find them to be tastier. Broccoli is high in calcium, which is essential for baby's rapid bone development during the second trimester. Pairing the broccoli with vitamin D–rich eggs supports optimal calcium absorption.

INGREDIENTS | SERVES 2

Tarragon chimichurri:
½ shallot
½ small jalapeño or serrano pepper, ribs and seeds removed
2 small garlic cloves, halved
¼ cup chopped fresh parsley
¼ cup chopped fresh tarragon
1 tablespoon chopped fresh chives
½ teaspoon sea salt
¼ cup red wine vinegar
¼ cup plus 2 tablespoons extra-virgin olive oil

Salmon and Broccoli:
110 grams leftover salmon (4 ounces)
½ cup chopped broccoli
1 tablespoon coconut oil, melted
½ teaspoon sea salt
Freshly cracked pepper
⅛ teaspoon red pepper flakes

Eggs:
3 free-range, organic eggs
2 tablespoons 2–3% organic goat milk, or unsweetened cashew milk
¼ teaspoon of salt
freshly cracked pepper
2 tablespoons grass-fed butter or vegan soy-free butter, plus extra for buttering bread
2 slices sourdough bread

DIRECTIONS | PREHEAT OVEN TO 400° F

1. Prepare the chimichurri: In a food processor, combine the shallot, serrano or jalapeño pepper, and garlic. Pulse until finely chopped. Add the herbs and salt and pulse again until the mixture is minced. Transfer to a jar with a tight-fitting lid, add vinegar and oil, and shake to combine. Set aside.

2. Prepare the broccoli: Toss together the broccoli, 1 tablespoon of coconut oil, ½ teaspoon of salt, a few cracks of pepper, and red pepper flakes on a parchment paper–lined baking sheet. Spread the broccoli evenly over the baking sheet and bake at 400° for 10–12 minutes or until it is al dente and the edges are crispy. (Cooking time will depend on how small you cut the broccoli.) Add the leftover salmon to the tray for the last 4–5 minutes of roasting to heat throughout.

3. While the broccoli is roasting, prepare the eggs: In a small bowl, whisk together the eggs, milk, ¼ teaspoon of salt, and a few cracks of pepper until fully incorporated. Set aside.

4. Butter the bread slices and toast them in the oven; remove when they are toasted to your liking.

5. With a few minutes to go on your broccoli and salmon, cook the eggs. In a medium, non-stick, non-toxic skillet, heat 2 tablespoons of butter or ghee over medium heat. When the butter starts to bubble, pour the eggs in the middle of the pan. Slowly stir the eggs and turn the heat to low. Gently fold the eggs over themselves until all the liquid has solidified. Remove and transfer to your plate.

6. Assemble the toast! Place a piece of toast on your plate and top with eggs, broccoli, and flakes of salmon. Drizzle with the tarragon chimichurri.

The leftover chimichurri will go great with any fish or vegetable dish!

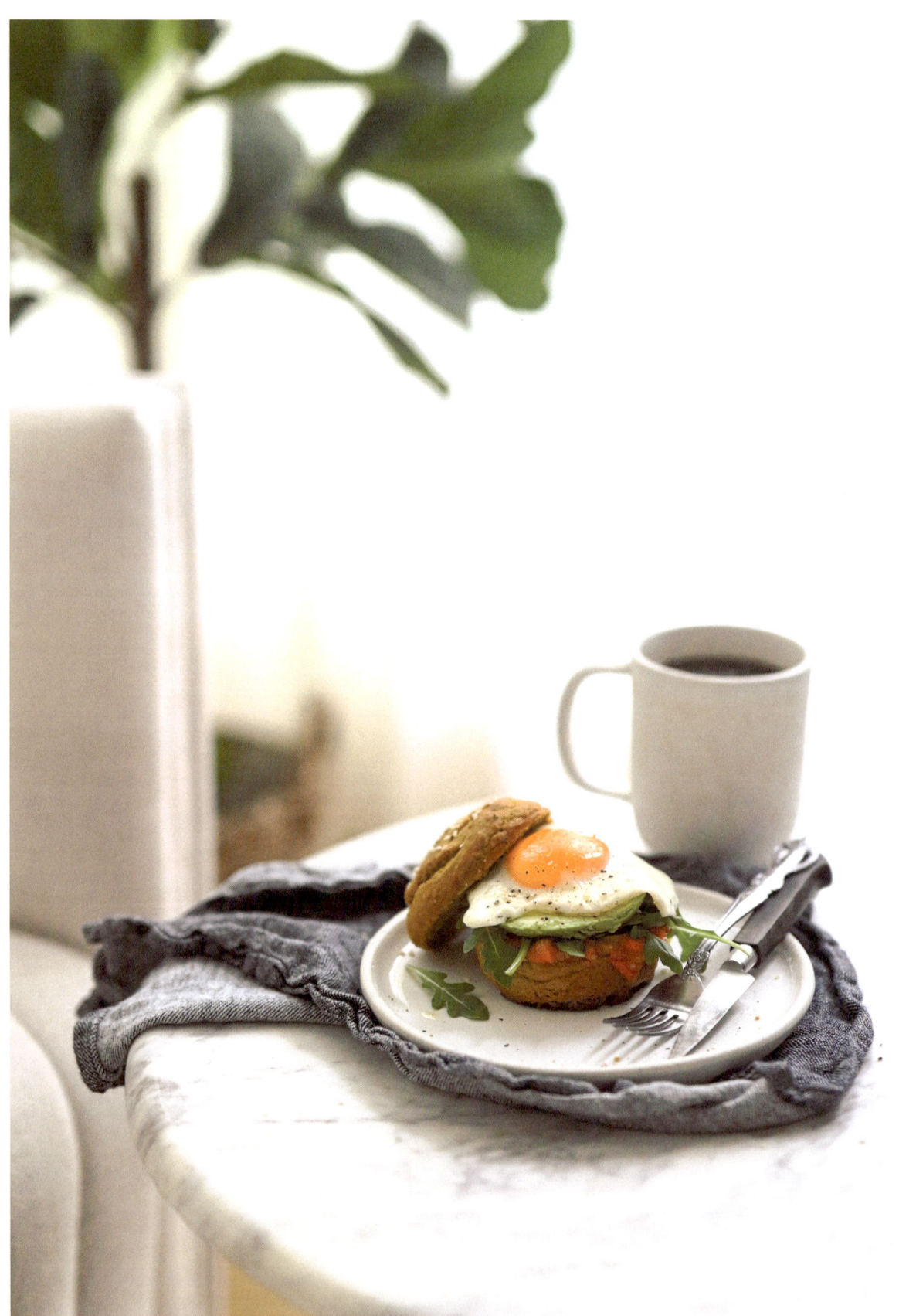

BUTTERNUT SQUASH BREAKFAST BUNS

WITH TOMATO JAM AND ARUGULA

Second-trimester aches and pains can be common as our uterus expands rapidly and the continued influx of relaxin affects our ligaments and bones. The hips, pelvis, lower back, and lower extremities are notorious areas of discomfort. Magnesium and calcium are heavy hitters in combating soreness throughout pregnancy. And vitamin C is amazing for connective tissue: it helps the body make the collagen needed for skin, ligaments, tendons, and blood vessels. This butternut squash breakfast bun offers a hearty start to the day, with the nutrients to feed a growing pregnant body.

INGREDIENTS | SERVES 4

Butternut squash buns:
2 free range, organic eggs
1 ½ tablespoons maple syrup
⅓ cup avocado oil
1 cup canned butternut squash purée
1 cup gluten-free flour blend
⅔ cup almond flour
1 ½ teaspoons baking powder
2 teaspoons salt
¼ teaspoon cumin
½ teaspoon thyme
½ teaspoon dried basil
½ teaspoon dried oregano
½ teaspoon garlic powder
¼ teaspoon white pepper

Eggs:
4 free range, organic eggs
½ teaspoon sea salt
Freshly cracked pepper

Sandwiches:
1 cup arugula
1 avocado, sliced, or organic cheddar or vegan cheddar

DIRECTIONS | PREHEAT OVEN TO 375° F

1. In a large bowl, stir together the eggs, maple syrup, avocado oil, and butternut squash purée.
2. In a medium bowl, combine the gluten-free flour blend, almond flour, baking powder, salt, cumin, thyme, basil, oregano, garlic powder, and white pepper.
3. Add the dry ingredients to the wet ingredients and stir to combine. Add the batter to 4 jumbo muffin silicone moulds, filling each one halfway.
4. Bake at 375° for 30 minutes.
5. While the buns cook, prepare the tomato jam. See the following page.
6. Remove the buns from the oven and let them cool before removing them from the silicone mould.
7. Turn the oven to 425° and place a small parchment paper-lined baking sheet in the oven to preheat before adding the eggs.
8. While the jam is cooking, prepare the eggs: Crack 4 eggs into a large jar or bowl. Remove the pan from the oven and quickly but carefully pour the eggs onto the warmed baking sheet. Sprinkle on the salt and pepper and return the eggs to the oven for 4–6 minutes, depending on when the yolks are cooked to your liking. Remove from the oven and cut out each egg.
9. Assemble the breakfast buns: Cut a bun in half, smear a bit of tomato jam on both sides, then fill with an egg, a few slices of avocado or cheese, and arugula. Enjoy!

You can wrap your breakfast bun in parchment paper without the arugula and store it in the fridge up to 5 days. Heat the sandwich, still wrapped in the parchment paper, in the oven at 350° F for 5 minutes. Add the arugula after baking.

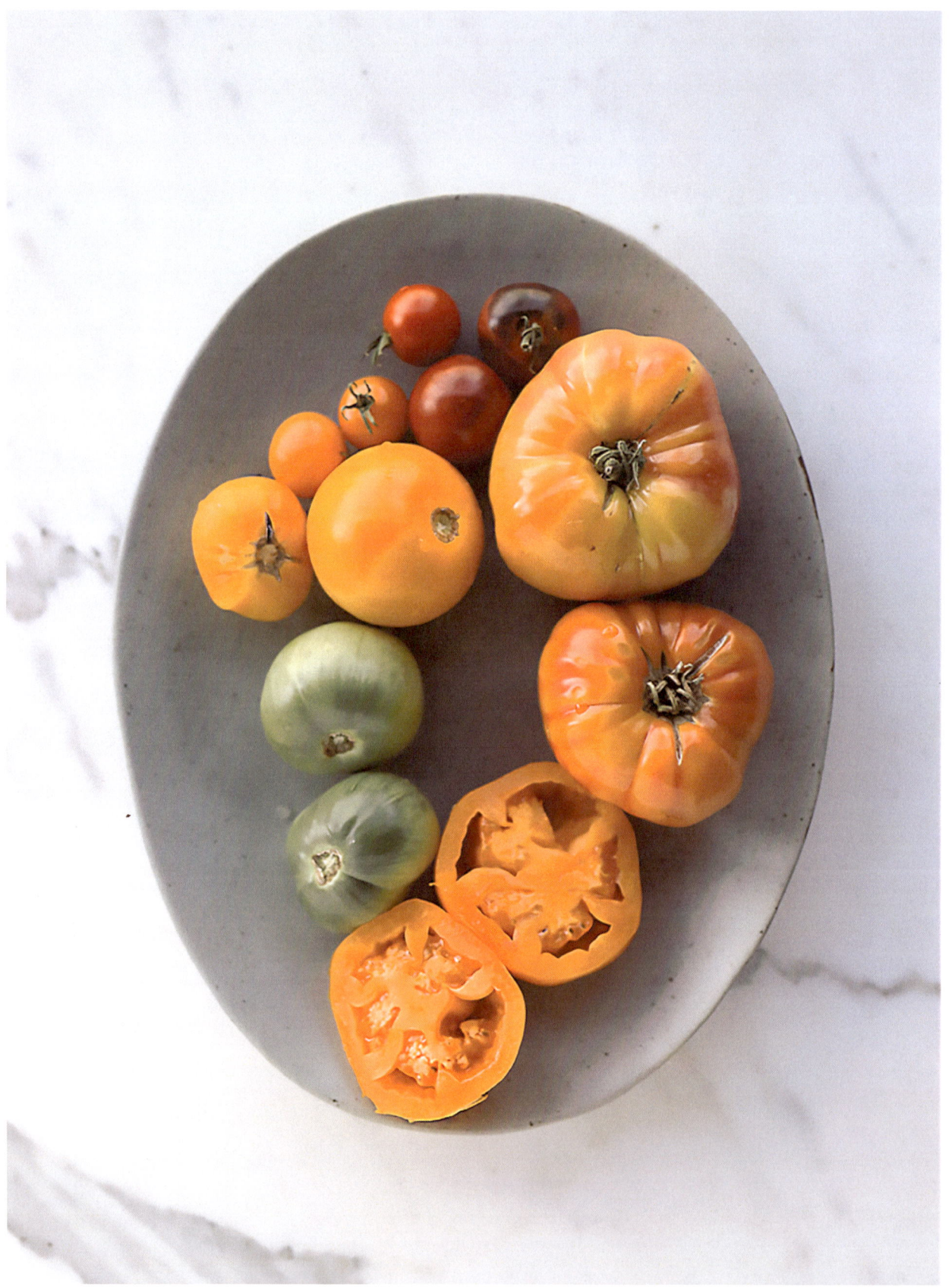

TOMATO JAM

CONTINUED

INGREDIENTS | YIELDS 1 ½ CUPS OF JAM

3 tablespoons coconut oil

¼ cup plus 2 tablespoons minced red onions

2 pints cherry tomatoes, halved or quartered

¾ teaspoon sea salt, divided

4 large pinches red pepper flakes

2 tablespoons maple syrup

1 tablespoon red wine vinegar (preferred) or apple cider vinegar

2 tablespoons fresh chopped chives

freshly cracked pepper

½ teaspoon hot sauce (optional)

DIRECTIONS

1. In a large non-stick frying pan over medium-low heat, sauté the coconut oil and red onions for 3–4 minutes until the onions are soft.
2. Add the cherry tomatoes, ½ teaspoon salt, red pepper flakes, and maple syrup.
3. Cook over medium-low heat for 15–20 minutes, stirring occasionally, until the tomatoes have cooked down and the sauce has thickened.
4. Remove from the heat and add red wine vinegar, chives, remaining ¼ teaspoon salt, and freshly cracked pepper. Stir, taste, and season with a little hot sauce if you like.

Keep the jam in an airtight jar for up to 7 days.

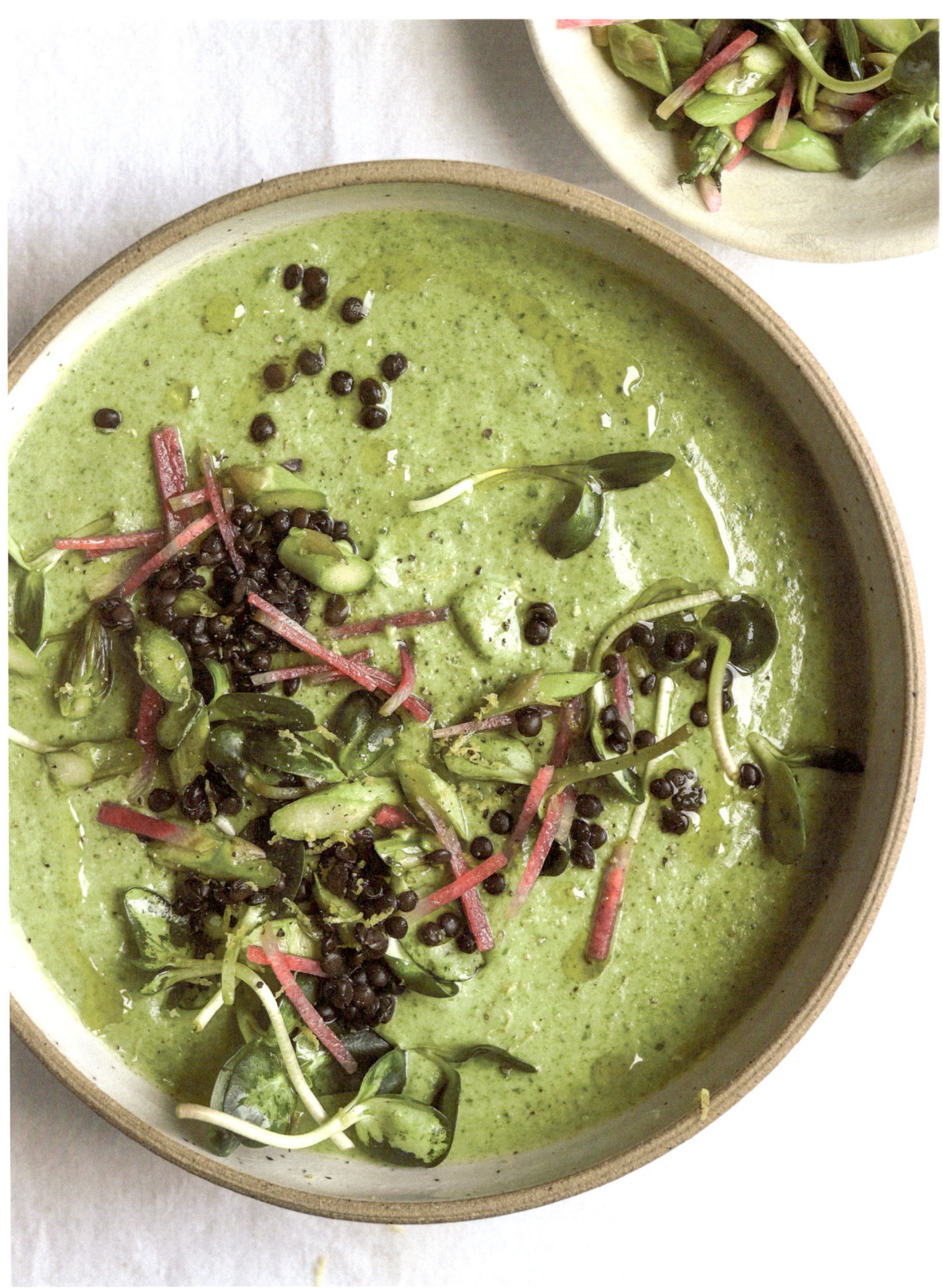

LEMON BROCCOLI SOUP

WITH MISO AND FRENCH LENTILS

In the cold fall and winter months, a warm soup nourishes the body and soul. Adding miso to soups, dressings, and sauces is a simple way to incorporate those much-needed probiotics for a healthy gut microbiome. This is beneficial not only for mom but for babe as well. It has been shown to reduce the risk of adverse pregnancy complications such as gestational diabetes, preeclampsia, digestive disorders, and autoimmune diseases. Including fermented products—such as kefir, tempeh, kombucha, miso, and sauerkraut—in your diet is like giving your gut a sprinkling of healthy fertilizer.

INGREDIENTS | SERVES 4

½ cup dry black lentils or beluga lentils
1 ¼ teaspoon sea salt, divided
1 tablespoon ghee or coconut oil
1 small yellow onion, chopped
1 celery stalk, chopped
4 cloves of garlic, chopped
4 cups chopped broccoli
2 thyme sprigs or 1 teaspoon dried thyme
3 cups chicken stock, vegetable stock, or bone broth
2 cups spinach, tightly packed
1 ½ tablespoons Italian parsley, tightly packed
2 tablespoons lemon juice
3 tablespoons white or shiro miso

Pea shoots, additional asparagus spears, sliced watermelon radish, avocado slices, or pumpkin seeds, for garnish (optional)

DIRECTIONS

1. Prepare the lentils: In a small saucepan, combine 1 ¾ cups filtered water, the dry black lentils, and ¼ teaspoon of the salt. Bring to a simmer, cover, and cook over medium-low heat for 20 minutes. Remove from the stove and drain any excess liquid. Set aside.

2. While the lentils cook, prepare the soup: In a medium saucepan, heat the ghee or coconut oil, onions, and celery over medium heat. Let the vegetables sweat for 5 minutes, stirring occasionally. Add the garlic and continue to cook until fragrant, approximately 1 minute. Add broccoli, thyme, and stock. Bring to a boil, cover, and reduce to a simmer for 12–15 minutes until the broccoli is very tender.

3. Remove from the heat, remove the thyme sprig and add spinach, parsley, lemon juice, the remaining teaspoon of salt, and miso. Stir until the spinach is wilted. Blend with an immersion blender, or transfer to a blender and blend until smooth. Taste and season with more salt and pepper if needed.

4. Top with lentils. Garnish with your choice of pea shoots, additional asparagus spears, watermelon radish, avocado, or pumpkin seeds.

This is a great recipe to double or even triple, freezing the extra for the third or fourth trimester—when you're exhausted! Storing hot liquids in plastic can increase the leaching of harmful chemicals into your food and water. If possible, replace plastic storage containers with glass or ceramics. This is especially important during pregnancy, as the growing babe can be more vulnerable to the negative effects of absorbed chemicals.

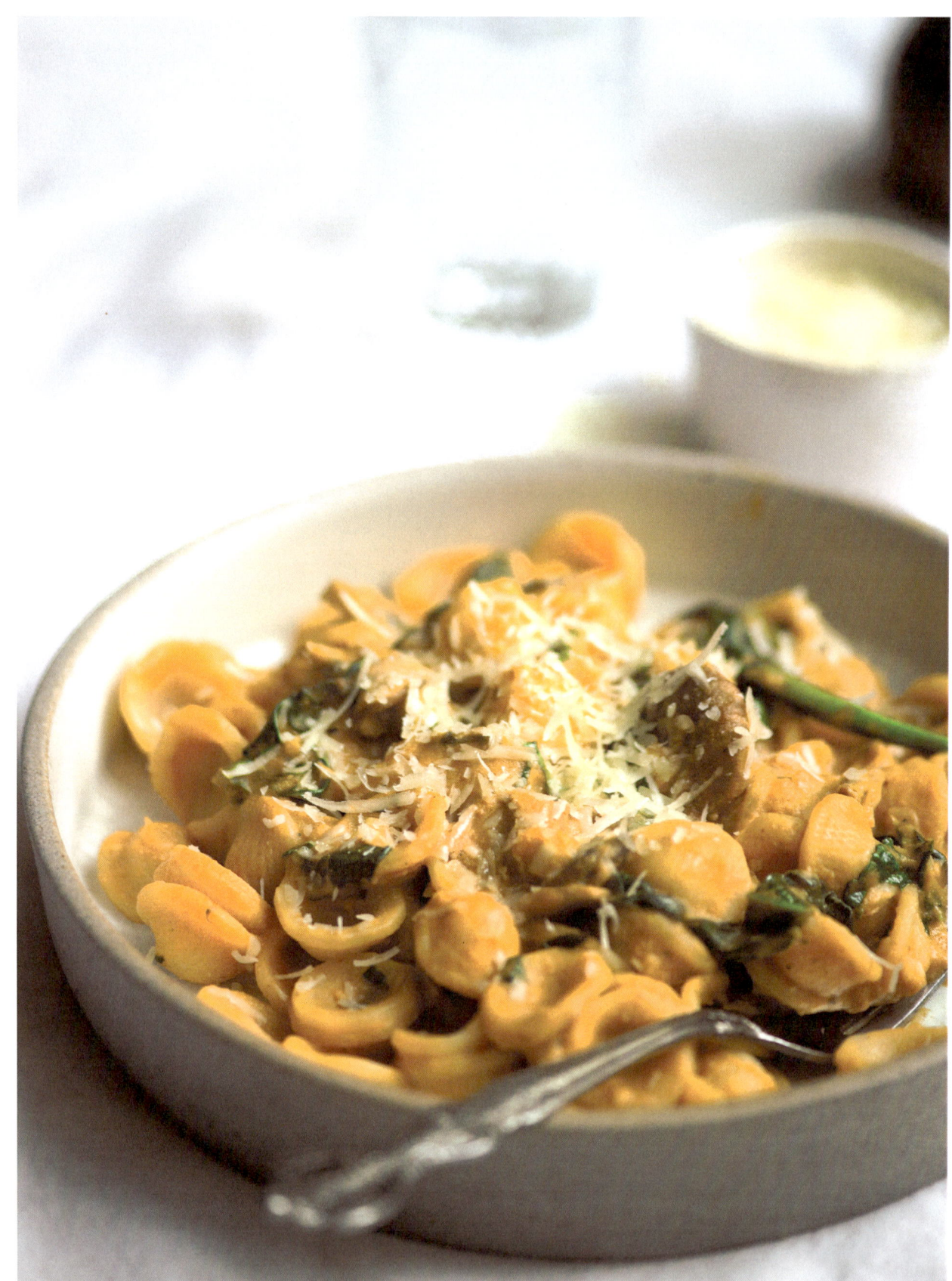

PUMPKIN TRUFFLE PASTA

WITH CHANTERELLES AND PARMESAN

As your babe continues to grow, you may experience sudden cravings and bursts of hunger. Whole-food, full-fat lunches with robust carbohydrates like this pumpkin pasta will set a pregnant mama up for success. Pumpkin provides vitamin C, potassium, and lots of fibre, which are ideal for second-trimester needs. Pre-make the sauce and you'll have an easy lunch for 2–3 days!

INGREDIENTS | SERVES 4

¼ cup minced yellow onions or shallots

2 ½ tablespoons freshly minced garlic

3 tablespoons ghee, avocado oil, or coconut oil, divided

225 grams cremini and chanterelle mushrooms, wiped clean with a paper towel and sliced or quartered (8 ounces)

500 grams whole grain, dried pasta (18 ounces)

¼ teaspoon truffle salt, plus more to taste

2 cups warmed chicken stock, vegetable stock, or bone broth, divided

1 cup puréed pumpkin

1 teaspoon sherry vinegar or apple cider vinegar

½ teaspoon sea salt

¼ cup truffle cashew cheese*

2 cups spinach, chopped

Shaved Parmesan (optional)

If you can't find truffle cashew cheese, a garlic cashew cheese or similar variety will also work well—just add a bit of truffle oil or truffle dust to create a richer truffle flavour.

DIRECTIONS

1. In a large Dutch oven or saucepan, sauté the onions and garlic with 1 tablespoon of ghee or oil over medium-low heat until soft, approximately 5 minutes. Add mushrooms and remaining 2 tablespoons of ghee or oil. Sauté the mushrooms, undisturbed, for 3–5 minutes until browned on one side. Stir and continue cooking for another 3–5 minutes until they are softened and brown on both sides.

2. While the mushrooms are browning, cook your pasta according to the package directions, making sure to salt the water generously. Drain, reserving ½ cup of the pasta water.

3. When the mushrooms are done, sprinkle with ¼ teaspoon of truffle salt and deglaze the pan with 1 cup of stock. Let the liquid reduce for a couple of minutes over medium heat. Add the remaining cup of stock, pumpkin purée, vinegar, and sea salt. Simmer for 5 minutes, turn the heat to low, and gently stir in the cashew cheese.

4. Stir in the spinach and ½ cup of salted pasta water. Flavour with more truffle salt to taste. (Every variety of truffle salt has a different intensity, so taste-test before adding too much!)

5. Stir the cooked pasta into the sauce and finish with freshly shaved Parmesan.

Cashew Cheese *is a plant-based alternative to dairy cheese. It is made from soaked cashews blended with spices, lemon, salt and sometimes active live cultures that yields a fabulously creamy texture with a zing of flavour. Think cream cheese meets dip! You can find this at your local health food or whole foods store.*

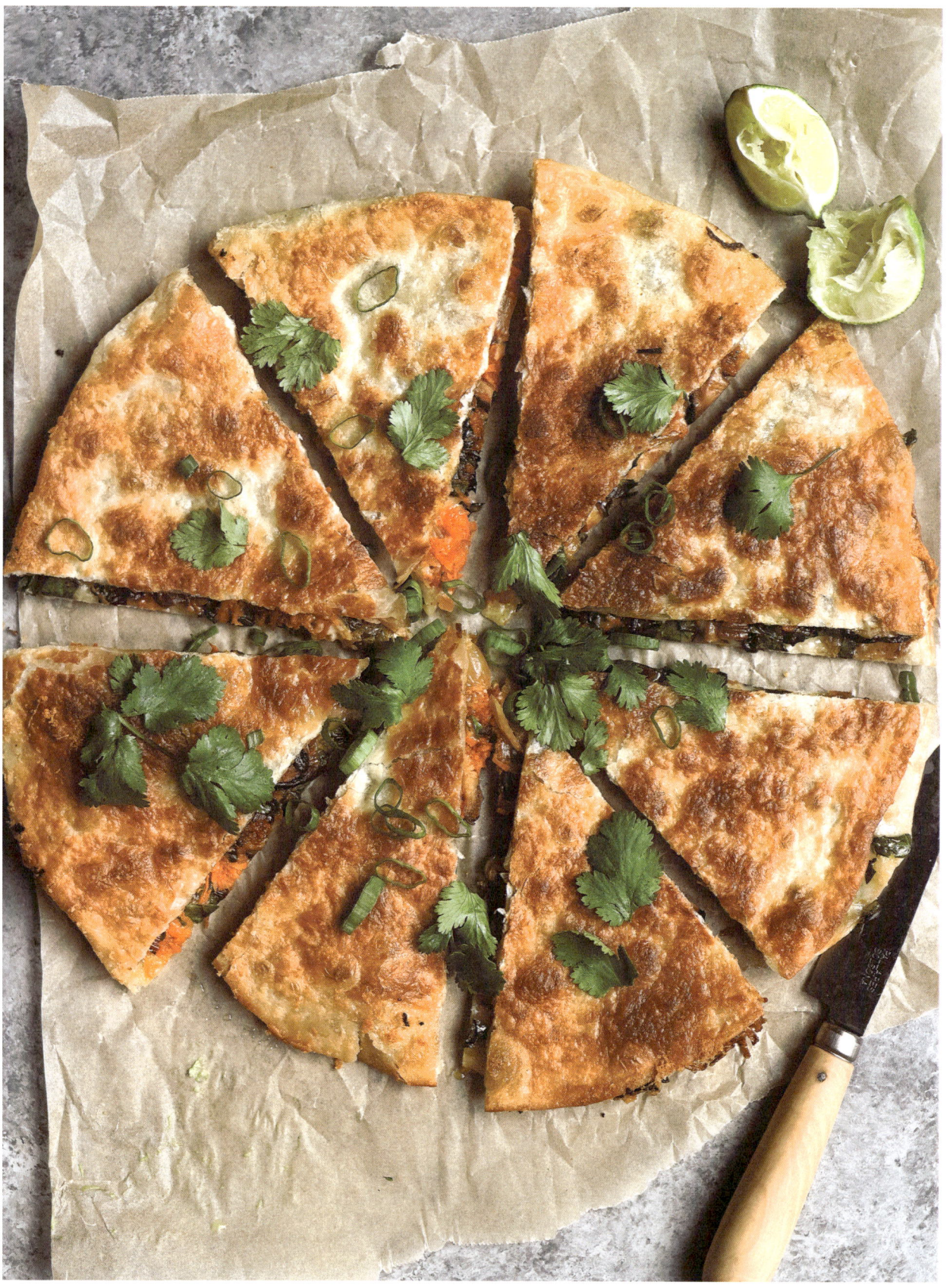

KIMCHI QUESADILLA

WITH SHIITAKES AND GREENS

This one is for the cheese lovers! You have to indulge in your favourites, especially during pregnancy. You need calcium this trimester to support babe's bone and tooth development and to maintain bone density. If you forgo the cheese in favour of vegan cheese, don't fret—leafy greens are a high source of calcium as well! This ooey-gooey quesadilla packs a punch with greens, carrots, kimchi for those much-needed probiotics, and green onions for prebiotics.

INGREDIENTS | SERVES 2

2 large whole-grain or gluten-free wraps

8 tablespoons ghee, avocado oil, or coconut oil, melted, divided

1 cup grated sharp white cheddar or vegan cheese, tightly packed

2 cups sliced shiitake mushrooms, wiped clean with a paper towel

¼ teaspoon sea salt

1 teaspoon tamari or soy sauce

¼ cup grated carrots

2 cups tightly packed chopped greens (e.g., spinach, kale, Swiss chard, or collards)

1 teaspoon sesame oil

¼ cup kimchi, drained

2 tablespoons chopped green onions (both white and green parts)

DIRECTIONS | PREHEAT OVEN TO 350° F

1. Place a piece of parchment paper on a baking sheet. Brush 1 tablespoon of oil on one wrap and lay the wrap, oil side down, on the parchment paper, ready for your toppings. Spread half the cheese on the wrap. Set aside the remaining cheese.

2. In a cast-iron skillet or non-stick, non-toxic frying pan, heat 4 tablespoons of ghee or oil over medium heat. Add the shiitake mushrooms and salt. Sauté for 3–4 minutes, stirring occasionally. Add the tamari and sauté for another 2 minutes until the mushrooms are soft.

3. Add 2 more tablespoons of ghee or oil to the pan with the mushrooms, and then add the carrots and greens. Sauté over medium heat, stirring occasionally, until vegetables are soft. Add sesame oil and stir to combine.

4. Spoon the mushroom and greens mixture on top of the cheese and spread out evenly.

5. Place the kimchi on top of the mushrooms and greens. Sprinkle green onions over the kimchi and top with the remaining cheese. Place the second wrap on top.

6. Brush the top with the remaining 1 tablespoon of ghee or oil. Bake at 350° for 10 minutes, turning over halfway through. If you do not want to bake the quesadillas, fry them in the same pan with a bit of coconut oil on each side until the cheese is melted and both sides are golden brown.

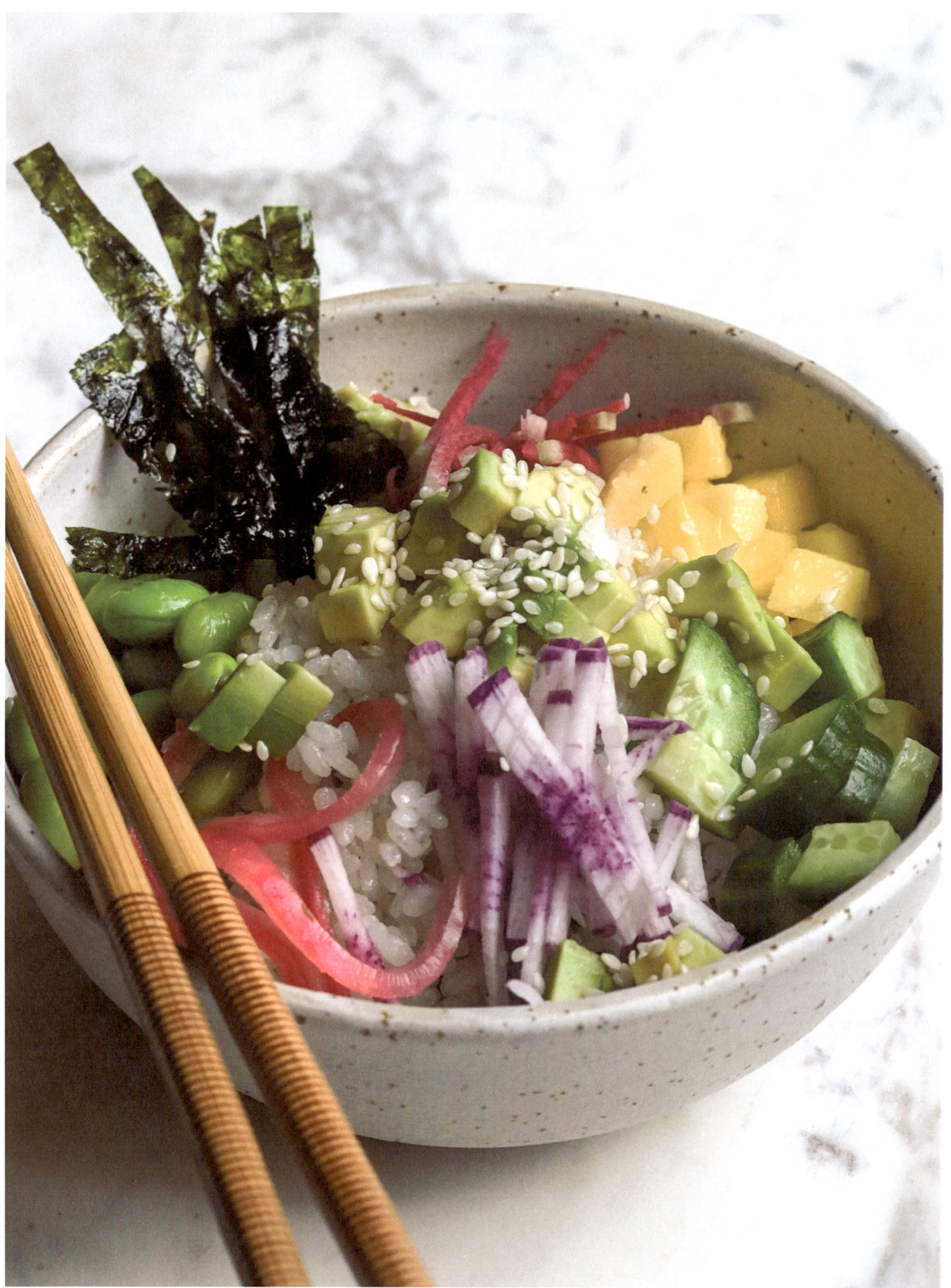

GINGER SOY SUSHI BOWL

WITH EDAMAME, AVOCADO, AND MANGO

This twist on sushi can help you quench pregnancy cravings without consuming raw fish. It is important to steer clear of raw fish, deli meats, and unpasteurized food while pregnant to prevent listeriosis. Mixing up a fresh bowl of this umami-packed, vegan take on sushi will leave you feeling very satisfied! Iodine, found in seaweed, is important for thyroid health. Iodine-rich foods such as seaweed can give maternal stores a much-needed leg up during the second trimester and help build a healthy thyroid for babe.

INGREDIENTS | SERVES 4

1 ½ cups sushi rice

½ teaspoon sea salt

½ cup cubed cucumber

1/2 cup cubed mango

r cubed

1 cup shelled edamame

3 watermelon radish and/or small purple daikon, shredded

2 avocados, sliced o

2 tablespoons sesame seeds (black or white)

Furikake or a sheet of dried seaweed torn into pieces

pickled red onions, optional

Dressing:

½ cup hempseed oil, flaxseed oil, or extra-virgin olive oil

⅔ cup tamari

2 tablespoons plus 2 teaspoons toasted sesame oil

¼ cup apple cider vinegar

4 teaspoons maple syrup

2 tablespoons lime juice

2 teaspoons minced ginger

¼ teaspoon chili flakes

DIRECTIONS

1. Rinse the rice thoroughly in a fine mesh sieve until the water runs clear. Place the rice in a large saucepan and cover with pure, filtered water. Cover and let it sit overnight.

2. The next day, drain the rice, rinse it thoroughly, and place it back in the saucepan with 3 cups filtered water and ½ teaspoon of salt. Bring to a boil, cover, turn the heat to low, and simmer for 15 minutes or until the rice is cooked through. (It shouldn't take too long after soaking overnight.) Remove from the heat but keep the lid on. Let it sit for 10 minutes untouched. Fluff with a fork and set aside.

3. While the rice is cooking, make your dressing: combine all the dressing ingredients in a jar with a tight-fitting lid and shake vigorously. Set aside.

4. In a bowl, layer your sushi bowl: rice, a bit of dressing, veggies, avocado, edamame, seeds, furikake or seaweed, and optional pickled red onions. Drizzle with extra dressing if desired and serve!

Kick this dish up a notch with a bit of "honey soy wild sockeye salmon bites": marinate 450 grams/1 pound of wild sockeye salmon chunks in 2 tablespoons of honey, 1 tablespoon of neutral oil, 1 tablespoon of sesame oil, 2 teaspoons freshly grated ginger, 2 tablespoons rice vinegar, and 1/4 cup tamari. Sauté in a fry pan with the sauce until cooked through.

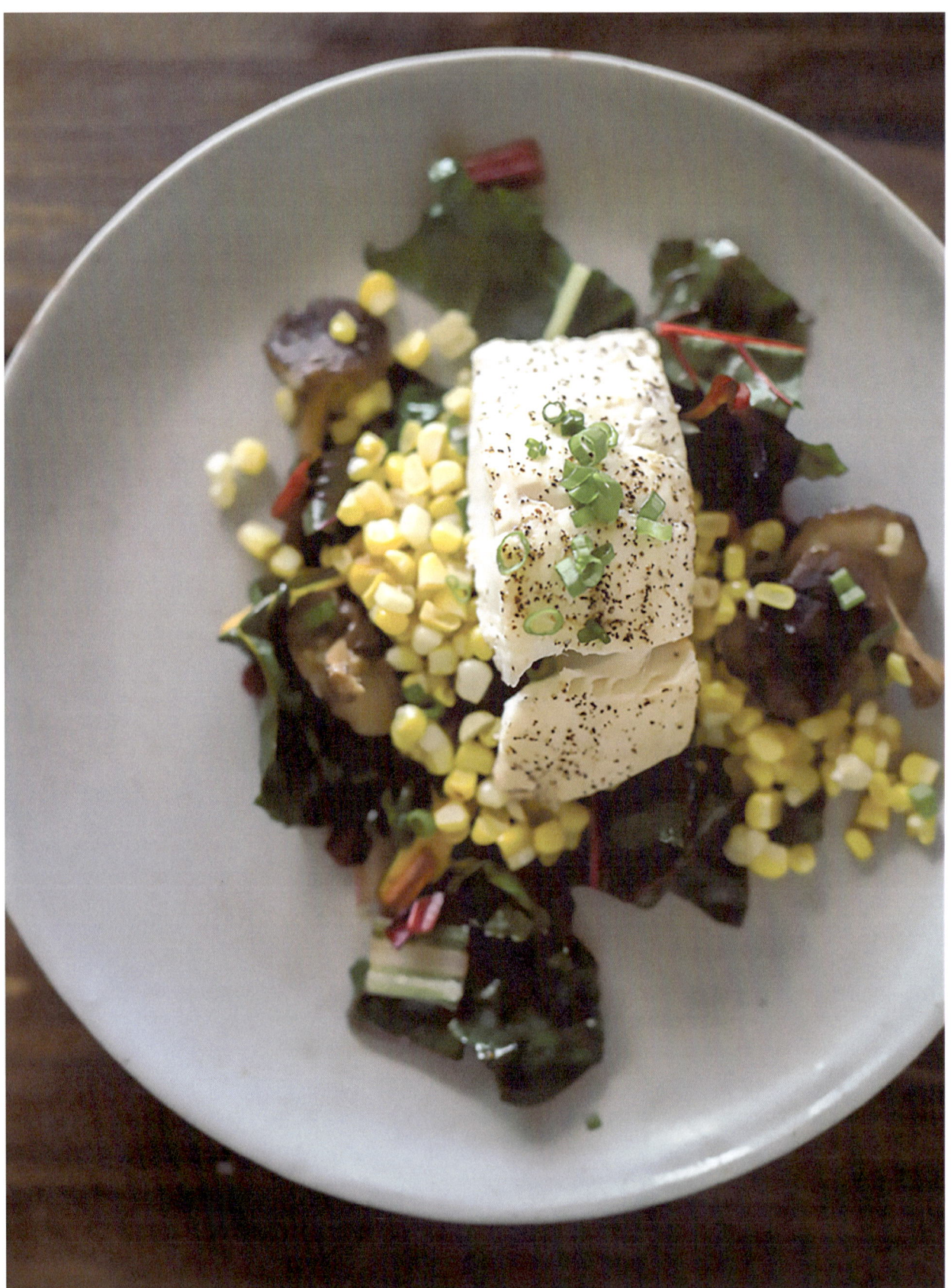

GRILLED LEMON HALIBUT

WITH MISO-CORN, SHIITAKES, AND SWISS CHARD

Adding a clean fish option to your weekly diet gives your body, and the growing baby, complete proteins and omega-3 essential fatty acids. Halibut is a light, flaky, and nutritious white fish that has low mercury levels. It is important to choose low-mercury fish during pregnancy, as high mercury levels—found in marlin, swordfish, and bluefin tuna—have been shown to have negative effects on the developing brain, auditory, and vision centres in the growing babe. You can double-check all fish options for mercury levels online; see the websites below.

INGREDIENTS | SERVES 4

- 4 cobs of corn, husks on
- 3 tablespoons ghee, avocado oil, or coconut oil, divided, plus more for rubbing corn
- ½ tablespoon freshly minced garlic
- ½ teaspoon minced ginger
- 5 green onions, sliced thin, green and white parts separated
- 250 grams shiitake mushrooms, each wiped clean with a paper towel (8.8 ounces)
- 1 tablespoon tamari or low-sodium soy sauce
- 3 tablespoons white or shiro miso
- 2 large bunches leafy greens (e.g., Swiss chard, collards, rapini, kale), ribs removed
- 450 grams wild halibut fillets (1 pound)
- Salt and pepper to season
- ½ lemon, to squeeze

It is important during pregnancy to choose fish that are low in mercury. Clean fish options can be found on these websites:

Oceanwise.ca

FDA.gov

DIRECTIONS

1. Preheat a ridged grill pan or grill to high. Once the grill is ready, place the corn, with the husks on, directly on the pan or grill for 10 minutes. Remove and let cool. Remove the husks and silk, rub the cobs with ghee or oil, and place back on the grill until the corn is charred. Remove from the grill and slice off the kernels. Set aside. (Alternatively, you can remove the raw kernels from the cob with a knife and sauté them on the stove in ghee or oil until charred.)

2. While the corn is roasting, heat a cast-iron or non-stick, non-toxic skillet over medium-low heat. Add 1 tablespoon of the ghee or oil, garlic, ginger, and the white parts of the green onion. Sauté for 1 minute over medium-low heat, stirring frequently to prevent burning. Add the mushrooms and another tablespoon of oil, stir to combine, and sauté over medium-low heat until soft, 4–5 minutes. Add tamari and toss to combine; sauté for 1 minute until the tamari soaks into the mushrooms. Add corn kernels and remove from heat.

3. Dissolve the miso into ⅓ cup hot (but not boiling) water. Add this to the corn and mushroom mixture over very low heat until the miso is dissolved and thoroughly combined. (Do not bring to a boil, as it will destroy the enzymes in the miso.) Set aside.

4. Prepare the greens: Roll the leaves lengthwise. Cut strips down the length of the roll, then cut one more time down the middle.

5. In a cast-iron or non-toxic, non-stick skillet, sauté the greens, 1 tablespoon of ghee or coconut oil, and salt and pepper over medium heat until the greens are wilted. Set aside.

6. Heat a grill pan to medium-high. Season the fish generously with salt and pepper on both sides. The salt on the skin will help it crisp. Place the halibut fillets skin side down on grill pan. Cover and cook for 3–4 minutes, then remove the lid and freshly squeeze the ½ lemon over the halibut. Cover again and continue cooking for 4–5 minutes, depending on the thickness of your halibut. The halibut should be tender and flaky, but not raw in the middle. Remove from the heat.

7. Divide the greens between each plate, top with the corn and mushroom mixture, and place a halibut fillet over top. Top with sliced green onions.

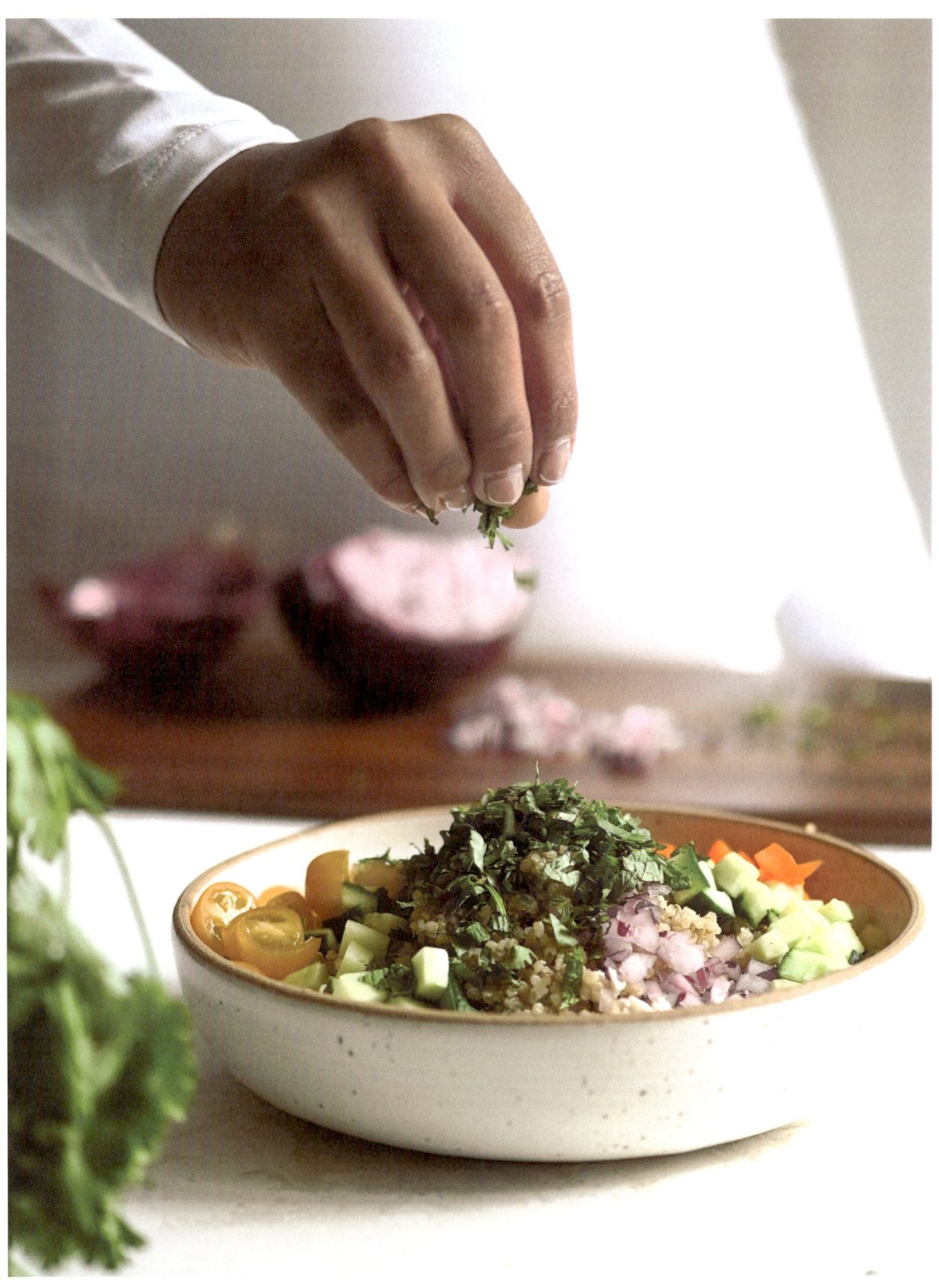

CHICKEN SOUVLAKI SALAD

WITH OLIVES, DATES, AND PARSLEY

This salad is a family favourite—it's quick and versatile, and the leftovers are perfect for weekday lunches. It's a balance of sweet and salty with olives, dates, and fresh herbs. Olives provide antioxidants, fats like oleic acid that benefit heart health, and vitamin E for skin health and elasticity (think stretch marks!). To make a great summer version, swap the cucumber for zucchini and grill it, along with the peppers and chicken, on the barbecue!

INGREDIENTS | SERVES 4

Chicken:
450 grams boneless, skinless chicken thighs, excess fat removed (1 pound)
2 tablespoons extra-virgin olive oil
2 tablespoons freshly squeezed lemon juice
4 teaspoons dried oregano
1 teaspoon dried marjoram or dried thyme
½ teaspoon cracked black pepper
¾ teaspoon sea salt
2 teaspoons freshly minced garlic

Salad:
1 pint cherry tomatoes, halved
¾ teaspoon sea salt, divided
¾ cup quinoa, uncooked
¼ cup minced red onions
1 small bell pepper, diced small
1 cup chopped cucumber
6 dates, pits removed, chopped
8 green olives, pits removed, chopped
¾ cup pasteurized sheep or goat feta cheese, crumbled
¼ cup fresh chopped mint
2 tablespoons fresh chopped parsley

Dressing:
4 tablespoons extra-virgin olive oil, hempseed oil, or flaxseed oil
1 teaspoon lemon juice
⅛ teaspoon freshly cracked pepper
¼ teaspoon sea salt

Tzatziki to serve (optional)

DIRECTIONS

1. Place the chicken in a large dish with the extra-virgin olive oil, lemon, oregano, marjoram, salt, pepper, and garlic. Mix well, and let the chicken marinate while you prepare the salad.

2. Place the halved cherry tomatoes in a large bowl and sprinkle with ½ teaspoon salt. Mix well and set aside for at least 10 minutes while you prep the rest of the salad.

3. In a medium saucepan, bring 2 cups water plus ¼ teaspoon salt to a boil. Add the quinoa. Cover, reduce heat to low, and simmer for 15 minutes. Remove from the heat, and let the quinoa stand, covered, for 5 minutes. Fluff with a fork and transfer to the tomato bowl.

4. Prepare the dressing: in a jar with a tight-fitting lid, mix together the dressing ingredients. Shake vigorously to combine and set aside.

5. Add the red onions, bell pepper, cucumber, dates, olives, feta, mint, parsley and reserved dressing to the tomato and quinoa bowl. Mix well.

6. Heat a grill pan over medium heat. Once hot, add the chicken. Cover and cook for 7–8 minutes, turning the chicken occasionally so it doesn't burn. Remove the cover and continue cooking to brown the chicken, approximately 2–3 minutes depending on the thickness of the chicken thighs.

7. Divide the salad into four portions and top with chicken and tzatziki

Labour and delivery are like a marathon, so let's train for them! Ina May Gaskin, the famed midwife, suggests vigorous hiking and upwards of 200 squats daily late into most pregnancies. Start slow, and level up as needed to keep your own personal fitness and flexibility in tip-top condition. Stay fuelled for exercise with a lunch like this quinoa salad.

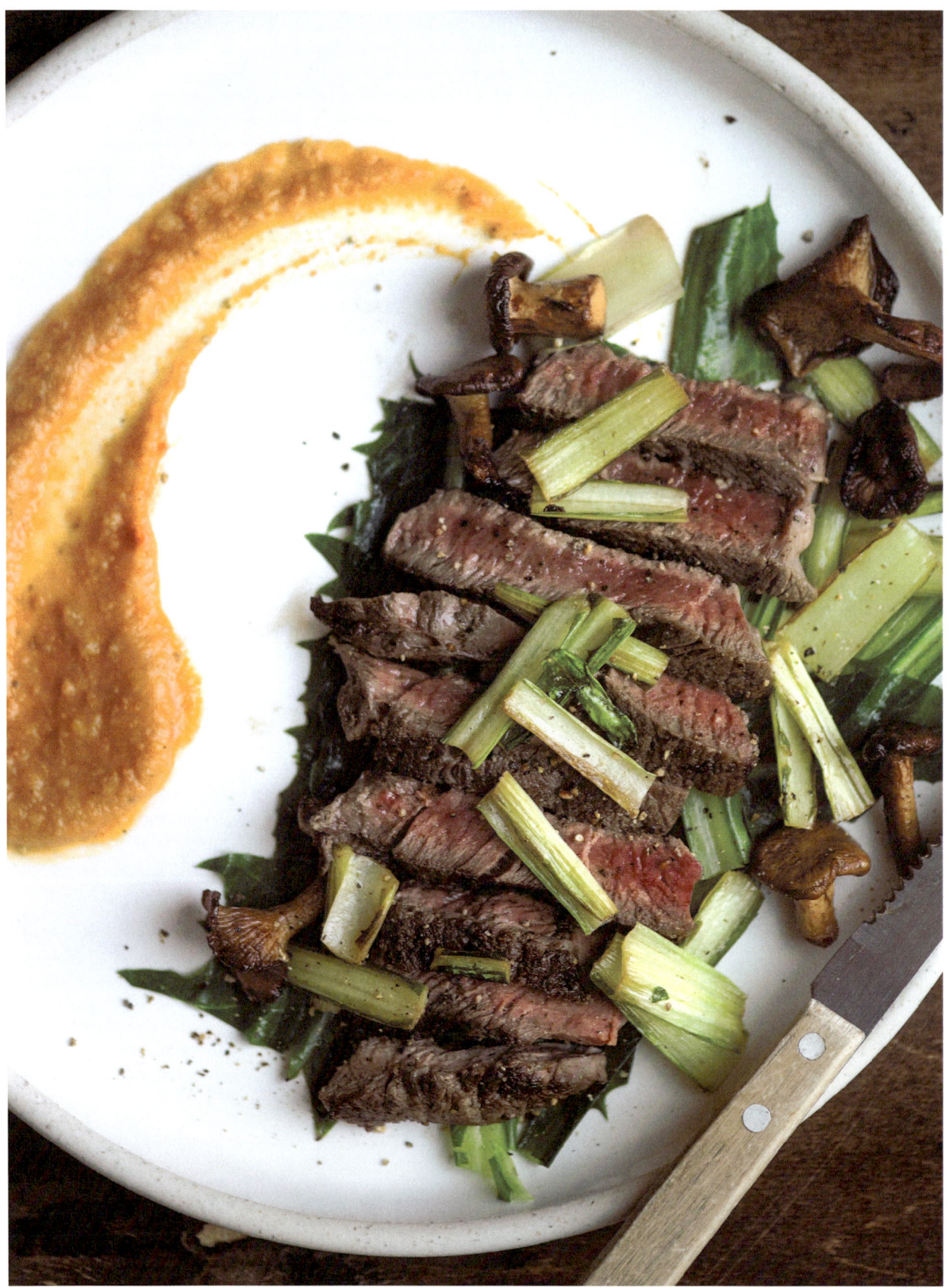

SEARED ELK STEAK

WITH GINGER CARROT SAUCE AND GREENS

There are so many benefits to wild game meat compared to factory-raised cows: higher omega-3 fatty acid content, no hormones or antibiotics, and a reduced carbon footprint, to name a few! Elk is higher in iron, protein, and B12 than beef. The beauty of this dish is that it combines iron-rich elk with vitamin C–rich carrots for optimal iron absorption. Greens are also high in iron and vitamin C! In the second half of pregnancy, the maternal requirement for protein doubles, and iron requirements also begin to increase, so grab seconds of this delicious dinner.

INGREDIENTS | SERVES 4

Steak:
450 grams elk flank steak (1 pound)
2 tablespoons rice vinegar
2 tablespoons avocado oil
2 garlic cloves, minced
1 teaspoon tamari or low-sodium soy sauce
1 teaspoon sea salt
1 teaspoon steak spice blend

Ginger carrot sauce:
¾ cup grated carrots
1 ½ tablespoons minced yellow onions
2 ½ tablespoons rice vinegar
½ tablespoon tamari
1 tablespoon maple syrup
3 tablespoons extra-virgin olive oil
2 teaspoons freshly grated ginger
⅛ teaspoon sea salt

Greens:
1 tablespoon ghee, avocado oil, or coconut oil
3 garlic cloves, sliced
1 bunch dandelion or rapini greens, chopped
⅛ teaspoon red pepper flakes
1 teaspoon balsamic vinegar

DIRECTIONS

1. In a glass dish, combine vinegar, oil, garlic, tamari or soy sauce, and salt and whisk to combine. Rub the whole flank steak with the spice blend and place it in the marinade. Flip to coat both sides with the marinade. Cover and let it sit in the fridge overnight.

2. Place all ginger carrot sauce ingredients in a food processor and purée. (You can make this in advance; store it in an airtight container in the fridge for 5–7 days.)

3. When you are ready to cook the steak, set the oven to broil and place the oven rack a few inches below the broiler. Set a wire rack on top of a baking sheet or use a broiler pan. Remove the steak from the marinade, shake off the excess, and set it on top of the wire rack. When the oven has come to temperature, place the pan with the steak in the middle of the oven. Broil for 4–6 minutes, flip, and broil for another 4–6 minutes.

4. While the steak is cooking, prepare your greens: heat ghee or oil in a sauté pan over medium-low heat. Add the garlic and let it sizzle for 20–30 seconds until it becomes aromatic, stirring so it doesn't burn or stick. Add the greens and red pepper flakes; sauté for 3–4 minutes until soft. Add the balsamic vinegar and stir to coat. Remove from the heat and set aside.

5. Check temperature of the steak by inserting an instant-read thermometer into the thickest part: 120–125° F for medium-rare, 130–135° F for medium, and 140–145° F for medium-well. Cooking an extra minute or two will raise the temperature by about 10 degrees. If it's becoming too crisp on the edges, turn the oven to "bake" at 400° F.

6. Transfer the steak to a cutting board and let it rest for 5 minutes before slicing. Slice against the grain.

7. While the steak is resting, heat the ginger carrot sauce. Place the carrot sauce on your plate, top with the steak, and serve with greens.

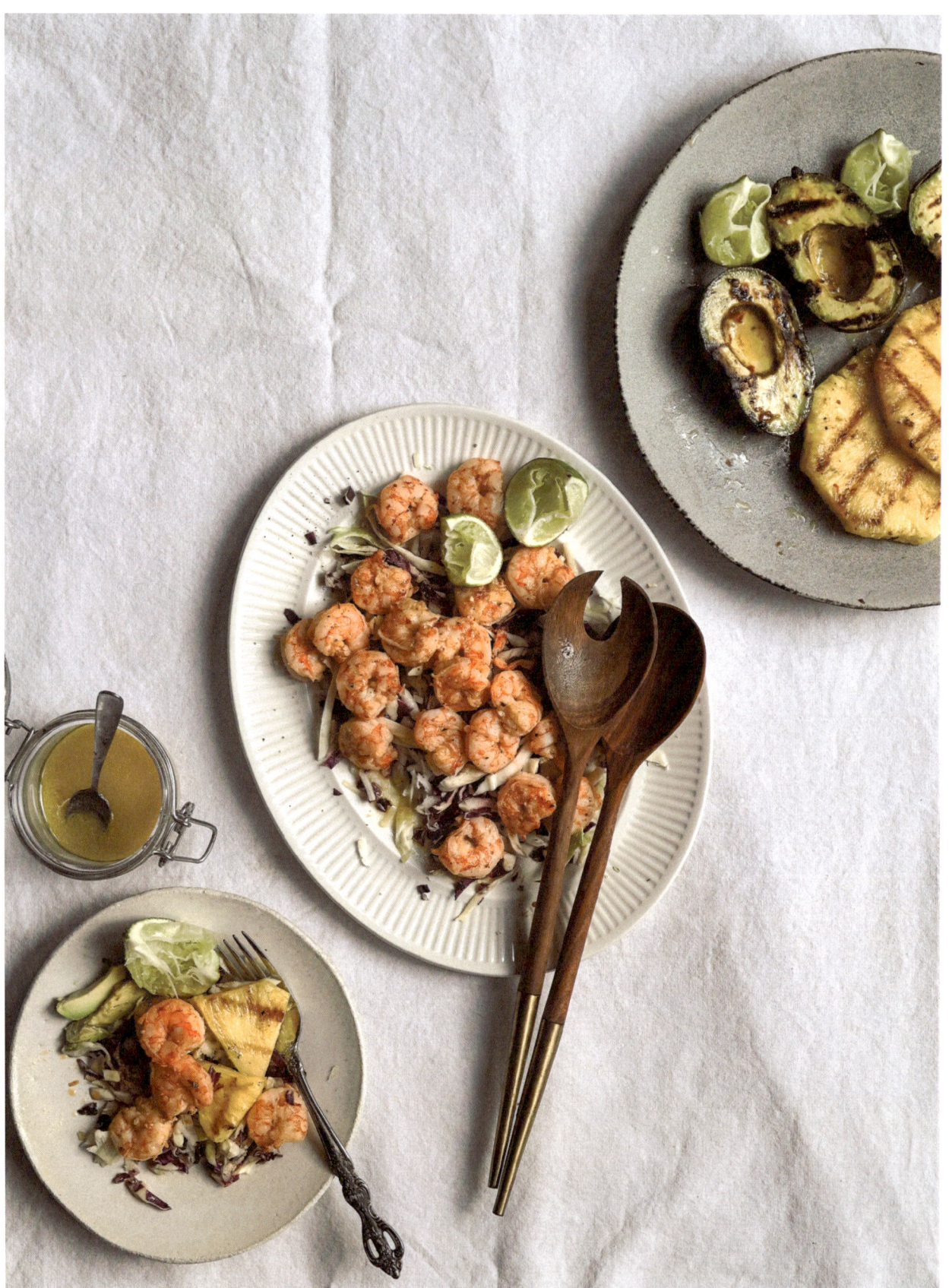

SPICY PINEAPPLE MISO SHRIMP

WITH GRILLED AVOCADO AND KOHLRABI SLAW

It's easy to fall into a routine of picking up the same vegetables at the grocery store, but next time you see kohlrabi, give it a try! It's a cross between a turnip and cabbage, so it's the perfect addition to slaw. The pineapple and lime give it a fresh twist while providing ample vitamin C and antioxidant goodness. Vitamin C not only helps iron absorption, it also supports the immune system and is integral to skin health in babe and collagen production in mama. And if you have never grilled an avocado … you're in for a real treat! You can also throw this dish into tortillas for a fun Taco Tuesday!

INGREDIENTS | SERVES 4

Pineapple miso shrimp:

3 tablespoons extra-virgin olive oil or avocado oil, divided
1 tablespoon sambal oelek*
1 ½ tablespoons white or shiro miso
280 grams raw, wild shrimp, preferably ocean-wise, peeled, deveined, and tails removed (10 ounces)
1 cup fresh pineapple chunks or rings
2 ripe avocados
1 ½ teaspoons lime juice or ½ a fresh lime

Slaw:

3 tablespoons pineapple juice
1 ½ tablespoons white or shiro miso
1 tablespoon extra-virgin olive oil
1 tablespoon lime juice
1 tablespoon rice vinegar
1 teaspoon pasteurized honey
1 ½ cups thinly sliced green cabbage (i.e., with a mandoline)
1 ½ cups grated kohlrabi
½ cup thinly sliced red cabbage, (i.e., with a mandoline)

DIRECTIONS

1. In a large bowl, combine 2 tablespoons of the oil, the sambal oelek, and the miso. Mash the miso with a fork or the back of a spoon until smooth and fully incorporated into the oil and sambal. Add the shrimp and pineapple and stir to coat them with the sambal-miso mixture. Set them aside to marinate while you prepare the rest.

2. Prepare the dressing for the slaw: In a food processor, combine the pineapple juice, miso, oil, lime juice, rice vinegar, and honey. Blend on low until smooth and fully combined.

3. In a large bowl, toss together the sliced cabbage, kohlrabi, and dressing. Set aside.

4. Halve the avocados and remove the pits. Using a pastry brush, brush the green flesh with a bit of the sambal/miso marinade from the bowl with the shrimp and pineapple. Set aside.

5. Heat a grill pan over medium heat and add the remaining 1 tablespoon of oil. Place the pineapple straight on the pan and grill for 4 minutes. (Using a splatter screen here really helps keep your kitchen counters clean!) Flip the pineapple and add the avocado halves, flesh side down. Grill for another 2 minutes.

6. Add the shrimp and grill over medium heat until they turn pink, for a total of about 3 minutes, flipping halfway through.

7. Remove the pineapple, shrimp, and avocado from the grill pan, sprinkle them with the lime juice, and set aside.

8. Divide the slaw between 4 plates and top with the shrimp and pineapple. Serve with half a grilled avocado on the side.

* If you can't find sambal oelek, red harissa, sriracha, or gochujang are suitable substitutes

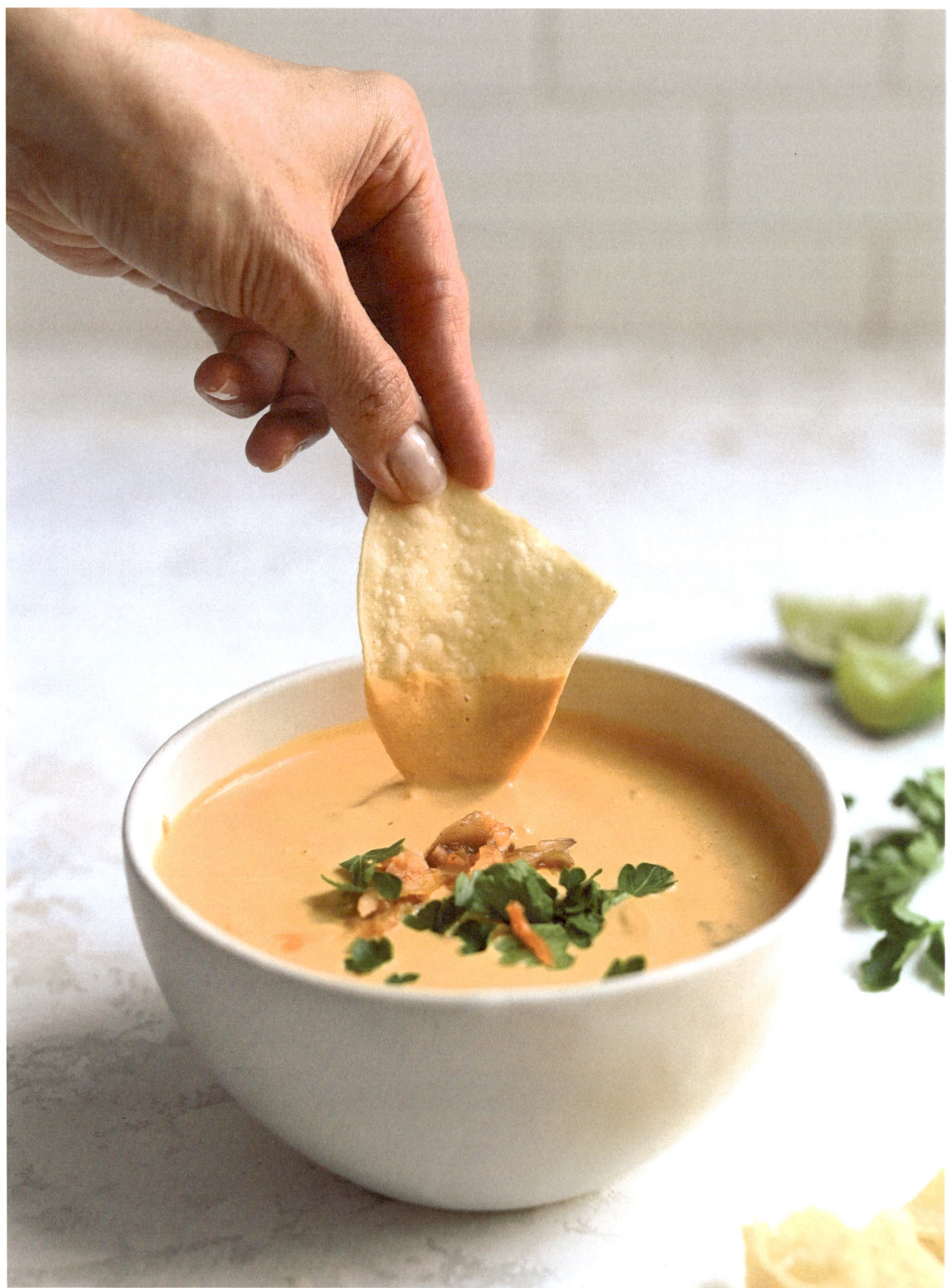

VEGAN KIMCHI "CHEEZ" DIP

WITH CARROTS AND POTATOES

Kimchi is a traditional Korean fermented food made of cabbage. Fermented foods are essential during pregnancy and for your gut microbiome. When moms have healthy microbial flora, babe is set up for success with their own healthy flora—which reduces their risk for allergies, eczema, and immune issues. This is an easy, versatile dip you can use with nachos, breakfast potatoes, or chips.

INGREDIENTS | YIELDS 4 CUPS

2 cups chopped carrots
3 cups chopped potatoes
1 teaspoon sea salt, divided
2 tablespoons diced yellow onions
4 tablespoons nutritional yeast
2 tablespoons lemon juice
¾ teaspoon garlic powder
4 tablespoons coconut oil
¾ cup drained kimchi, chopped, plus 1 tablespoon kimchi juice
Tortilla chips or roasted veggie chips to serve

DIRECTIONS

1. Place carrots and potatoes in a medium saucepan. Add enough water to cover plus ¼ teaspoon salt. Bring to a low boil, cover, and simmer for 12 minutes. Add the onions and simmer for another 2 minutes or until the potatoes and carrots are fork-tender.

2. Remove vegetables from the heat and drain through a sieve, reserving at least 2 tablespoons of the cooking liquid. Transfer the potatoes, carrots, and onions to a blender along with the 2 tablespoons of the cooking liquid.

3. Add the remaining ¾ teaspoon salt, nutritional yeast, lemon juice, garlic powder, and coconut oil to the blender. Blend on high until smooth and fully combined.

4. Pour the sauce into a bowl and stir in the kimchi and kimchi juice.

5. Enjoy with tortilla chips or roasted veggie chips, or incorporate into other dishes like burrito bowls or nachos!

Nutritional yeast is a vegan, natural cheese flavouring derived from deactivated and dried yeast, typically in the form of flakes. It is reminiscent of a malty, parmesan rind and can be used on anything from popcorn to mashed potatoes to sauces to give a cheese-like flavour. You actually get more protein per calorie than cheese and most brands supplement with vitamin B12, a vitamin naturally occurring in animal protein that supports a healthy nervous system.

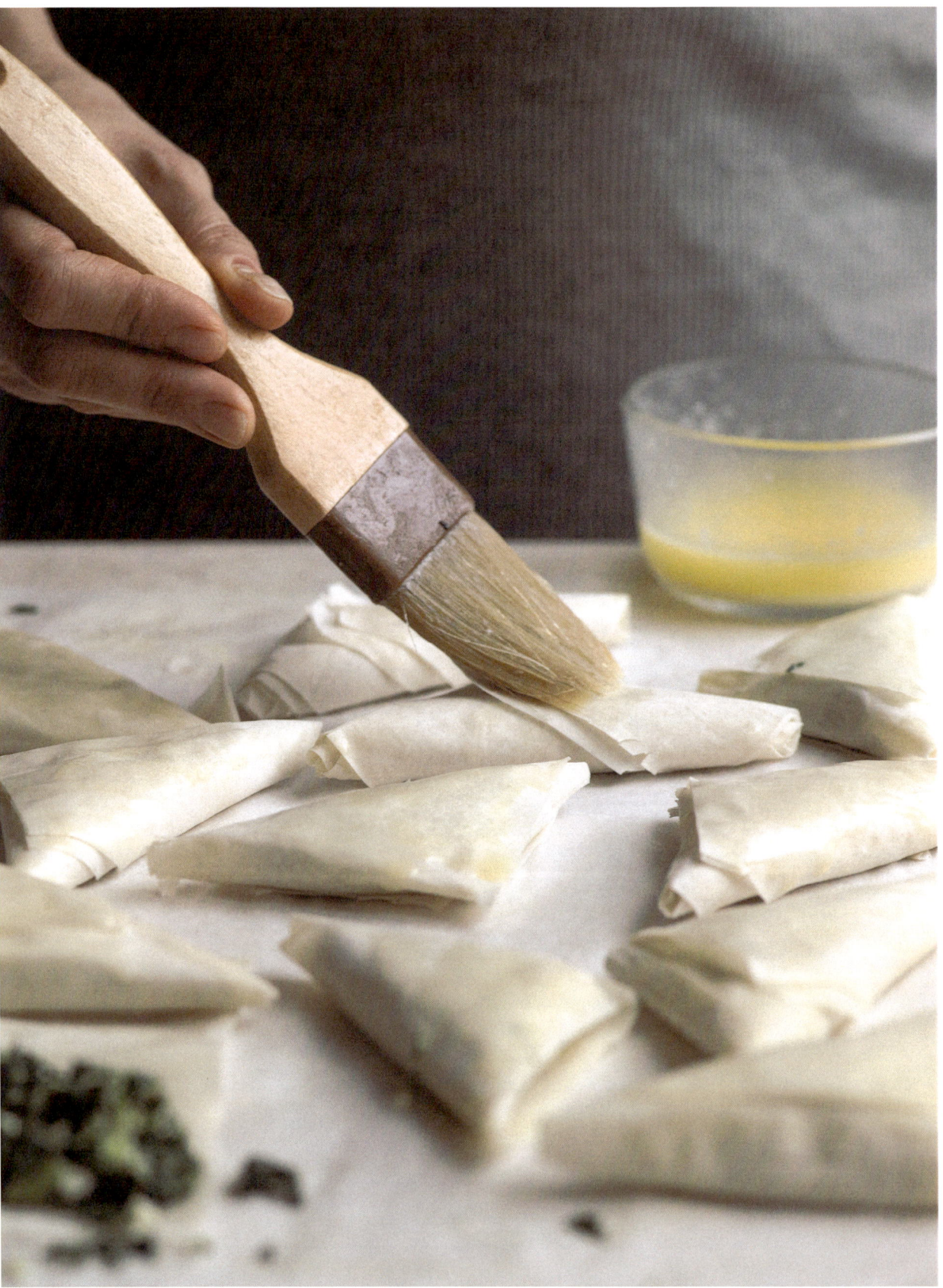

SPANIKOPITA

WITH SPELT PHYLLO AND DANDELION GREENS

Varying the produce you buy is key to a balanced diet with an array of micronutrients. Instead of always reaching for kale or spinach, switch it up with something different like beet greens, rapini, or dandelion greens as we have used here. Incorporating fresh greens into recipes is key—they offer blood-building folic acid and iron. Combined with the B12-packed cheese in this tasty appetizer, you can feel great about snacking your way to healthy red blood cell levels.

INGREDIENTS

1 package frozen spelt phyllo dough
2 cups chopped fresh dandelion leaves, tightly packed
283 grams frozen spinach, thawed, drained of all water (10 ounces)
1 ½ cups assorted shredded, organic pasteurized cheese (e.g., sharp cheddar, Parmesan, Swiss, or pasteurized feta)
2 teaspoons freshly minced garlic
2 teaspoons minced yellow onions
1 tablespoon fresh lemon juice
2 tablespoons fresh chopped parsley
1 teaspoon dried dill
¼ teaspoon sea salt
Freshly cracked pepper
1 free range, organic egg, beaten
2 tablespoons grass-fed butter, ghee, or coconut oil

DIRECTIONS | PREHEAT OVEN TO 350° F

1. Place the frozen phyllo dough in the fridge to thaw overnight. (If you wish, you can make the filling ahead of time while the dough is thawing out.)
2. Bring a saucepan of salted water to a boil. Add the dandelion greens and simmer on low for 7–8 minutes until soft. Drain thoroughly and add to a medium mixing bowl.
3. Add the spinach, cheese, garlic, onions, lemon juice, parsley, dill, salt, and pepper to the bowl. Mix well to combine. Add the egg and stir well to combine.
4. Gently remove the phyllo dough from the package and lay it flat on the counter.
5. Melt the butter, ghee, or coconut oil in a small glass container in the oven. Remove and set the container on the counter to cool.
6. Gently separate one sheet of phyllo dough from the stack and lay it on the counter. Brush the butter, ghee, or coconut oil sparingly onto the dough. Lay another piece on top of the buttered layer and brush this piece the same as the first.
7. Cut the phyllo dough down the middle vertically, then cut each strip down the middle vertically again. You should have 4 long, skinny strips of phyllo dough.
8. Place roughly 1 ½ tablespoons of the greens-and-cheese mixture on the edge of one strip of dough. Fold over into a triangle shape, then fold down into another triangle shape. Continue folding until you reach the top of the strip. The aim is to capture the mixture in a little triangular pocket. Practice your folding technique with a strip of paper - it's really quite easy when you get the hang of it!
9. Line a baking sheet with parchment paper and arrange your spanakopita on the tray. Brush with excess butter or oil.
10. Bake at 350° for 25–30 minutes until golden brown.

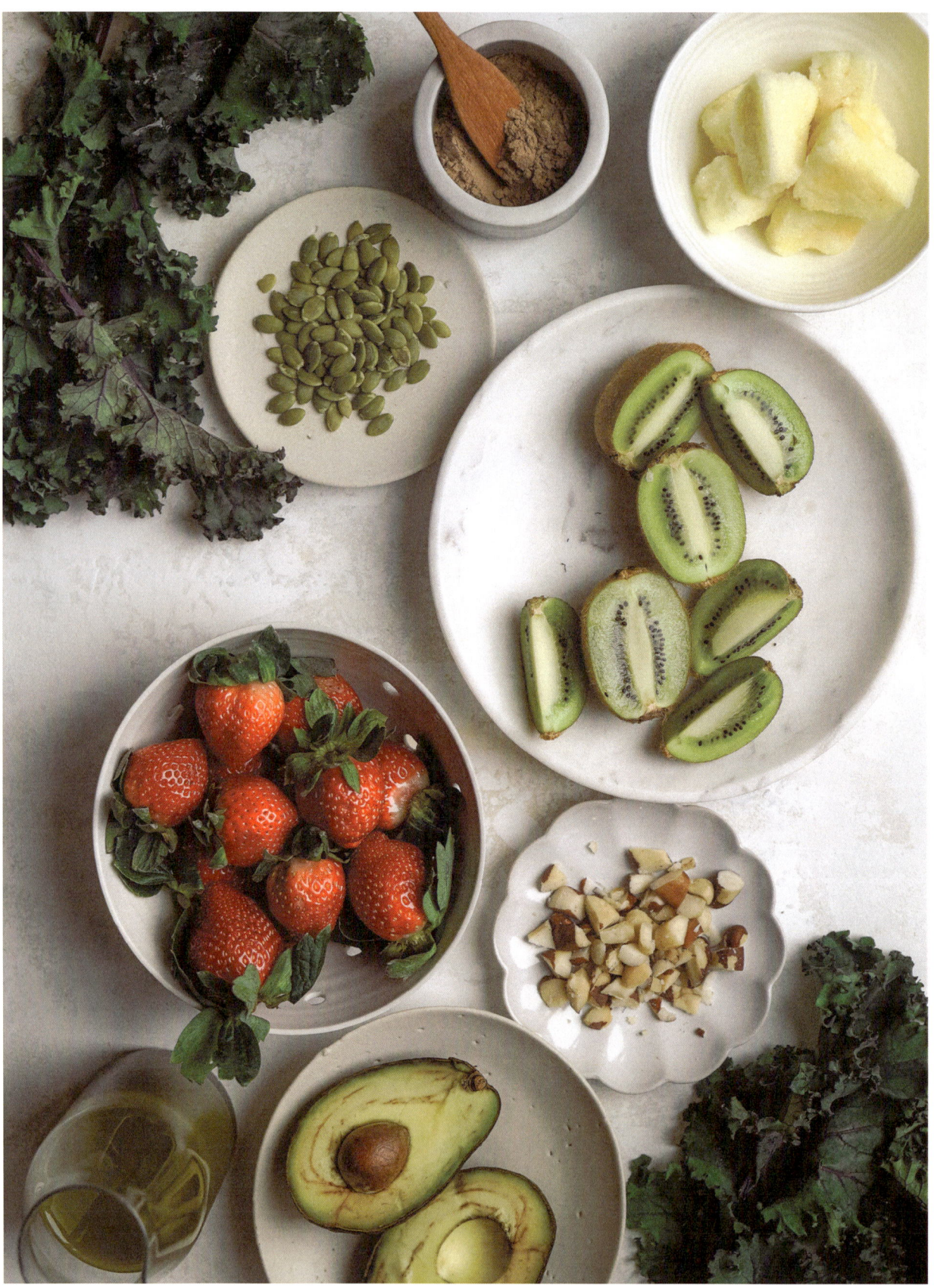

SMOOTH SKIN SMOOTHIE BOWL,

TWO WAYS

A smoothie bowl that combats stretch marks and is good for the gut? Yes, please! These smoothie bowl ingredients are high in selenium, vitamin E, vitamin A, vitamin C, and zinc, all of which benefit skin health, elasticity, and collagen production. Did you know that two Brazil nuts contain your daily recommended amount of selenium and help with skin elasticity and inflammation? Selenium is a powerful antioxidant that works well with zinc and vitamin E, which are also beneficial for skin health and tissue and wound healing. Finally, we've added camu camu—this fruit boasts the highest concentration of vitamin C in the world, which helps promote collagen and elastin levels. We have provided two options for the smoothie base so you can switch it up!

INGREDIENTS

Smoothie base #1:
½ cup raspberries
¾ cup strawberries
¼ cup frozen mango, pineapple, or papaya chunks
½ cup coconut or vanilla kefir
⅓ cup orange juice
1 tablespoon milled flaxseed
1 tablespoon camu camu powder
¼ avocado

Smoothie base #2:
⅓ cup plus 2 tablespoons fresh pressed green juice, no sugar added
¼ cup avocado
½ cup spinach, kale, or greens of your choice, ribs removed
1 ½ cups frozen pineapple, mango, or papaya chunks
½ cup coconut or vanilla kefir
½–1 tablespoon spirulina
1 tablespoon camu camu powder
1 tablespoon milled flaxseed

Toppings:
1 tablespoon chia seeds
1 tablespoon hemp hearts
1 tablespoon crushed Brazil nuts
1 tablespoon pumpkin seeds
1 tablespoon shredded coconut
Raspberries or sliced strawberries
1 kiwi, diced
¼ cup granola

DIRECTIONS

1. Blend all smoothie base ingredients in a blender. Transfer to a bowl.
2. Add your toppings and enjoy with a spoon!

The quality of spirulina you use makes a huge difference in the health benefits. Chat with your local whole-foods store to discover what's available. Anise uses frozen spirulina cubes by SpiraVeg. The taste is strong, so start with a little bit and add more if possible.

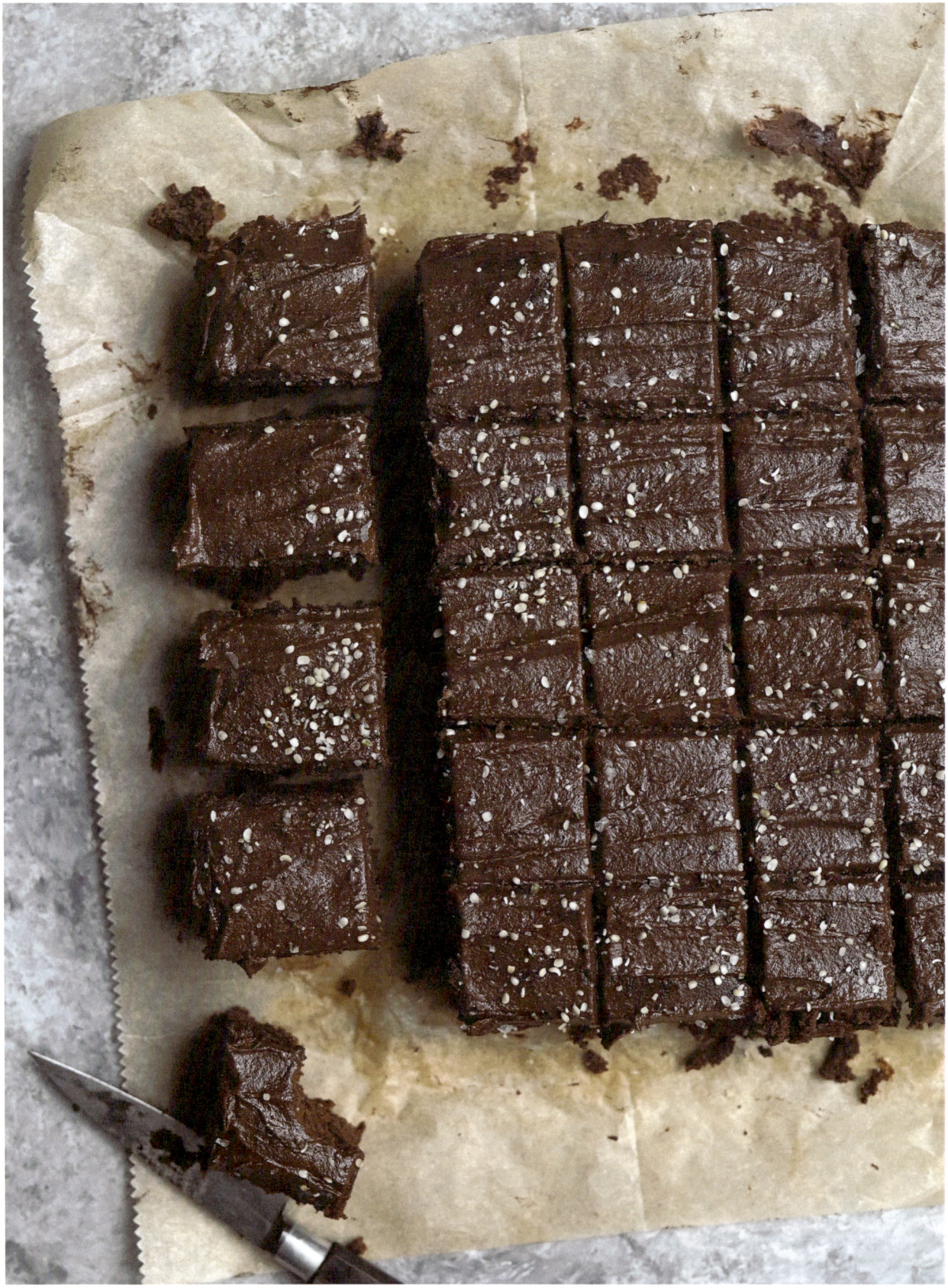

CHOCOLATE AVOCADO BROWNIES

WITH DATE AND CACAO FROSTING

This recipe came to Anise when she was trying to sneak more healthy fats into her kids' snacks. Whenever she makes a batch of these brownies, they are typically gone before she can even enjoy one herself! Dark chocolate is high in antioxidants, iron, magnesium, potassium, and B vitamins. Chocolate containing more than 75 percent cacao can improve cholesterol, blood pressure, overall heart health, and cognition. Blended with bananas and avocado, it gives us an energy boost with whole-food, plant-based fats and carbohydrates.

INGREDIENTS | YIELDS 25 SMALL BROWNIES

1 cup mashed bananas
1 cup mashed avocado, tightly packed
2 free range, organic eggs
½ cup maple syrup
½ teaspoon vanilla
¾ cup cacao powder
¼ cup coconut sugar
¾ teaspoon baking soda
¼ teaspoon sea salt
2 tablespoons Dandy Blend (optional)
1 ½ cups almond flour
¼ cup crushed walnuts

Frosting:
8 medjool dates, pits and stems removed
¼ cup plus 2 tablespoons cacao powder
1/2 cup mashed ripe avocado
¼ cup plus 1 tablespoon maple syrup
⅛ teaspoon sea salt

DIRECTIONS | PREHEAT OVEN TO 350° F

1. Line a 9 x 9" glass baking dish with parchment paper.
2. Add the banana, avocado, eggs, maple syrup, and vanilla to a high-speed blender and blend on low until combined.
3. Add cacao powder, coconut sugar, baking soda, sea salt and Dandy Blend, if using. Pulse lightly to combine. (If you have run out of room in your blender for additional ingredients, combine these ingredients in a medium bowl. Add the banana-avocado mixture to the bowl of dry ingredients and stir again until fully combined.)
4. Stir the almond flour and walnuts into the blender mixture until fully combined and transfer the batter to the lined baking dish. Smooth the top with a spatula. If you aren't using the frosting, you can top the brownies with additional nuts, chocolate chips, or even fresh raspberries!
5. Bake at 350° for 45 minutes.
6. While the brownies are baking, prepare the frosting: In a food processor, add dates and enough boiling water to cover. Let the dates sit for 10 minutes to soften. Drain the water and add the cacao powder, avocado, maple syrup and salt. Blend until smooth.
7. Remove the brownies from the oven and let them cool completely before frosting and slicing. (They may seem mushy until they have cooled, so try to be patient!)
8. Using a spatula, spread the frosting over the brownies. Slice into squares and keep in an airtight container at room temperature for up to 5 days—if they last that long!

Anise has also included the option of adding Dandy Blend, a dandelion root powder that tastes similar to coffee but also aids in digestion and immunity, supports kidney and liver function, and boasts antioxidants and anti-inflammatory properties.

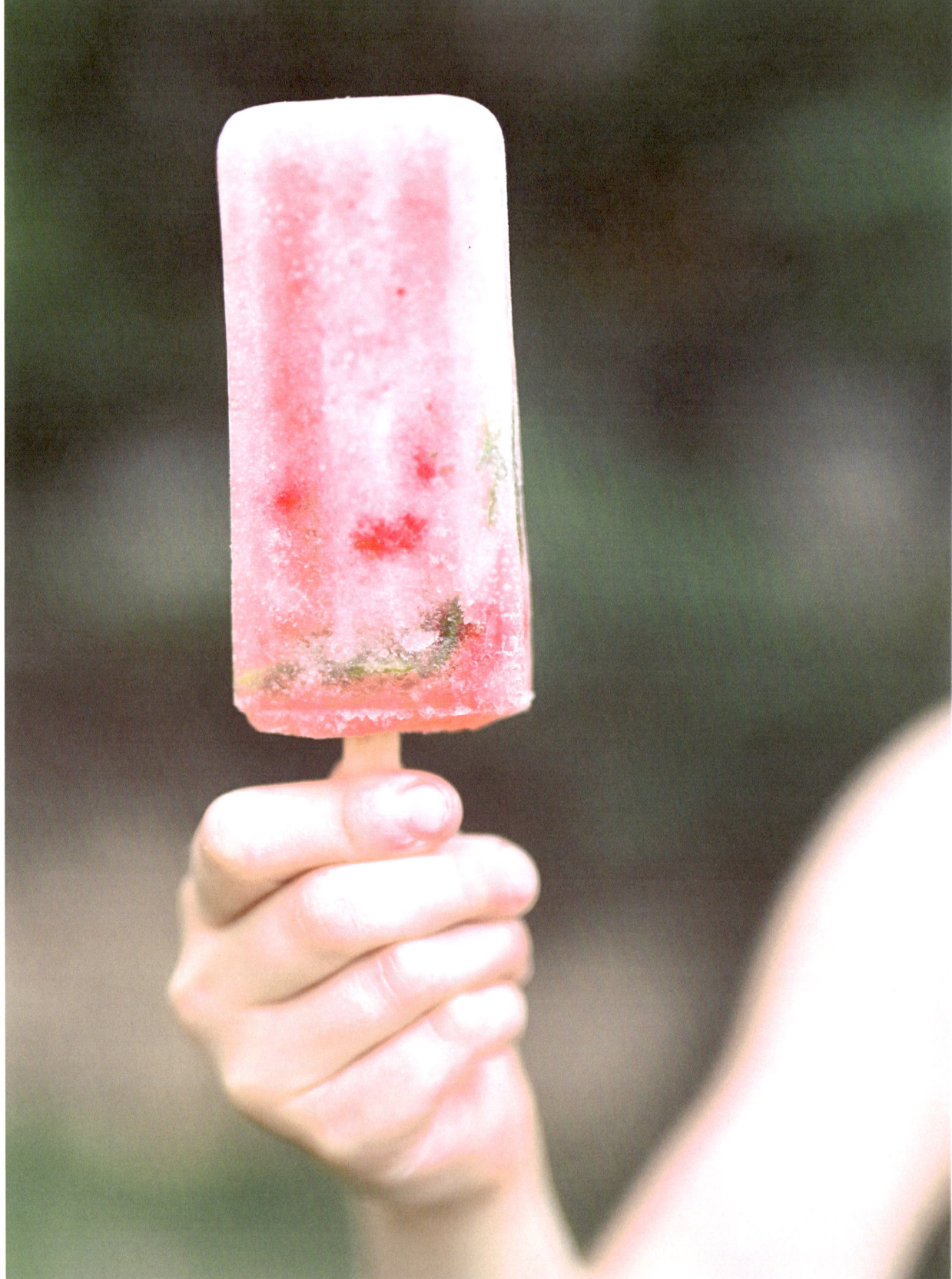

GUAVA KOMBUCHA FREEZIES

WITH RASPBERRIES AND CHIA SEEDS

These easy and refreshing popsicles are perfect for those days when you need a little something special. Kombucha is a fermented tea that provides probiotics for optimal gut health. However, kombucha is unpasteurized to keep its healthy microorganisms intact, so if you have never had it before, check with your midwife or doctor before trying. If you were drinking kombucha regularly before pregnancy, you can continue drinking this magical tea throughout pregnancy. You can find kombucha in a variety of flavours. Anise has suggested guava here, but this recipe works well with any fruity flavour.

INGREDIENTS | SERVES 6

2 cups plus 12 frozen raspberries
1 cup guava kombucha
¼ cup pasteurized honey
¼ cup chia seeds

DIRECTIONS

1. In a blender, purée 2 cups of raspberries, kombucha, and honey. Mix in the chia seeds.
2. Pour into Popsicle moulds. Add a few whole raspberries to each popsicle and place in the freezer for 6–12 hours.

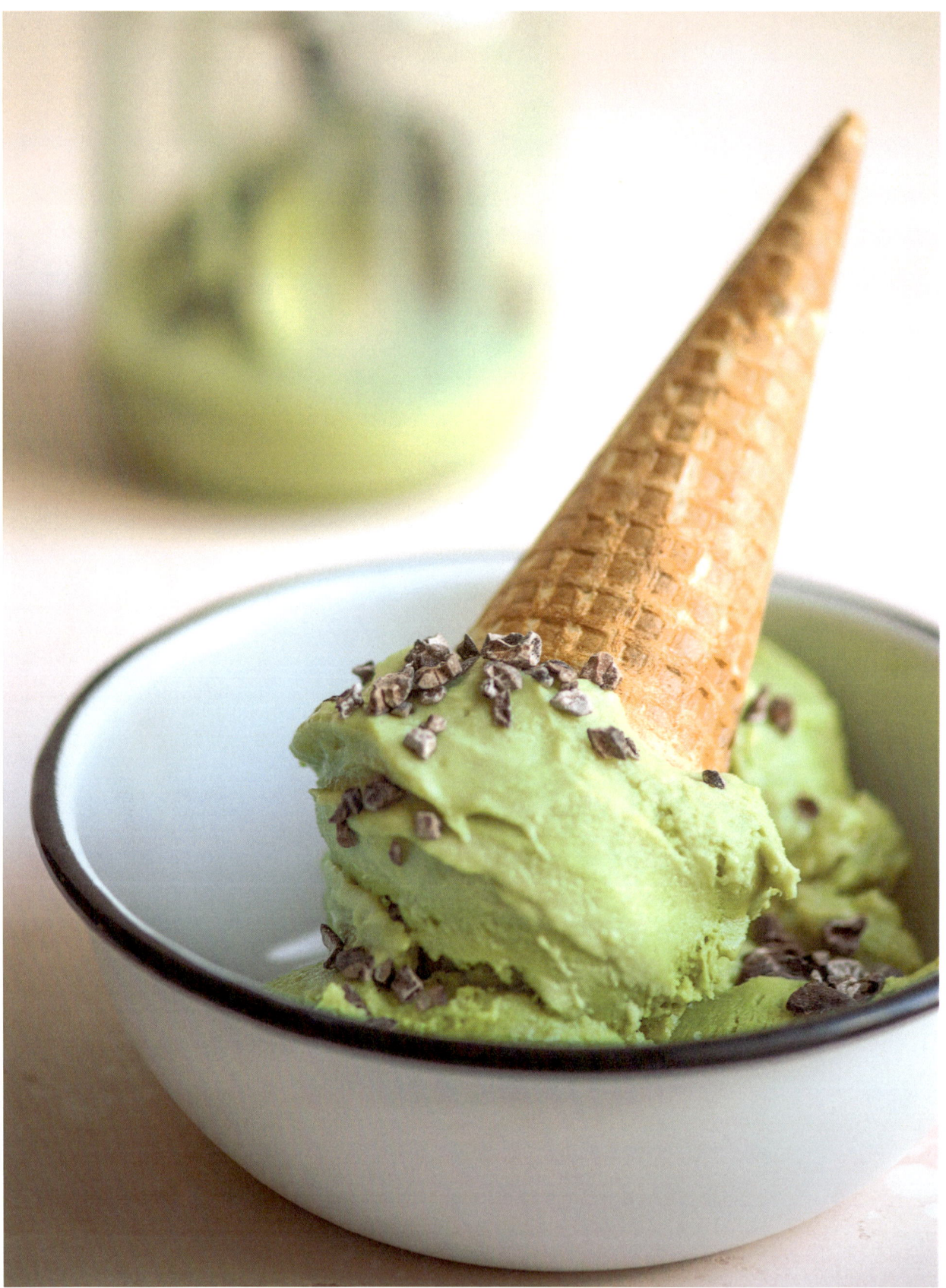

MINT CHOCOLATE NICE CREAM

WITH CACAO NIBS

Avocado and coconut are loaded with healthy mono- and polyunsaturated fats—perfect for building much-needed fat stores in Mama's body for proper growth and development in babe. You are finally feeling kicks and flips at this point, and this delicious dessert will have you both dancing to the freezer for a sweet and satisfying treat.

INGREDIENTS | SERVES 2

1 (400-ml) can full-fat coconut milk (14 ounces)
1 (400-ml) can coconut cream (14 ounce)
1 large ripe avocado
1 cup spinach
1 tablespoon nut milk
6 tablespoons maple syrup
3 ½ teaspoons vanilla extract
2 teaspoons peppermint extract
½ cup dark chocolate or vegan carob chips
¼ cup cacao nibs

Optional superfood add-ins:
2–3 tablespoons collagen or 1 tablespoon spirulina. You could also add 1 tablespoon matcha in the fourth trimester!

DIRECTIONS

1. Pour 1 can of coconut milk and 1 can of coconut cream into 2 ice cube trays and freeze for at least 6 hours or overnight. (You should be able to fit one can into one tray, but you will need only 9 out of the 12 cubes.)

2. The next day, in a high-speed blender (like a Vitamix or a Ninja), blend the avocado, spinach, nut milk, maple syrup, vanilla, and peppermint. Once those are fully incorporated, add 9 of the frozen coconut milk cubes and 9 of the frozen coconut cream cubes and blend until well combined. (You will have to use the blender attachment—and some elbow grease—to push the cubes into the blade, but slowly it will start to come together like ice cream.)

3. Once the mixture is fully blended, stir in the chocolate or carob chips and cacao nibs and serve immediately. The longer this blends or sits, the more it will soften into a thick smoothie.

4. The nice cream can also be stored in the freezer: pour the mixture back into the ice cube trays, then re-blend when you are ready to eat.

For another fun way to use this recipe, arrange popsicle sticks on a parchment paper–lined baking sheet. Plop a bit of the nice cream at the top of the popsicle stick and let it spread out into a fat pancake. Place in the freezer for a couple of hours until hard. Remove, dunk in melted chocolate, and pop back in the freezer. Enjoy anytime as a fun treat!

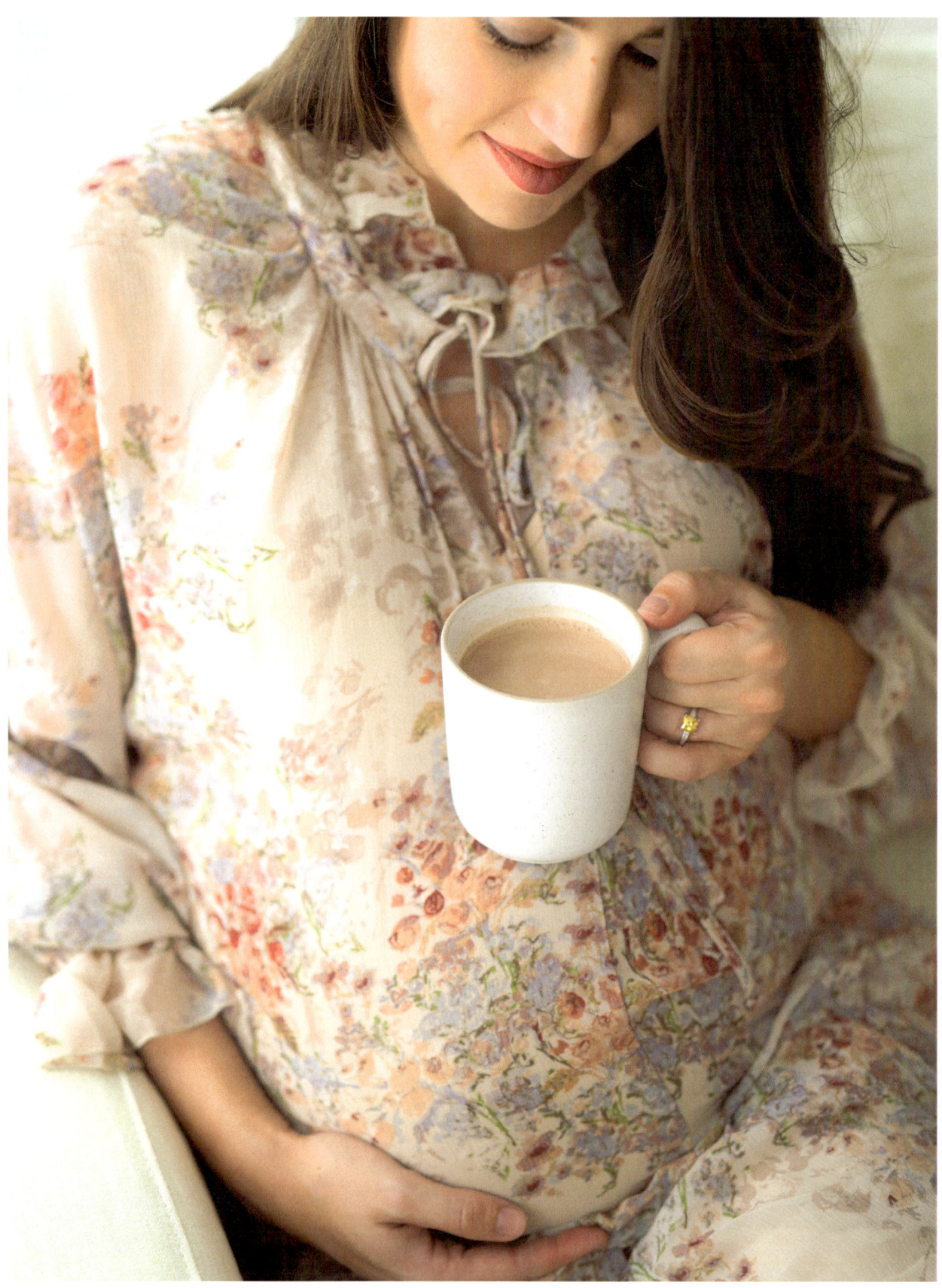

THIRD TRIMESTER

HOME "STRETCHING"!

Time is moving so fast—yet crawling—as we anticipate meeting our precious baby. Mama's belly is expanding and stretching, making room for an increasingly chubby and adorable newborn. This massive growth in mom and sprout can make the third trimester the most challenging for women physically, mentally, and emotionally. Pesky symptoms like heartburn, pelvic pain, varicose veins, constipation, hemorrhoids, high blood pressure, and sciatic pain—even conditions like preeclampsia and gestational diabetes—can plague mommas right until the end. Meanwhile, babe has switched gears from organ development to putting on weight and fine-tuning their cellular maturation.

You still need to keep nutrition high to allow babe to store extra energy for childbirth and the postpartum stage. You should continue to eat more than you did pre-pregnancy, adding about an extra 350 to 450 calories daily than pre-pregnancy—often now in smaller meals because babe is pressing up and kicking into the stomach. Make them count by always combining protein, fat, and carbs to get you through.

This trimester we focus on magnesium to ease those sore muscles and combat constipation; omega-3s and protein for proper cellular development; plenty of whole-food fibre; and iron and vitamin C to build baby's stores before birth.

The third trimester can bring on a roller coaster of emotions. Anxiety about labour, delivery, and the changes to come in your lifestyle and relationships can trigger mood shifts during these final months. Luckily, your growing belly comes with a growing heart that expands to accept all the physical and mental changes. Lean into these last weeks with grounding exercises and anxiety-reducing meditations. Allow yourself to connect with babe on a walk in nature, in a warm bath, or in a prenatal yoga class.

This is also a great time to start building your community and postpartum support toolbox: ask for help with postpartum meal prep (cue all the soup recipes from these final 2 trimesters!) or meet some new mom friends at an aquatics or birthing class. Perhaps consider having a friend throw you a "Mother's Blessing." Historically, this began as a Blessing Way that celebrates a women's transition into motherhood within the Navajo community. Deriving inspiration from this beautiful tradition, a "Mothers Blessing" typically includes activities that honour the mother, such as bringing poems and letters with good wishes from each attendee, a birth affirmation flag banner to have at birth, beads from everyone set with an intention that can be turned into a bracelet, or henna on the belly. There are many unique ways to honour you as the momma-to-be and your transition into motherhood.

This is the last time you and your baby's heartbeat will share one body… Take some extra time to breathe into the changes and ground yourself in your innate maternal strength.

LABOUR PREP BY DR. CARRIE

BIRTH OF A BABY | BIRTH OF A MOTHER

The last days of pregnancy are a place in between. Waiting, wanting, impatience, anxiety, the great unknown. It's a longing to meet your beloved babe, all while knowing your life will change completely.

Although moms-to-be are often eager for the labour to start, the last few weeks and days of pregnancy are a biological and physiological event that is important and sacred.

Shift your mind frame from feeling anxious or discouraged to allowing yourself one last push to rest, nourish, sleep, connect with a partner, and fully bloom into the mother you are becoming. Arriving into labour and childbirth rested and nourished will give you much-needed energy and mental strength for the feat ahead.

Late pregnancy is also an amazing time to add botanicals and food-as-medicine to encourage a smooth labour transition. But remember to always check with your health care providers to ensure these are the right choices for you!

RED RASPBERRY LEAF TEAS OR TINCTURES

Red raspberry leaf tones the uterus, preparing it for labour and delivery. It also helps prevent postpartum hemorrhage from an overly relaxed or atonic uterus. It eases the pain of delivery and enriches breast milk. It has a rich concentration of vitamin C, vitamin E, calcium, and iron. Raspberry leaves also contain vitamins A, B complex, and many minerals including phosphorus and potassium. Drink 1–2 cups daily!

DATES

What a lovely way to reduce the need for induction and encourage a speedier childbirth with fewer complications—all with a few dates a day. Studies show that consuming up to 6 dates a day for 4 weeks before the estimated due date significantly improves birth outcomes. Dates can be eaten whole or added to your daily meals and snacks.

EVENING PRIMROSE OIL / GLA

The therapeutic effects of this powerful oil are amazing in the last month before birth. Taking evening primrose oil orally, or via vaginal suppository if recommended by your health team, encourages ripening of the cervix and can decrease the chance of going past your due-date. Studies have also shown benefits in babies' health directly postpartum. Those are huge wins for an easy addition to your third-trimester routine.

PERINEAL MASSAGE

Gentle massage and stretching of the perineal tissue and musculature can help prepare for the crowning and birth of your baby. A massage from a partner, or self-massage, performed daily during the last weeks of pregnancy, can reduce tearing, lower the incidence of episiotomy, reduce the duration of the "pushing" phase of labour, and ease postpartum healing. Use a mild vegetable or massage oil and be sure to ask your midwife, pelvic floor physiotherapist, naturopathic doctor, or other health care provider for more support if needed.

SQUATS!

An old midwives tale states, "Squat 300 times a day, and you are going to give birth quickly." While 300 squats might be a bit much, squatting can prepare our muscles for childbirth and generate greater pelvic mobility in late pregnancy. Start with 25 squats a day, and add more if it feels right for you!

HOMEOPATHICS

EZ Birth is a combination homeopathic remedy that uses energetic medicine to encourage a healthy and happy labour and birth.

LABOUR-AID

During labour we exert quite a bit of energy! Drinking a concoction like this Labour-Aid will replenish electrolytes and fluids while giving you energy for the marathon of childbirth!

INGREDIENTS

1 cup coconut water
1 cup filtered water
¼ cup plus 2 tablespoons fresh lemon or lime juice
¼ cup maple syrup
Liquid mineral/magnesium supplement that aims for 250 mg/dose (Trace Minerals Research is a good option)
½ teaspoon sea salt
15 drops Bach Rescue Remedy (optional—for handling stress and calming nerves)

RESEARCH ARTICLES

Dates:
https://pubmed.ncbi.nlm.nih.gov/21280989/#:~:text=It%20is%20concluded%20that%20the,non%2Dsignificant%2C%20delivery%20outcome
and https://www.ncbi.nlm.nih.gov/pmc/articles/PMC5637148/

Evening primrose oil:
https://www.ncbi.nlm.nih.gov/pmc/articles/PMC9947258/

Perineal massage:
https://pubmed.ncbi.nlm.nih.gov/32399905/

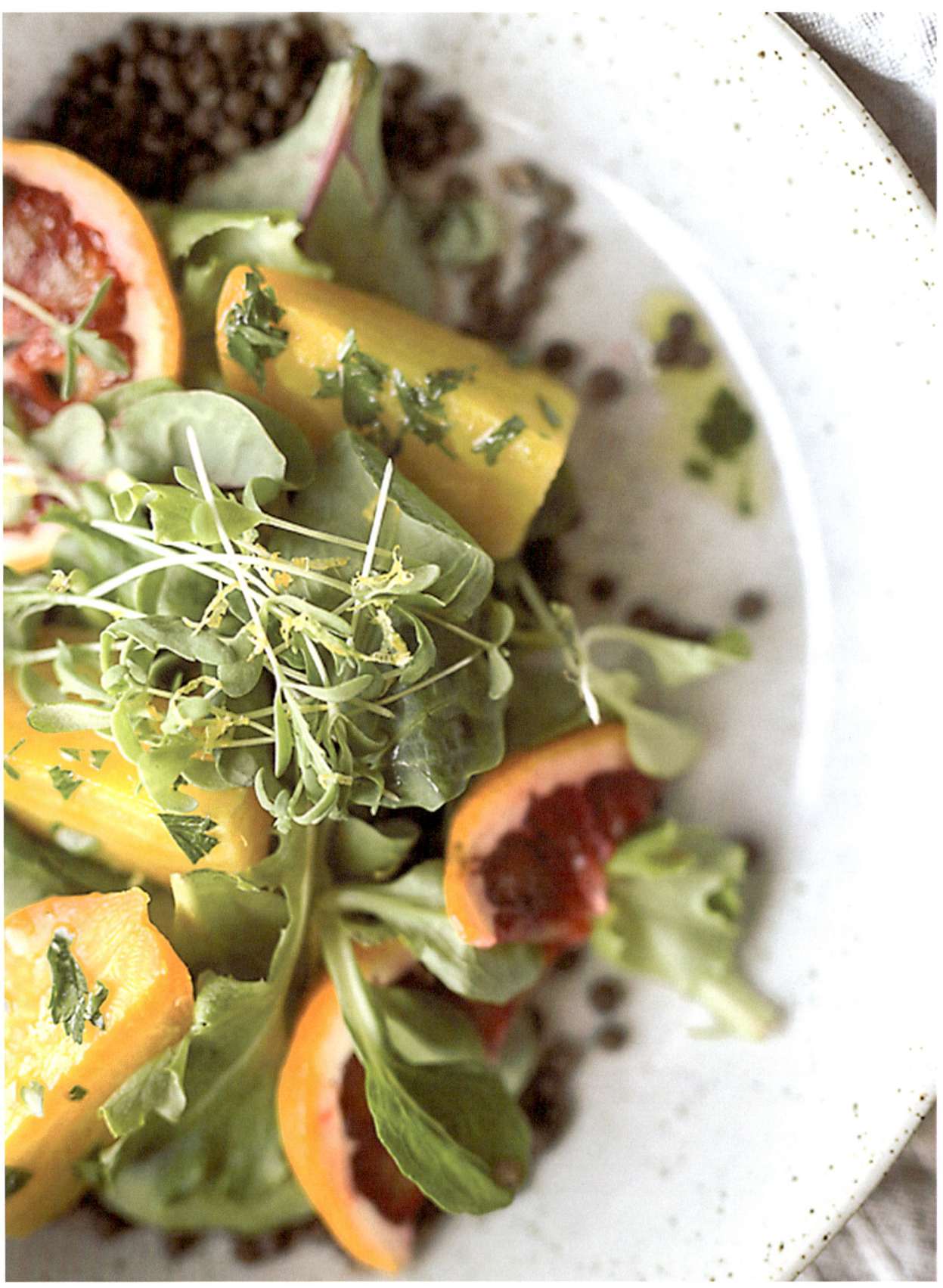

THIRD TRIMESTER

TABLE OF CONTENTS

BREAKFAST
Shakshuka with Beans and Greens 101
Tropical Bircher Muesli with Quinoa, Papaya, and Kiwi..103
Superhero Pancakes with Vanilla Coconut Sauce 105
Pumpkin Caramel Smoothie with Coconut and Dates 107

LUNCH
Beet, Citrus, and Lentil Salad with Citrus Gremolata 109
Sesame Ginger Soba Noodles with Mango and Avocado..111
Mediterranean Quinoa Salad: with Feta, Artichokes, and Mint 113
Cauliflower Fried Rice with Shredded Chicken and Veggies 115

DINNER
Mulligatawny with Apples, Lentils, and Rice 117
Bison Borscht with Beets, Cabbage, and Potatoes..119
Dairy-Free Salmon Chowder with Celery Root and Tarragon 121
Shepherd's Pie with Elk and Eggplant 123

SNACKS AND SWEETS
Red Raspberry Leaf Mojito with Kombucha, Strawberries, and Mint..........................125
Avocado and Corn Salsa with Swiss Chard Stems 127
Hot Cacao: Relaxing and Magnesium-Rich 129
Beet Dip with Mint and Lemon 131
Red Raspberry Bites: Dr. Carrie's "Ripe and Ready" Snacks 133
Bliss Balls with Banana, Walnut, and Figs 135
Labour Prep Chocolate Pudding with Dates, Avocado, and Chia Seeds......................137
Chocolate Brittle with Peanut Butter and Cinnamon..139

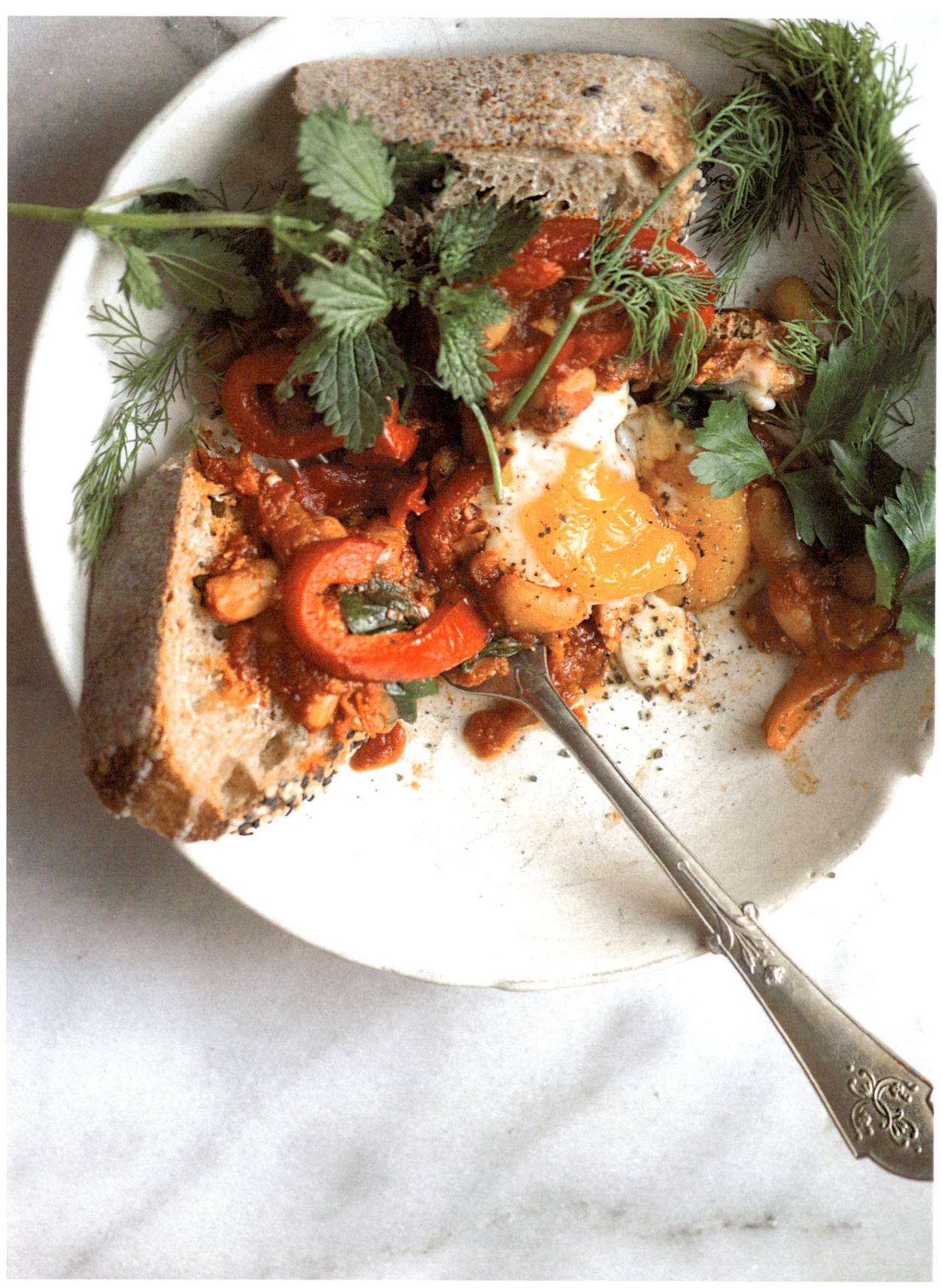

SHAKSHUKA

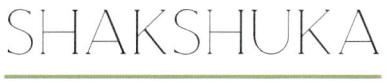

WITH BEANS AND GREENS

Shakshuka, meaning "mixture," is a warm and comforting breakfast originating in North Africa and the Middle East. It consists of eggs poached in a bubbling mixture of tomatoes, onions, chilies, and spices. It is so satisfying you may want it for lunch and dinner too. Common third-trimester symptoms include varicose veins and other vascular changes, due to the drastic increase in blood volume—up to 50 percent!—during pregnancy. This delicious combo of eggs, tomatoes, and greens offers vein-strengthening biotin, vitamin E, vitamin K, and B vitamins.

INGREDIENTS | SERVES 4

- 2 tablespoons grass-fed butter, ghee, or coconut oil
- 1 medium onion, sliced thin
- ¾ teaspoon sea salt
- 2 bell peppers, sliced thin
- 3 garlic cloves, minced
- 3 sprigs fresh thyme or ½ teaspoon dried thyme
- 1 ½ teaspoons ground cumin
- 2–3 pinches red pepper flakes
- Freshly cracked pepper
- ¼ teaspoon paprika
- 1 (796-ml) can chopped tomatoes, or 5 cups chopped fresh tomatoes (28 ounces)
- 3 pinches saffron
- 2 cups chopped greens of your choice, rinsed and ribs removed
- 1 (398-ml) can cannellini beans, drained and rinsed (14 ounces)
- 6 free-range, organic eggs
- Cilantro for garnish
- Fresh sourdough, to serve

DIRECTIONS

1. In a deep skillet or sauté pan with a lid, heat ghee or oil over medium-low heat and add onions and ¼ teaspoon salt. Sauté for 3–4 minutes until soft.
2. Stir in bell peppers and garlic. Sauté over medium-low heat for 5–6 minutes until bell peppers are soft.
3. Turn up the heat to medium and stir in thyme, cumin, red pepper flakes, remaining ½ teaspoon of salt, pepper, and paprika. Let the spices become fragrant, 1–2 minutes, then add the tomatoes. Stir, cover, and simmer over medium heat for 10 minutes.
4. While the tomatoes and peppers are simmering, prepare a saffron "tea": Warm water in a kettle, but do not bring it to a boil. Pour ¼ cup of the warm water into a small dish. Add 3 large pinches of saffron. Let this steep while the tomato and peppers simmer.
5. When the tomato and peppers have finished simmering, remove the thyme sprigs, and add the saffron "tea," drained beans, and chopped greens to the tomatoes and peppers. Stir to combine.
6. With a spoon, make 6 little pockets in the skillet mixture and crack your eggs into the holes. Cover the skillet and continue cooking for another 10 minutes, or until the eggs are cooked to your liking. Remove from the heat and sprinkle with fresh cilantro. Serve with crusty sourdough.

Saffron takes this dish to a whole new level. Try to find high quality saffron threads at your local specialty kitchen store or spice store. However, if you can't find them, the dish will still be delicious!

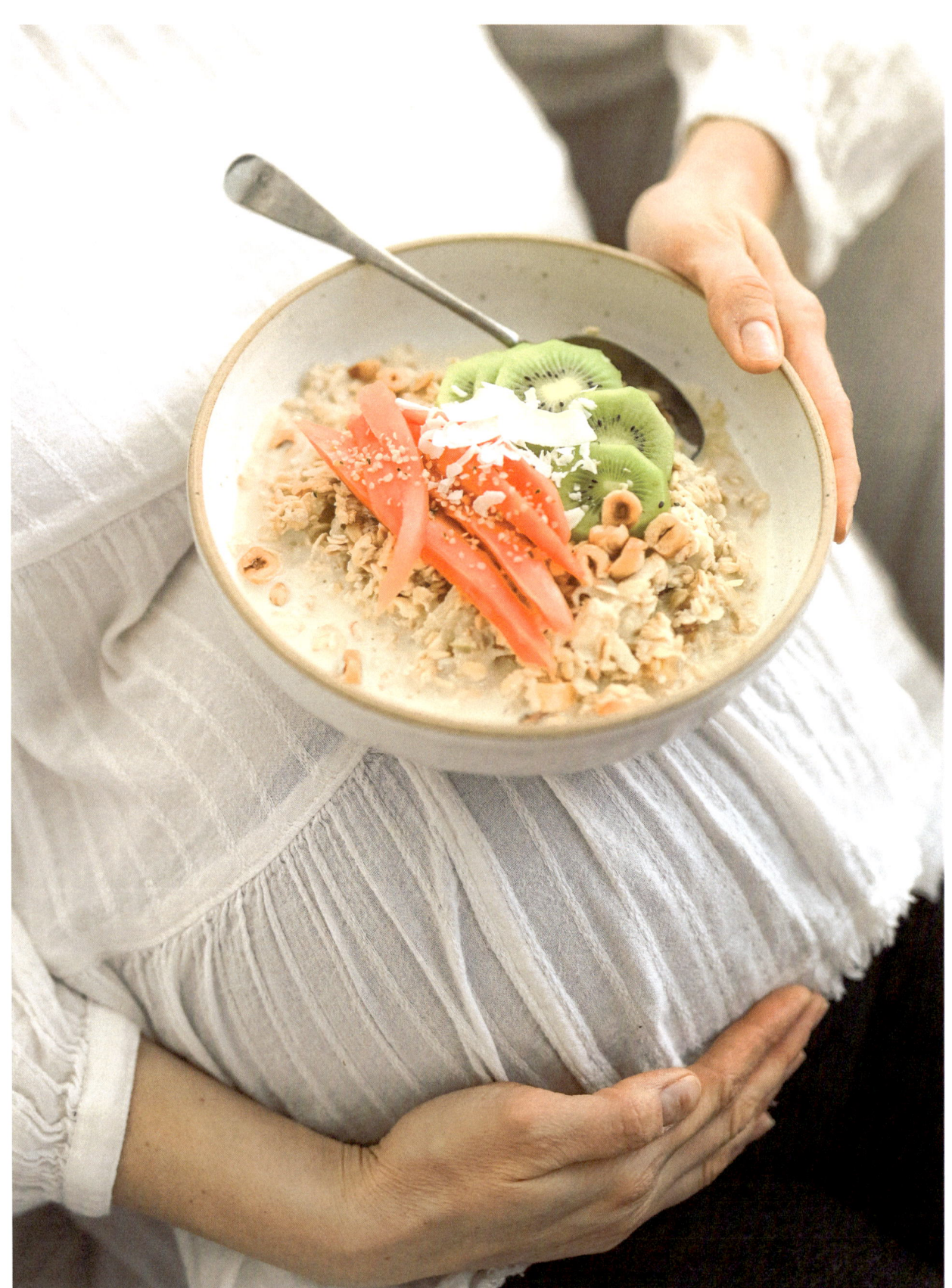

TROPICAL BIRCHER MUESLI

WITH QUINOA, PAPAYA, AND KIWI

The pregnant body is amazing and beautiful in all forms, but for some, stretch marks are one of the less desirable changes that occur as the baby grows. A nutrient-dense diet that promotes collagen production gives the skin more strength and elasticity during the beautiful bloom of pregnancy. Pumpkin seeds are high in zinc, vitamin E, and amino acids that support vibrant skin tissue. Allow yourself to stretch and grow while giving your body what it needs to stay strong and resilient.

INGREDIENTS | SERVES 4-6

1 cup rolled oats
1 cup quinoa flakes*
2 tablespoons macadamia nuts, crushed
2 tablespoons sliced almonds
2 tablespoons pumpkin seeds
2 tablespoons chia seeds
¼ cup diced dried apricots
2 ¼ cups light coconut milk or cashew milk
¼ cup plus 2 tablespoons coconut kefir or yogourt (plain or vanilla)
¾ teaspoon lemon juice
2–3 tablespoons maple syrup

Toppings:
(amounts are per serving)
1 kiwi, sliced or chopped
½ cup chopped papaya plus juice
2 tablespoons shredded coconut
1 tablespoon crushed macadamia nuts
1 tablespoon hemp hearts

* If you don't have quinoa flakes, you can substitute an extra cup of rolled oats. Just add an extra ½ cup of milk and another ¼ cup kefir or yogourt.

DIRECTIONS

1. In a container with a lid, mix together the oats, quinoa flakes, nuts, seeds, apricots, coconut or cashew milk, kefir or yogourt, lemon juice, and 2 tablespoons of the maple syrup.

2. Taste and adjust for sweetness. Depending on the yogourt or kefir you use, you may need to add another tablespoon of maple syrup.

3. Cover with the lid, and let the mixture sit overnight in the fridge.

4. In the morning, top with kiwi, papaya and its juice, coconut, macadamia nuts, and hemp hearts.

Feel free to add or substitute whatever nuts, seeds, and dried fruit you have on hand!

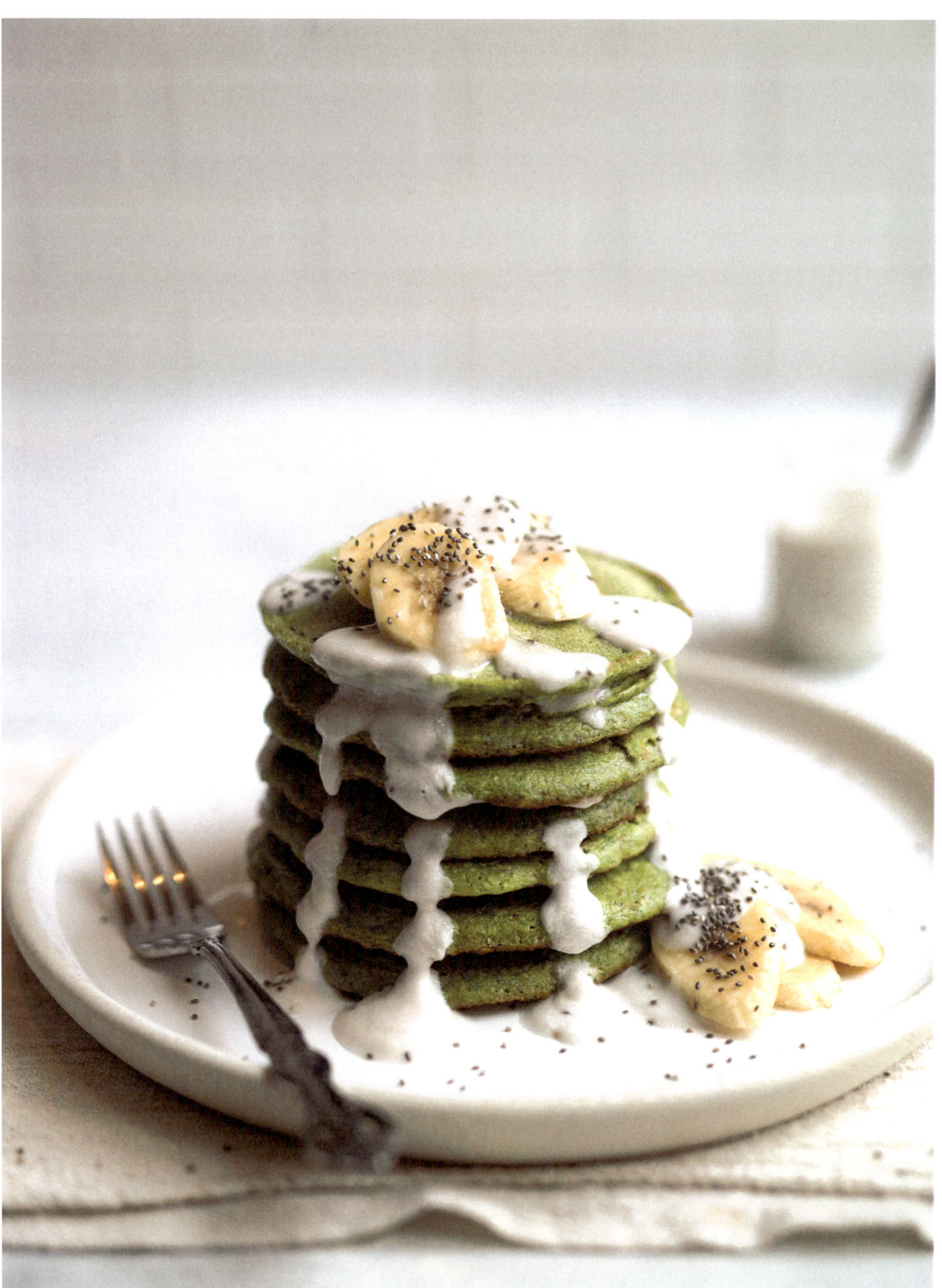

SUPERHERO PANCAKES

WITH VANILLA COCONUT SAUCE

These bright-green superhero pancakes are a hit for mamas and kiddos alike. Anise and Dr. Carrie have been making versions of these since they started having babies. They call them "superhero" pancakes for their green colour—and to entice the little ones! Packed with fibre, iron, omegas, and antioxidants, these crowd-pleasing pancakes are perfect for big family breakfasts, and the recipe can be doubled to satisfy hungry hands throughout the day. Constipation and hemorrhoids can worsen in the late stages of pregnancy. To keep your digestive tract moving, boost your fibre and magnesium with ingredients like oats, banana, spinach, and flax.

INGREDIENTS | YIELDS 10 MEDIUM PANCAKES

4 free range, organic eggs
1 tablespoon milled flaxseed
1 small ripe banana
1 cup spinach
2 tablespoons avocado oil
1 ½ teaspoons vanilla extract
1 tablespoon coconut sugar
⅛ teaspoon sea salt
1 teaspoon baking powder
¼ cup oat flour, spooned and levelled
¼ cup almond flour, spooned and levelled
¼ cup coconut flour, spooned and levelled
4–6 tablespoons coconut oil or grass-fed butter for frying the pancakes

Vanilla coconut sauce (optional):
1 can coconut cream
2 teaspoons maple syrup
1 teaspoon vanilla

Optional Toppings:
Maple syrup
Bananas
Pomegranate seeds
Berries
Chia or hemp hearts

DIRECTIONS

1. Prepare the vanilla coconut sauce: In a food processor, combine the coconut cream, maple syrup, and vanilla. Purée until smooth. Set aside.
2. In a blender, combine the eggs, flaxseed, banana, spinach, oil, vanilla, sugar, and salt. Blend on medium until fully combined.
3. Add the baking powder and blend on the lowest setting to incorporate.
4. Add in the flours and blend on the lowest setting to incorporate.
5. Heat a large cast-iron skillet or stainless-steel frying pan to medium.
6. Add 2 tablespoons of oil or butter to the pan.
7. Once the oil is sizzling, pour in the pancake batter to make any size pancakes you like.
8. Cook over medium heat for about 3 minutes or until bubbles begin to appear. Then flip and cook for another 2 minutes.
9. Repeat with the remaining pancake batter and add additional oil if needed.
10. Serve with vanilla coconut sauce, bananas, berries, pomegranate seeds, hemp hearts, or whatever you like!

Choosing non-toxic cookware is as important as choosing high-quality ingredients. As we cook, the materials in the cookware get imparted into the food. If we are cooking with a cast-iron skillet, we get the added benefit of iron, but if we choose cookware containing sub-optimal materials like PFAS, lead, cadmium, or mercury, those chemicals get absorbed into the food—and into our bodies, where they can create hormone disruptions and imbalances in everything from our nervous system to our gut. Do your research and choose wisely! Our favourites are cast iron and All-Clad.

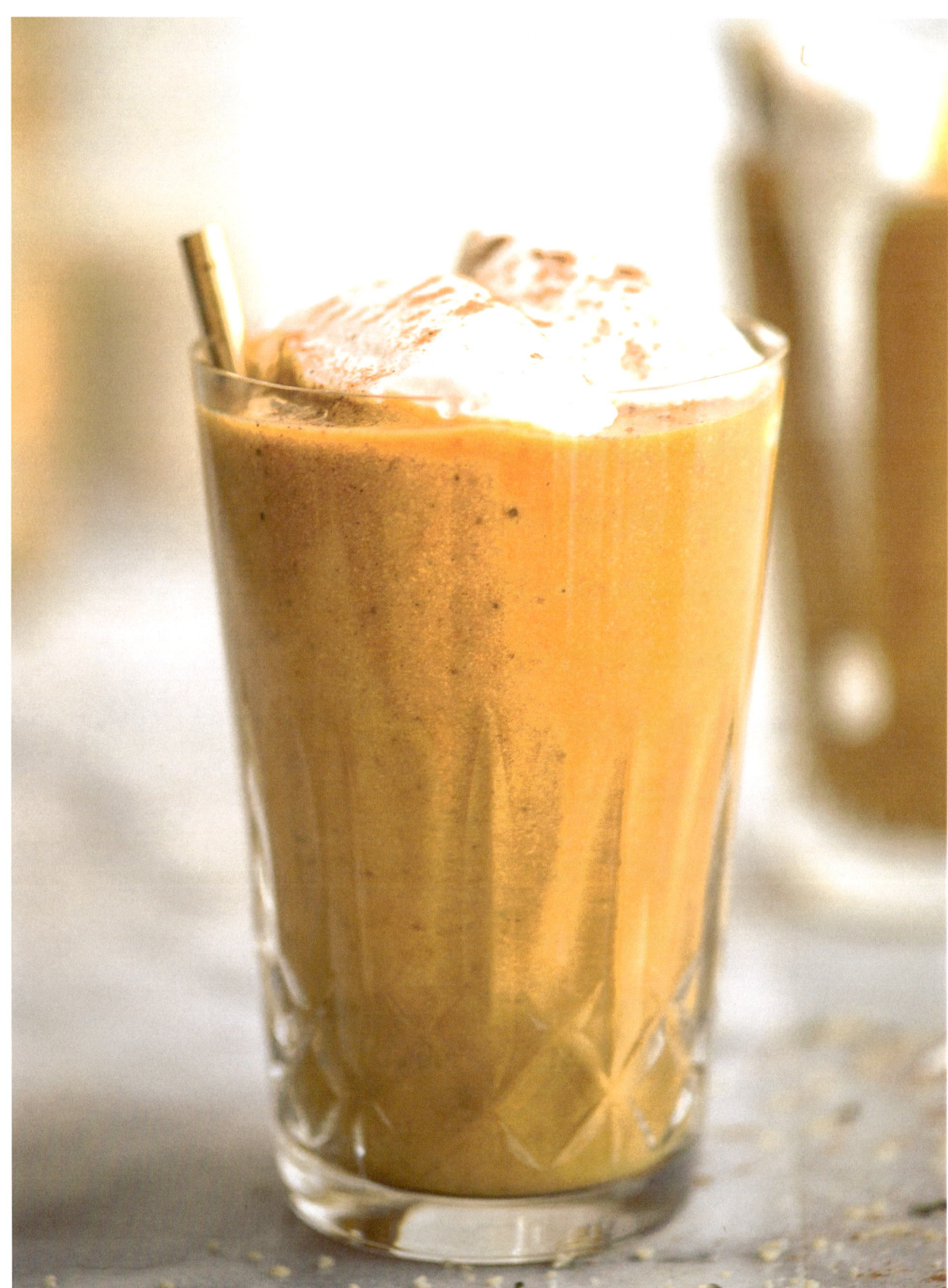

PUMPKIN CARAMEL SMOOTHIE

WITH COCONUT AND DATES

A smaller breakfast, like this pumpkin caramel smoothie, is perfect when the belly gets bigger, organs move up and around, and the space for larger meals shrinks. Easy breakfasts are great for mamas on the run or those who crave something lighter. Some mamas want to drink smoothies all day, so add this one to your arsenal when you're ready for something different!

INGREDIENTS | SERVES 2

¾ cup light coconut milk
½ cup canned pumpkin purée
¼ cup nut milk or vanilla coconut kefir
½ teaspoon vanilla extract or paste
1 teaspoon pumpkin pie spice
½ banana
2 ½ tablespoons almond butter
2 tablespoons milled flaxseed*
2 dates, pits removed
Pinch salt

Optional:
Coconut whip
Extra almond butter
Coconut flakes

DIRECTIONS

1. Combine all ingredients and a handful of ice in a blender. Blend until smooth.
2. Top with coconut whip, drizzled almond butter, and/or coconut flakes!

*If you can't find milled flaxseed, make sure the flaxseed is blended all the way, since the body has difficulty breaking down the whole seed.

Feeling nauseated? Add as much fresh ginger as you can stomach!

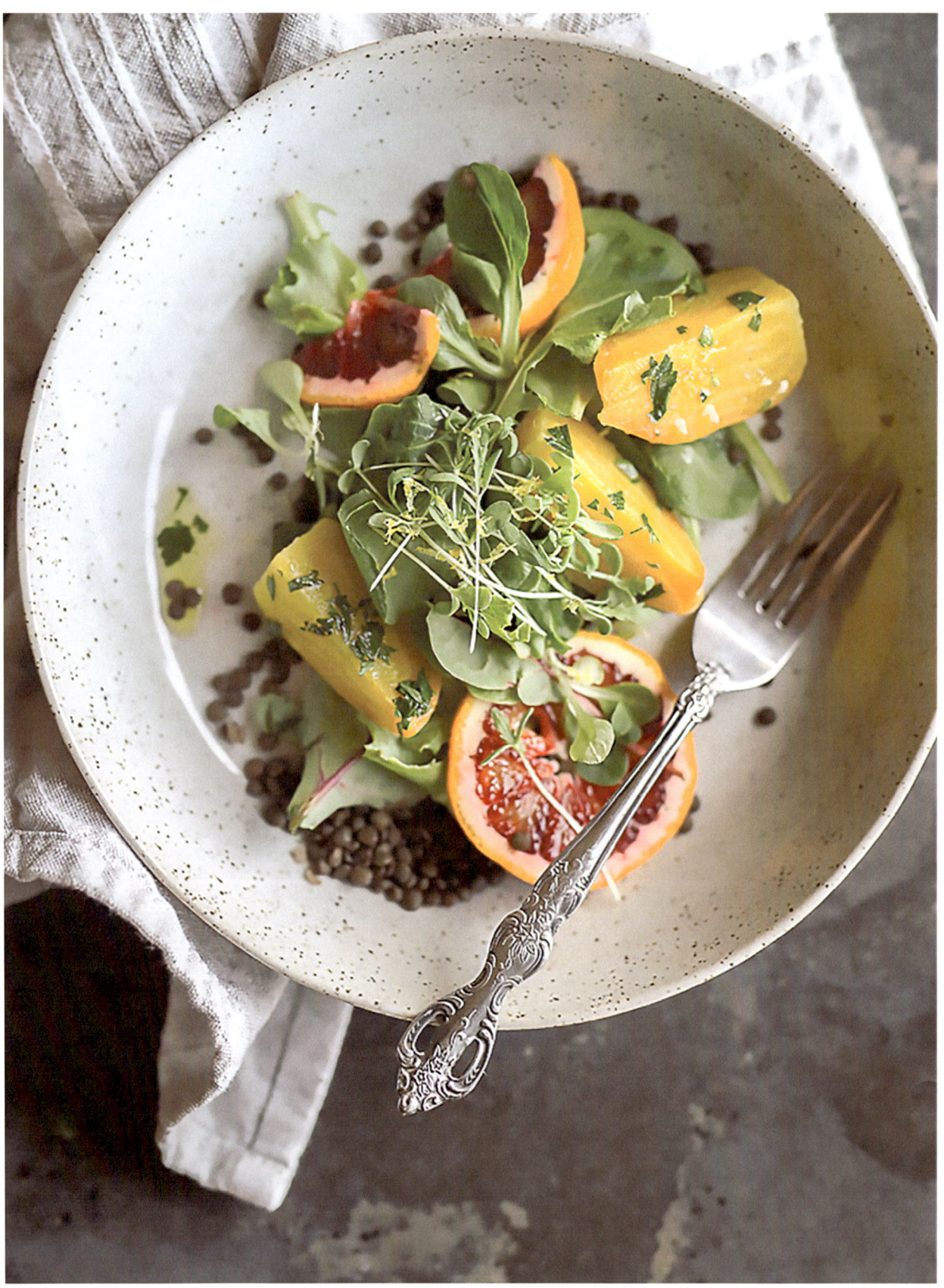

BEET, CITRUS & LENTIL SALAD

WITH CITRUS GREMOLATA

This plant-based meal is packed with zinc, magnesium, and protein: all key elements to keep preeclampsia at bay. During pregnancy, preeclampsia—a condition of late pregnancy involving high blood pressure and swelling—can be linked to low levels of protein, zinc, magnesium, and vitamin D. Take care and pride in nourishing your body and babe with meals like this.

INGREDIENTS | SERVES 2

4 medium-to-large golden beets
⅓ cup French lentils or beluga lentils
¼ teaspoon sea salt
1 cup arugula
1 cup mixed tender greens, like baby Swiss chard and mâche
1 blood orange, sliced, skin removed
2 tablespoons basil or mint, chiffonade

Citrus Gremolata dressing:
1 garlic clove, finely minced
½ teaspoon orange zest
½ teaspoon lemon zest
1 ½ tablespoons fresh minced parsley
2 tablespoons freshly squeezed orange juice
1 tablespoon apple cider vinegar
1 tablespoon extra-virgin olive oil, flaxseed oil, or hempseed oil

DIRECTIONS

1. Prepare the dressing: Combine all dressing ingredients in a mason jar with a tight-fitting lid, and shake to combine. (Alternatively, you can place all ingredients in a bowl, and whisk to combine.) Set aside.

2. Prepare the beets: If the beets are still attached to the greens, remove the beet greens and wash the beets vigorously until all dirt is gone. (Reserve the beet greens for another time by wrapping the cut ends in a wet paper towel and keeping them in the fridge crisper drawer. You can use them as you would Swiss chard, kale, or collards.) Scrub the beet roots until clean and cut off the stub end where the greens were attached.

3. Place beets in a medium saucepan and add enough water to cover plus 2 inches. Bring to a boil, then cover and lower the heat to a simmer. Cooking time will vary depending on the size of your beets. Medium beets will need to cook for approximately 30 minutes. You can test them by sliding a knife into a beet; if it goes in easily, they are finished. Cooking them in an Instant Pot or buying precooked organic beets is also an option.

4. While the beets cook, prepare the lentils: In a small saucepan, combine ⅔ cup filtered water, dry black lentils, and salt. Bring to a simmer, cover, and cook over medium-low heat for 20 minutes. Remove from the stove and drain any excess liquid. Set aside.

5. When the beets are finished cooking, remove them from the water and let cool. Remove the beet skin by rubbing the edge of a spoon along the beet; the skin should easily slide off with a bit of rubbing.

6. Cut the beets into quarters, toss with half the dressing, and set aside.

7. Assemble the salad: Divide the arugula and mixed greens over two plates and top with the lentils, beets, and oranges. Drizzle with the remaining dressing and sprinkle on the basil or mint.

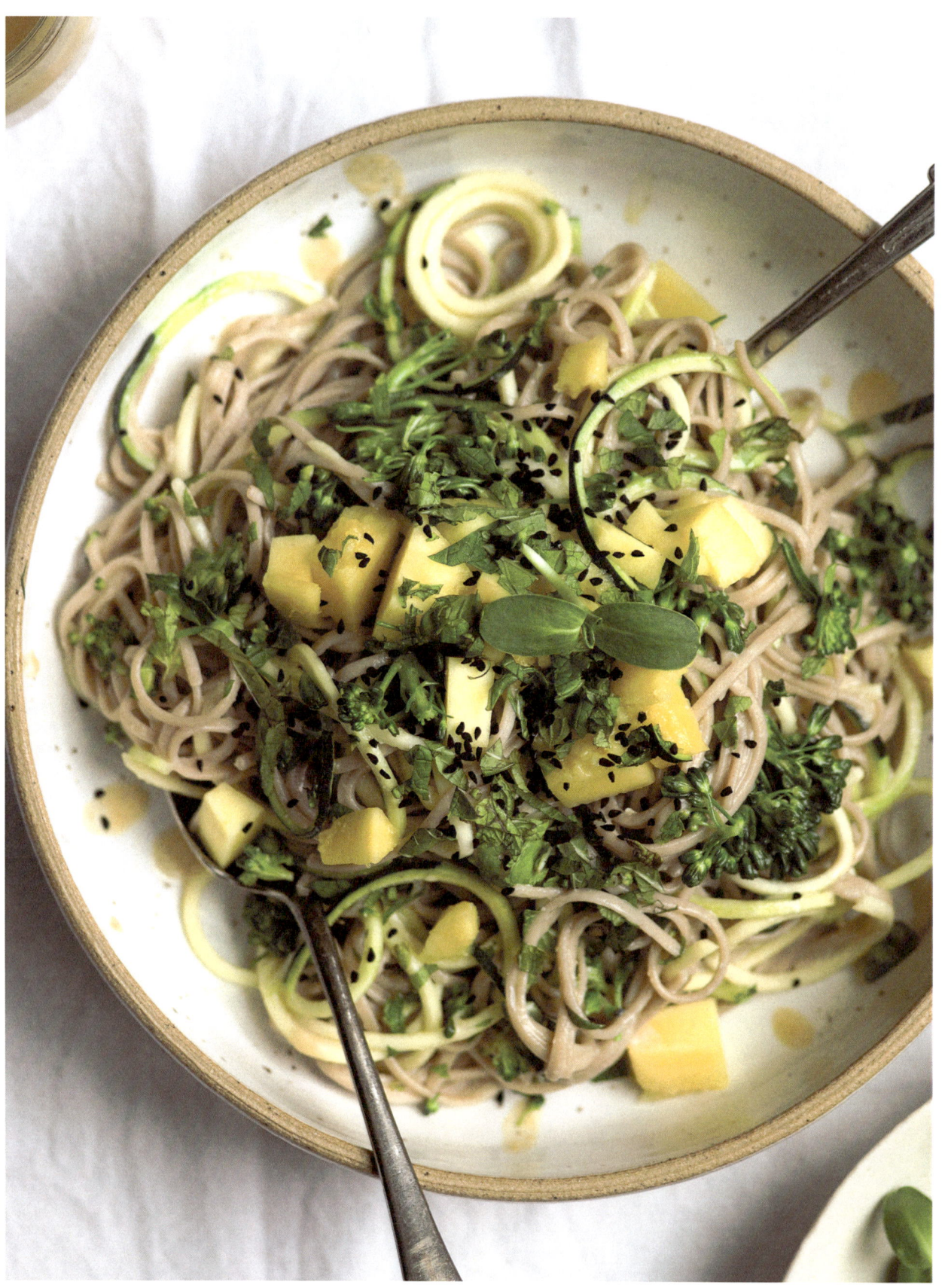

SESAME GINGER SOBA NOODLES

WITH MANGO AND AVOCADO

As baby packs on the weight, most pregnant mamas start to feel heartburn after eating certain foods or larger portions. This is an awesome time to try nutrient-dense, fat- and veggie-based salads for the midday meal. Eating smaller, more frequent meals is the key to feeling more comfortable in the third trimester, so pack a big portion of this delicious lunch and snack on it throughout the afternoon. The star of this dish is the dressing, so feel free to switch up the vegetables if you don't have the ones below on hand. This dish works really well with fresh bell peppers and purple cabbage, but try to keep the edamame and mango!

INGREDIENTS | SERVES 4

Dressing:
1 (2 inches by ½ inch) knob of ginger
2 medium garlic cloves
½ cup toasted sesame oil
¼ cup tamari
¼ cup rice vinegar
1 tablespoon pasteurized honey or maple syrup
1 tablespoon almond butter
½ teaspoon red pepper flakes
1 teaspoon lime juice

Salad:
1 cup shelled edamame
1 teaspoon sea salt
340 grams buckwheat soba noodles (12 ounces)
1 small cluster broccolini, cut into small chunks
1 small-to-medium zucchini, spiralized
1 small ripe mango, cubed
2 avocados, pits removed, cubed
1 cup tightly packed fresh herbs such as mint, cilantro, and/or Thai basil
Black or white sesame seeds for garnish

DIRECTIONS

1. In a food processor, chop the ginger and garlic until very fine. Add the remainder of the dressing ingredients and purée until smooth. Set aside. You can store the dressing in a mason jar in the fridge up to 10 days.

2. If the edamame beans are frozen, place them in a large colander under running water for a minute or two to defrost. Set aside.

3. Bring a large saucepan of water to boil and add 1 teaspoon of salt. Drop the noodles into the boiling salted water and cook for 4 minutes. Add the broccolini and edamame, return to a boil, and continue cooking with the noodles for another 3 minutes. Drain in the large colander you used for the edamame. Run cold water over the colander for 1–2 minutes, tossing the mixture with your hands to cool the noodles and stop them from cooking further.

4. Transfer the noodles and vegetables to a large bowl. Add the spiralized zucchini. Toss with as much dressing as you like. (You can save the rest for quinoa bowls or salads!)

5. Top with chopped mango, avocado, fresh herbs, and sesame seeds.

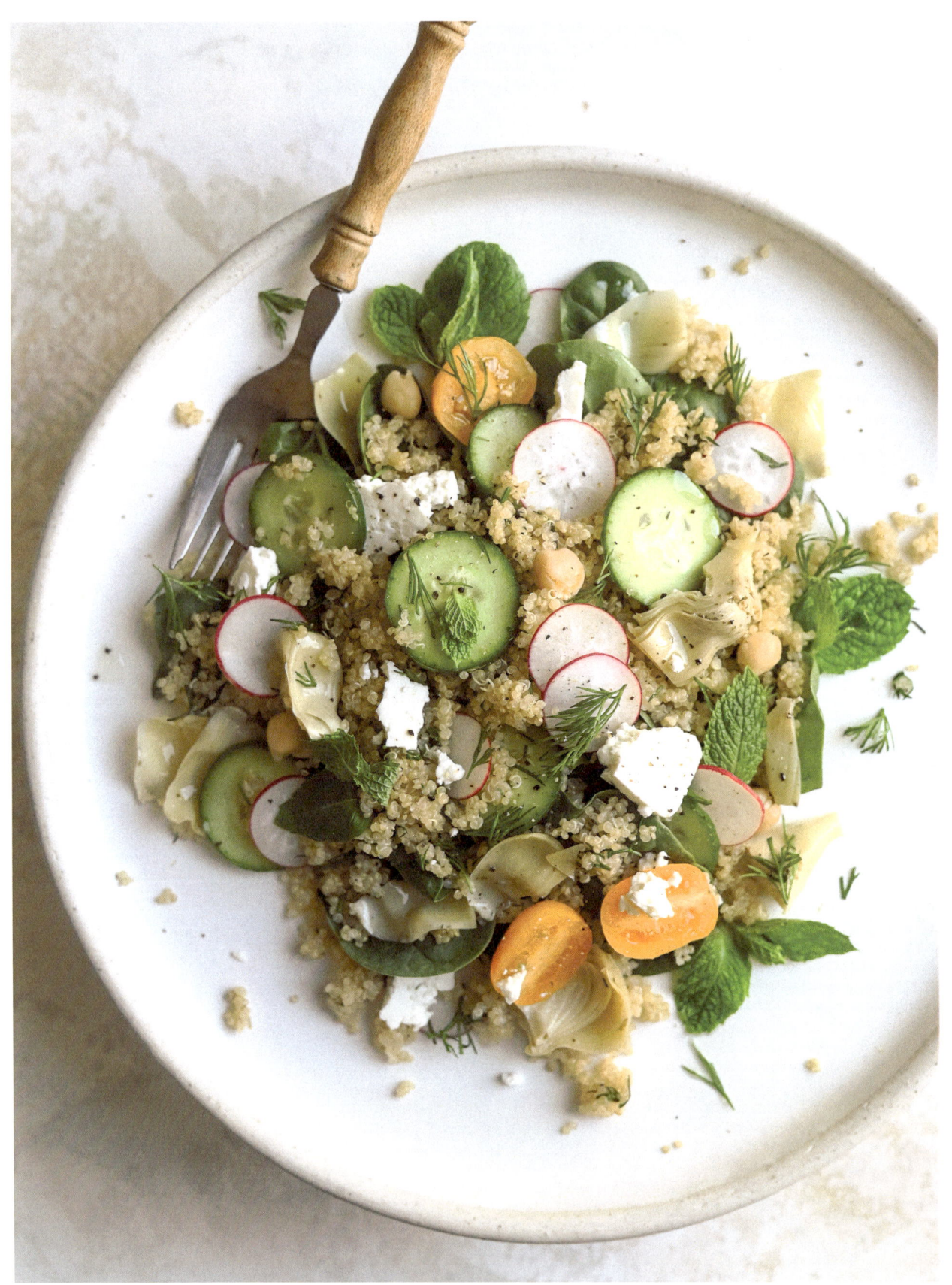

MEDITERRANEAN QUINOA SALAD

WITH FETA, ARTICHOKES, AND MINT

If Anise were to have a signature salad, this would be it. She has made this countless times over the past fifteen years: for Mother's Blessings, birthday parties, potlucks and just to have on hand for easy lunches. Every time it is on the table, at least one person asks for the recipe, so it would seem wrong not to include it in this cookbook! The complex carbs, protein from the quinoa and chickpeas, fat from the pistachios and feta, and prebiotics from the green onions and artichokes make it the perfect salad to have on hand!

INGREDIENTS | SERVES 6

1 cup quinoa
1 ⅛ teaspoon sea salt, divided
1 large Roma tomato, chopped
2 small green onions, sliced thin
1 (400-ml) can whole hearts of palm, cut in half lengthwise and sliced thin (14 ounces)
1 (170-ml) jar marinated artichoke hearts, quartered, liquid reserved (6 ounces)
1–1 ½ cups finely chopped fresh spinach
1 mini cucumber, sliced
½ (400-ml) can of chickpeas, drained and rinsed (14 ounces)
2 tablespoons lemon juice
Freshly cracked pepper
½ cup chopped fresh mint
¼ cup crumbled sheep or goat feta
¼ cup crushed pistachios
optional: sliced radishes to garnish

DIRECTIONS

1. Rinse the quinoa thoroughly with cold running water through a fine mesh sieve. In a medium saucepan, bring 2 cups water plus ½ teaspoon sea salt to a boil. Add the quinoa. Cover, reduce heat to low, and simmer for 15 minutes. Remove from the heat, and let the quinoa stand for 5 minutes, covered. Fluff with a fork and set aside.

2. Add the chopped tomatoes to a large bowl and sprinkle with ⅛ teaspoon of salt. Gently stir to combine.

3. Add the cooled quinoa, sliced green onions, sliced hearts of palm, quartered artichoke hearts, chopped spinach, sliced cucumber and chickpeas. Stir to combine.

4. Add 5–6 tablespoons of the reserved artichoke heart marinade (this should be the entire jar), the lemon juice, ½ teaspoon salt, and a few cracks of pepper. Stir to combine.

5. Add the mint, give the salad a good toss, and top with the crumbled feta, crushed pistachios, and sliced radishes.

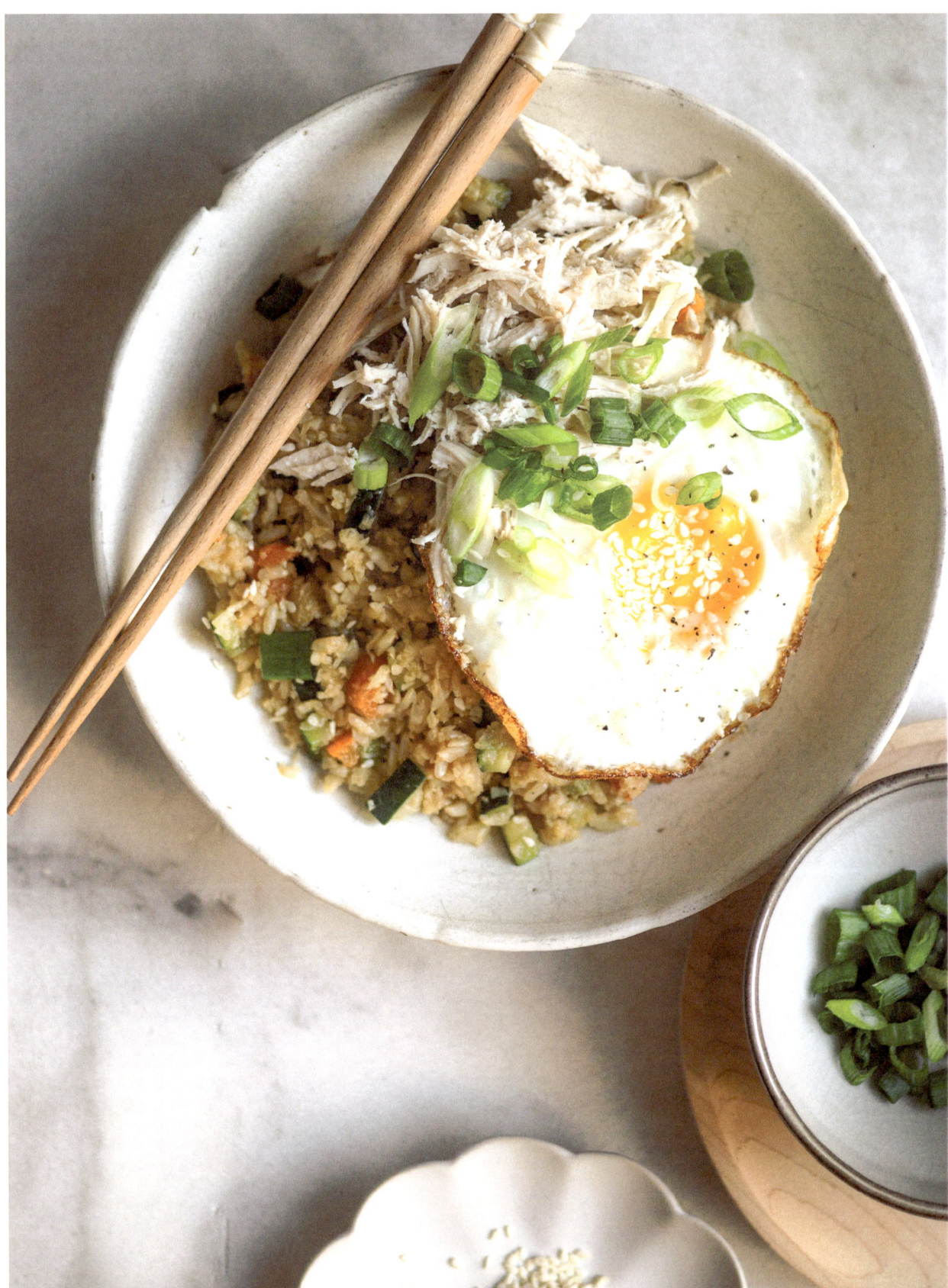

CAULIFLOWER FRIED RICE

WITH SHREDDED CHICKEN AND VEGGIES

We know energy levels can be up and down in the third trimester, so lighten the load by doubling recipes and choosing easier options in the kitchen. Plan to make this when you have leftover chicken in the fridge. Most grocery stores will have pre-cut and washed veggies, like mirepoix, and you can find cauliflower rice in the frozen section. A few handy life hacks will be so helpful as you move into the postpartum period!

INGREDIENTS | SERVES 4

Chicken:
4 chicken breasts or 6 thighs, boneless and skinless, excess fat removed
1 tablespoon lemon juice
¼ teaspoon sea salt
Freshly cracked pepper

Cauliflower fried rice:
8 cups cauliflower chunks (or 6 ½ cups cauliflower rice)
5 tablespoons avocado oil, coconut oil, or ghee, divided
1 small yellow onion, diced
½ teaspoon sea salt, divided
2 tablespoons freshly minced garlic
1 tablespoon freshly minced ginger
3 cups diced vegetables (I used carrots, celery, zucchini, and mushrooms)
2 tablespoons sesame oil
4 tablespoons tamari
2 tablespoons liquid aminos (I use Braggs)
2 free range, organic eggs
2 green onions, sliced thin
Sesame seeds to garnish

*If you have leftover brown rice you can also substitute half the cauliflower rice for brown rice.

DIRECTIONS

1. *If you aren't using leftover chicken:* Preheat the oven to 400º F. Place the chicken, lemon juice, salt, and pepper into a parchment paper packet, folding around the edges to close. Place on a baking sheet and bake in the oven for 20 minutes.

2. Set the chicken aside and shred once cooled.

3. Prepare the cauliflower rice: In a large food processor, or in batches in a small food processor, pulse the chunks of cauliflower until they resemble rice. (You can also grate on a cheese grater or buy pre-riced cauliflower to save time!) Set aside.

4. In a large Dutch oven or large deep skillet, heat 3 tablespoons of oil or ghee over medium-low heat. Add onions and ¼ teaspoon of salt. Sauté over medium-low heat until the onions begin to soften. Add the garlic and ginger and sauté until fragrant, about 1 minute.

5. Turn the heat to medium and add another tablespoon of oil or ghee, the diced vegetables, and another ¼ teaspoon of salt. Sauté over medium heat until the vegetables are soft, about 5 minutes or so depending on their size. Add additional oil and lower the temperature if they begin to stick.

6. Once the vegetables are soft, add the cauliflower rice and the last tablespoon of oil. Sauté over medium heat for 2 minutes, stirring occasionally.

7. Finally, add sesame oil, tamari, and aminos. Stir together until fully combined.

8. Turn heat to medium-low and make a little hole in the middle of the rice mixture. Crack your eggs into the hole. Whisk raw eggs together and then incorporate into the cauliflower rice. Let the eggs slowly cook into the mixture for 2 minutes. (You can also fry the eggs separately and add them to the cauliflower rice at the end).

9. Taste and adjust seasoning if necessary, adding more tamari or aminos if desired.

10. Top with shredded chicken, green onions, and sesame seeds.

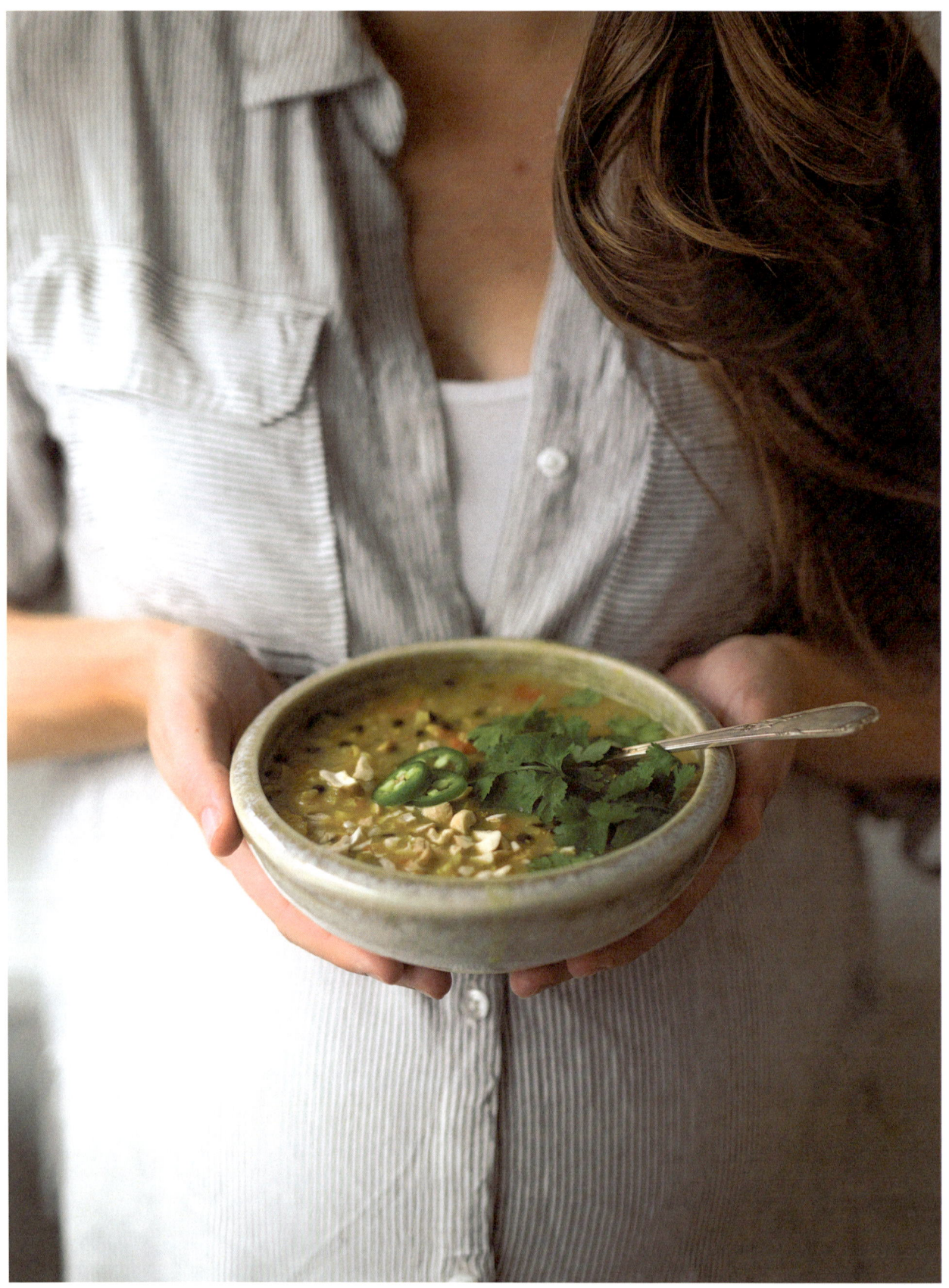

MULLIGATAWNY

WITH APPLES, LENTILS, AND RICE

During the last 4–6 weeks of pregnancy, many mamas feel a welcome surge of energy in their eagerness to meet babe. Lean into this lovely energetic shift, but stay present for your developing babe. This mulligatawny is bursting with flavour and perfect for cozying up and giving ourselves abundant nourishment and care. We have provided a few soups this trimester to help you stock your freezer, and this one will reheat perfectly in a couple of months' time.

INGREDIENTS | SERVES 4-6

4 tablespoons ghee, grass-fed butter, or avocado oil, divided

1 medium yellow onion, diced

1 ½ teaspoons sea salt, divided

2 tablespoons freshly minced garlic

3 teaspoons freshly minced ginger

2 tablespoons curry powder or Madras curry powder

1 ¼ teaspoons cumin

½ teaspoon coriander

1 teaspoon cinnamon

½ teaspoon turmeric

Freshly cracked pepper

450 grams boneless, skinless chicken thighs, excess fat removed, cut into bite-sized pieces (1 pound)

1 cup diced carrots

2 cups chopped apple (Pink Lady or another tart and flavourful variety)

1 cup chopped Roma tomatoes

4 cups chicken stock

1 cup French or black beluga lentils

¾ cup canned coconut milk

1 ½ cups cooked brown basmati rice*

Cilantro, cashews, and jalapeños to garnish

DIRECTIONS

1. In a large Dutch oven or stockpot, heat 3 tablespoons of the ghee or oil over medium-low heat, then add the onions and ¼ teaspoon of salt. Sauté for 3–4 minutes until onions are soft, stirring frequently to avoid burning. (Turn down the heat or add additional ghee or oil if they begin to burn.)

2. Once the onions have softened, add the remaining 1 tablespoon of ghee or oil, garlic, ginger, curry powder, cumin, coriander, cinnamon, turmeric, ½ teaspoon of salt, and about 10 cracks of pepper, stirring to coat the onions with the spices. Turn the heat to medium and cook for about 1 minute until the spices become fragrant.

3. Add the chicken, carrots, apple, and tomatoes. Stir to coat everything with the spices and sauté over medium heat for 2–3 minutes or until the vegetables have softened.

4. Add the chicken stock, lentils, and another ½ teaspoon salt. Bring to a low simmer, cover, and turn the heat to medium-low. Let everything simmer for 15–18 minutes or until lentils are al dente.

5. Stir in the coconut milk, the last ¼ teaspoon of salt, and the cooked rice; bring back to a simmer to quickly warm the rice. Taste and add more salt and pepper if needed.

6. Serve the soup topped with cilantro, chopped cashews, and sliced jalapeños.

*Precook the rice as it takes much longer to cook than the other ingredients.

You can use an Instant Pot and complete steps 2–3 on the sauté function. Once you have added the stock and lentils, set the Instant Pot to manual for 8 minutes and use the quick release carefully. Finish with steps 5 and 6.

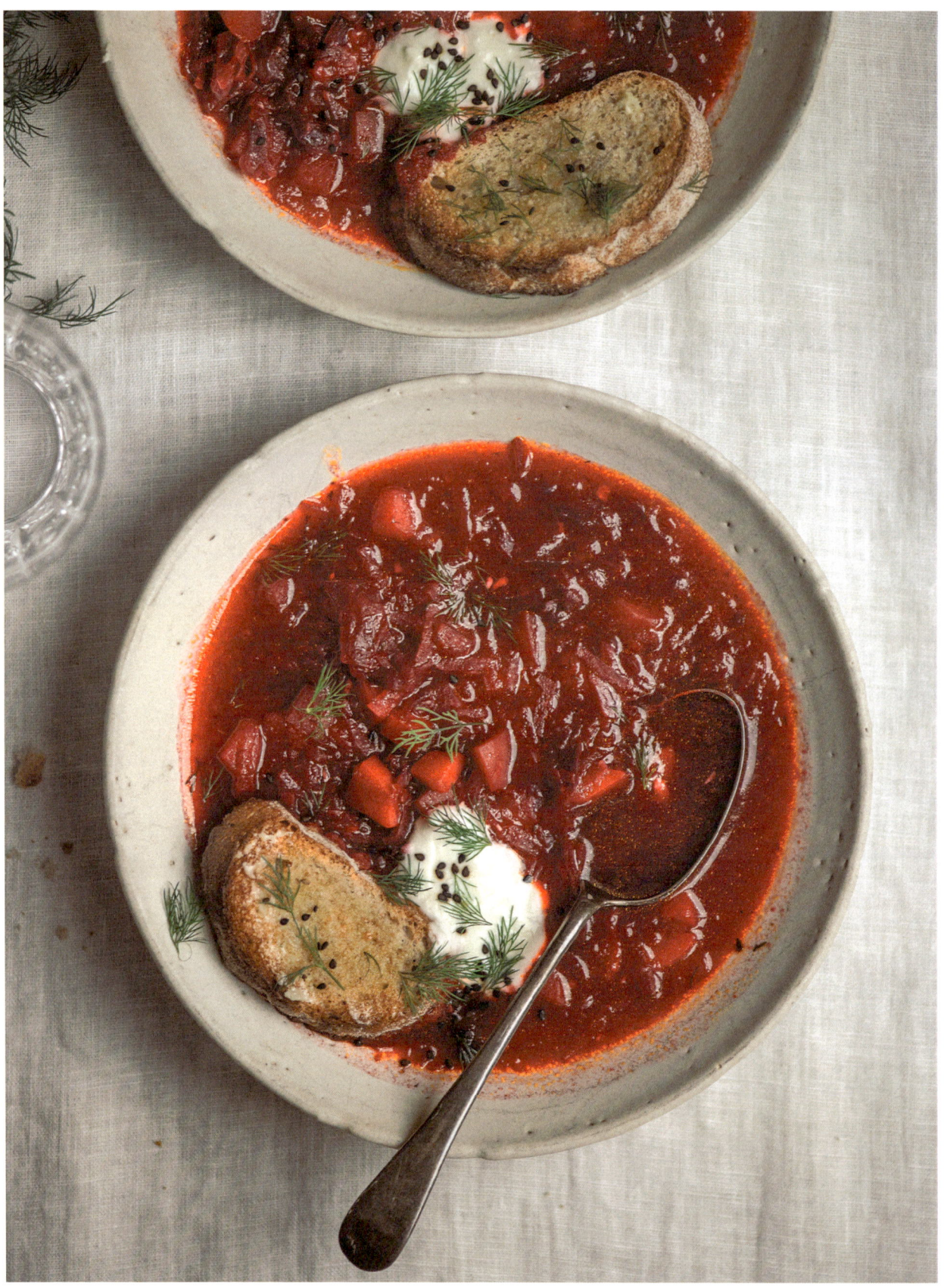

BISON BORSCHT

WITH BEETS, CABBAGE, AND POTATOES

Antioxidants are great during any trimester, but they are amazing at protecting the placenta and growing babe during the last stretch of pregnancy. Anytime you switch to a vegetable with colour, you gain antioxidants, bioflavonoids, vitamins and minerals. This beet borscht feels so wholesome with its iron-building and antioxidant-rich ingredients; make sure you make a double or even triple batch for your fourth-trimester freezer!

INGREDIENTS | SERVES 4

3 tablespoons ghee, coconut oil, or avocado oil, divided
1 large yellow onion, chopped
1 ¾ teaspoons sea salt, divided
450 grams bison stir-fry pieces (1 pound)
1 ½ tablespoons freshly minced garlic
4 tablespoons tomato paste
7 cups beef broth
1 ½ cups diced carrots
4 cups shredded raw beets
2 cups shredded cabbage (red or green)
2 cups diced potatoes
2 bay leaves
1 teaspoon dried dill
Freshly cracked pepper
3 tablespoons apple cider vinegar or sauerkraut brine
2 tablespoons fresh dill

DIRECTIONS

1. In a large Dutch oven or stockpot, heat 3 tablespoons of the ghee or oil over medium-low heat. Add the onions and ¼ teaspoon of salt, and sauté for 3–4 minutes, stirring frequently, until the onions are soft. (Turn down the heat or add additional ghee or oil if the onions begin to burn.)

2. Add the bison stir-fry pieces and garlic and sauté for 1–2 minutes until the bison is browned.

3. Add the tomato paste, broth, carrots, beets, cabbage, potatoes, bay leaves, dried dill, 1 ½ teaspoons of salt, and a few cracks of pepper. Simmer for 15–18 minutes until the potatoes and carrots are soft.

4. Add the vinegar or sauerkraut brine, and fresh dill. Taste and season with additional salt and pepper if needed.

You can also use an Instant Pot. Complete steps 1 and 2 on the sauté function, and step 3 on manual mode for 6 minutes. Quick release carefully. Continue with step 4.

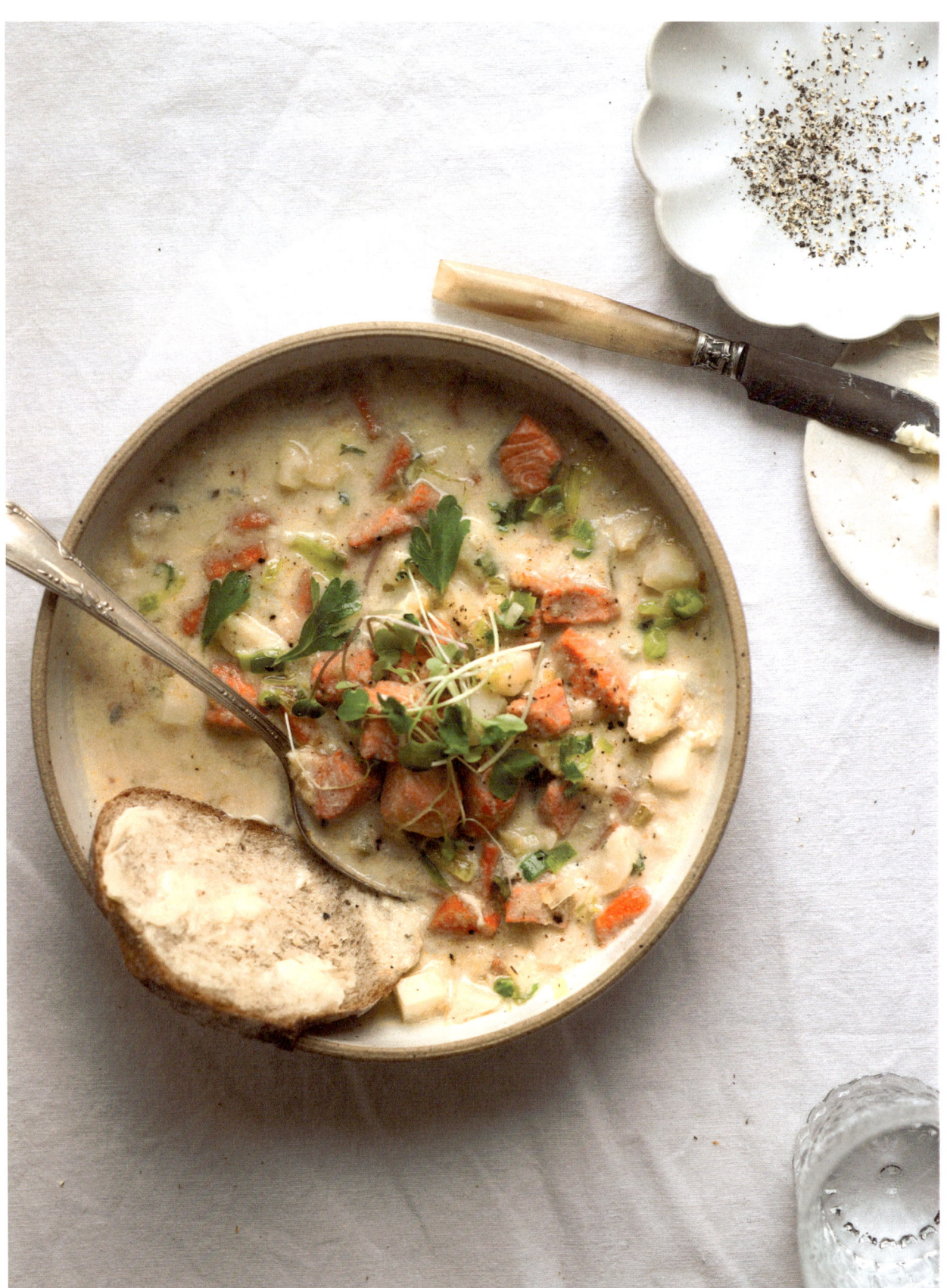

DAIRY-FREE SALMON CHOWDER

WITH CELERY ROOT AND TARRAGON

The third trimester is a massive brain-development chapter for babies. The baby's brain is tripling in weight, forming neuron connections and wiring. Their eyes are also maturing, getting ready to open to the world. It's not by chance that foods rich in essential omega-3 fatty acids, like salmon, are craved by Mama and babe this trimester, as they are the critical building blocks of the baby's brain and eyes. The most biologically active forms of omega-3s come from marine sources, so you can feel great nourishing yourself and your baby's growing brain with this delicious salmon chowder.

INGREDIENTS | SERVES 4

Cashew cream:
¾ cup raw unsalted cashews
⅛ teaspoon salt
¼ teaspoon lemon juice

Chowder:
3 tablespoons ghee, grass-fed butter, or coconut oil
2 cups chopped leeks, white and light green parts only
2 cups diced carrots
1 cup diced celery
¾ teaspoons sea salt, divided
5 cups peeled, chopped celery root and/or parsnips
4 cups clam juice
6 fresh thyme sprigs
2 bay leaves
Freshly cracked pepper
450-565 grams wild sockeye salmon, bones and skin removed, cut into large chunks (1- 1 ¼ pounds)
2 tablespoons roughly chopped fresh tarragon, tightly packed
2 tablespoons roughly chopped fresh parsley, tightly packed
Juice from ½ lemon

DIRECTIONS

1. Make the cashew cream: Soak cashews in pure, filtered water overnight. In the morning, drain the cashews, rinse thoroughly under cold water, and transfer to a high-speed blender. Add ¼ cup plus 2 tablespoons of pure filtered water and blend on high until smooth and creamy. Add salt and lemon juice. If you are not using a high-speed blender like a Vitamix, which creates an extra-smooth cream, strain the cashew cream through a fine-mesh sieve. Set aside.

2. In a large Dutch oven or stockpot, melt the ghee or oil over medium-low heat. Add the leeks, carrots, celery, and ¼ teaspoon salt. Cook for 5 minutes or until vegetables are soft.

3. Add the celery root, parsnips, clam juice, thyme sprigs, bay leaves, ½ teaspoon of salt, and a few cracks of pepper. Bring to a boil, cover, lower to a simmer, and cook until the vegetables are soft, about 15 minutes.

4. Gently fold the salmon, cashew cream, tarragon, and parsley into the soup. Simmer on low, being careful not to bring the soup to a boil, until the salmon is cooked through, about 5 minutes.

5. Add the lemon juice, taste, and season with additional salt and pepper if desired. Remove the thyme sprigs and bay leaves before serving.

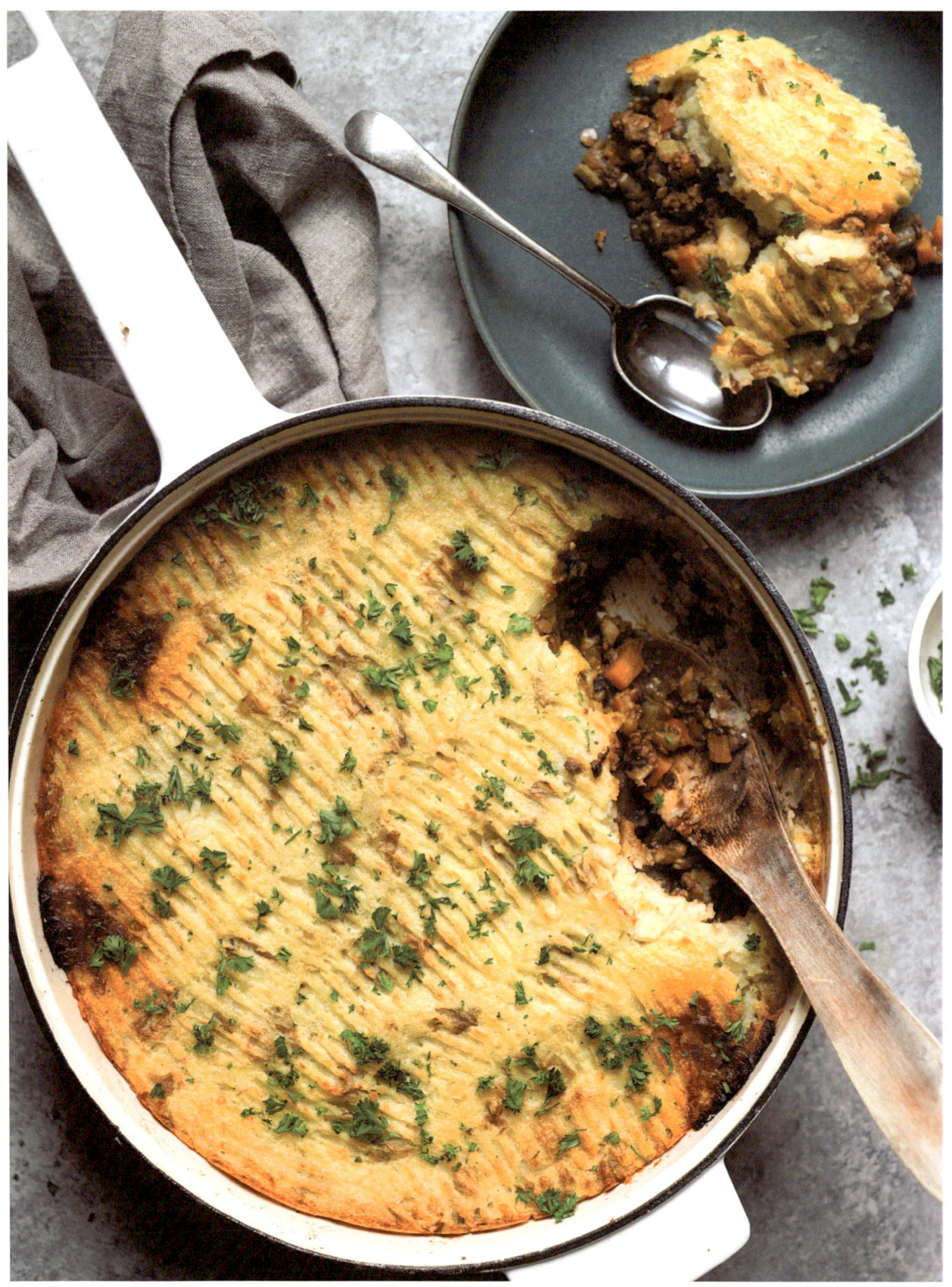

SHEPHERD'S PIE

WITH ELK AND EGGPLANT

Food for thought: mineral status is correlated with pregnancy length as well as childbirth outcomes. There is also a positive correlation between pregnancy micro-nutrition (or "vitamin and mineral content") and postpartum health outcomes for the mother. Game meat is especially high in zinc, iron, and selenium because the animals feast on natural vegetation rather than grain feed. Consuming wild meat also allows you to avoid steroids and hormones. There's no better time than pregnancy to steer clear of toxins and load up on vitamin- and mineral-rich foods.

INGREDIENTS | SERVES 4

Potato topping:
4 cups peeled and chopped parsnips and/or celery root
1 teaspoon sea salt, divided
3 ½ cups chopped potatoes
½ cup grass-fed butter, ghee, or vegan soy-free butter

Pie filling:
5 tablespoons avocado or coconut oil, divided
450 grams ground elk (1 pound)
1 teaspoon sea salt, divided
Freshly cracked pepper
¾ cup minced onions
¾ cup grated carrots
225 grams cremini mushrooms, wiped clean and diced (8 ounces)
2 tablespoons minced fresh garlic
8 sprigs of thyme
1 bay leaf
2 cups peeled and chopped eggplant
2 ½ tablespoons tomato paste
1 ½ tablespoons Worcestershire sauce
2 cups beef bone broth or beef stock

DIRECTIONS | PREHEAT OVEN TO 350° F

1. In a large saucepan, combine the parsnips, celery root, and ½ teaspoon salt. Add enough water to cover plus about 4-5 inches (you will need enough water once you add the potatoes). Bring to a low boil, cover, turn heat to low, and let simmer for 5 minutes. Add the potatoes and continue cooking for another 10–12 minutes until the vegetables are fork-tender. Drain the vegetables and return them to the saucepan. While they are still hot, add the butter and last ½ teaspoon of salt. Mash with a potato masher until fully combined and smooth.

2. While the vegetables are simmering, heat 3 tablespoons of the oil in a large, deep sauté pan on medium-high heat. Add the ground meat, ¼ teaspoon salt, and a few cracks of pepper, and sauté for 2–3 minutes.

3. Stir in the onions, carrots, mushrooms, garlic, thyme, and bay leaf, and cook for 3–4 minutes until the onions and mushrooms have softened.

4. Add the eggplant, ½ teaspoon salt, and the last 2 tablespoons of oil or butter, and cook for another 2–3 minutes until the eggplant has softened slightly.

5. Add the tomato paste, Worcestershire sauce, and bone broth or stock. Simmer for about 5-7 minutes, stirring frequently, until the sauce has thickened.

6. Taste, and add the last ¼ teaspoon of salt and a few extra cracks of pepper if desired. Remove the thyme sprigs.

7. Spoon the meat-and-eggplant mixture into the bottom of a large ovenproof dish (or use the pan you cooked the meat in, if it is ovenproof).

8. Using a spatula, layer the mash generously on top of the filling.

9. Fluff up the mashed potatoes with a fork to make rough peaks.

10. Bake in the oven at 350° for approximately 20 minutes until bubbling and golden brown. Remove the bay leaf as you portion the pie out.

You can substitute black beluga lentils for the ground game meat, or use half and half for the added fibre!

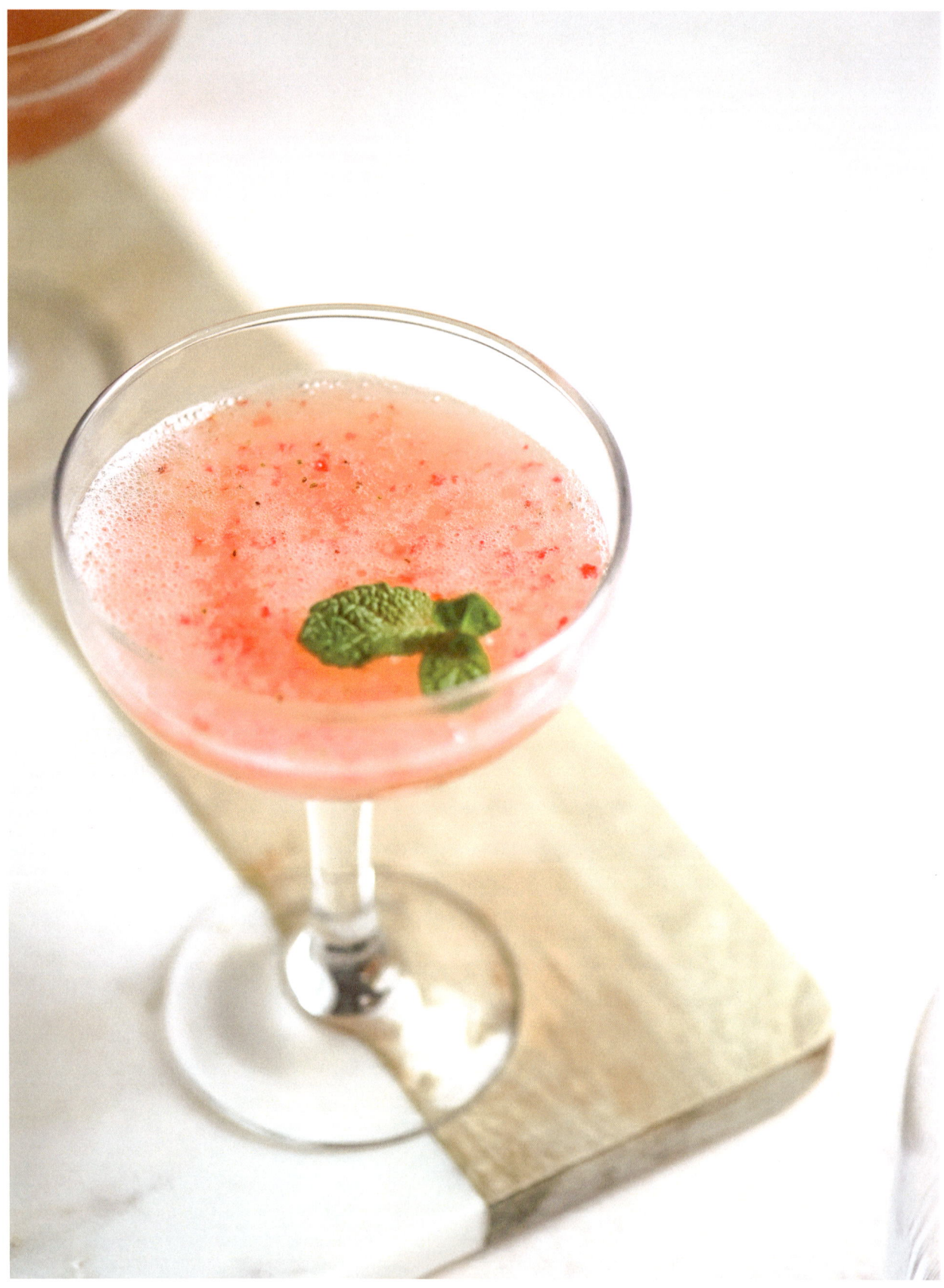

RED RASPBERRY LEAF MOJITO

WITH KOMBUCHA, STRAWBERRIES, AND MINT

This herbaceous and bubbly drink is perfect to quench your thirst, build your gut flora, and tone and strengthen the muscles of your uterine lining. Red raspberry, or Rubus idaeus, has been used for centuries as a botanical labour preparation medicine. It is traditionally used in the third trimester, but it can taste a bit earthy, so mix it up with this refreshing mojito!

INGREDIENTS | SERVES 1

2 organic red raspberry leaf tea bags
1 cup chopped fresh strawberries
2 tablespoons fresh lime juice
1 ½ tablespoons pasteurized honey, divided
¼ cup fresh mint, tightly packed
¼ cup kombucha

DIRECTIONS

1. Steep the raspberry leaf tea bags in 1 cup of boiling water for at least 10 minutes. Discard the tea bags.

2. While the tea is steeping, combine the strawberries, lime juice, and 1 tablespoon of honey in a food processor. Pulse until puréed smooth. Add the mint, and pulse quickly to incorporate.

3. Combine ¼ cup of the strawberry purée, the kombucha, and the tea in a glass. Taste, and add the remaining ½ tablespoon of honey if desired. (Save the leftover strawberry purée in a jar with a tight-fitting lid.)

4. Add ice, and enjoy!

Drink 2–3 cups of red raspberry tea daily in the last 3–4 weeks of pregnancy to help tone the uterus and prepare for birth.

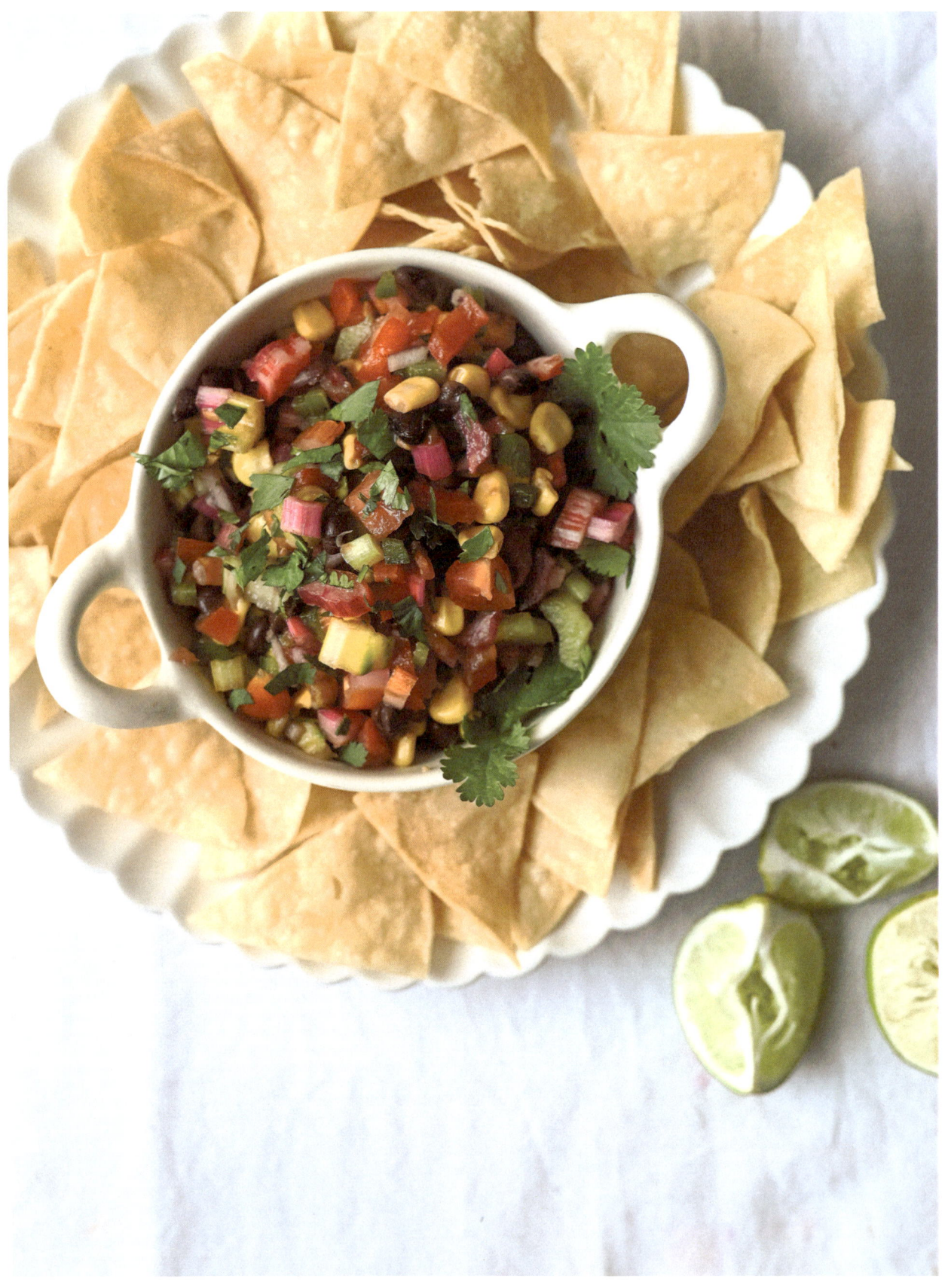

AVOCADO AND CORN SALSA

WITH SWISS CHARD STEMS

This phytonutrient-rich salsa will taste better and better as the week goes on. Phytonutrients are the powerful antioxidants found in plants, especially fresh vegetables like the ones in this yummy salsa. Snacking in the third trimester is a way of life for pregnant mamas. Babe is getting bigger and taking up lots of mom's stomach space, so small nutritious snacks are a perfect way to get adequate nutrition without feeling too uncomfortable.

INGREDIENTS | YIELDS 4 CUPS

1 tablespoon coconut or avocado oil, divided
1 ½ cups finely diced Swiss chard stems
1 cup fresh or frozen corn
¼ teaspoon sea salt
¾ cup cooked or canned black beans, drained
1 ¼ cups diced Roma or cherry tomatoes
3 tablespoons minced red onions
3 tablespoons chopped fresh cilantro
1 jalapeño, ribs and seeds removed, minced
1 medium-large avocado, cubed
Tortilla chips, to serve

Dressing:
4 tablespoons extra-virgin olive oil
3 tablespoons lime juice
2 tablespoons pasteurized honey
½ teaspoon paprika
1 teaspoon cumin
Pinch or two of cayenne pepper
½ teaspoon sea salt

DIRECTIONS

1. In a skillet, melt 1 tablespoon of coconut or avocado oil over medium-low heat.
2. Add the Swiss chard stems, the corn, and ¼ teaspoon of salt. Sauté, stirring occasionally, for 3–4 minutes until the stems are soft. (If the vegetables begin to burn or stick, add a bit more oil and/or turn down the heat.)
3. Transfer Swiss chard stems and corn to a bowl.
4. Add the black beans, tomatoes, red onions, cilantro, and jalapeño. Stir to combine.
5. In a small bowl or jar with a lid, combine all the dressing ingredients. Stir vigorously or shake in the jar to combine. Pour over the salsa and toss to combine.
6. Before serving, add the avocado and stir gently to combine.
7. Serve with tortilla chips and enjoy!

Substitute mango for the black beans for a fresh salsa to throw over grilled fish.

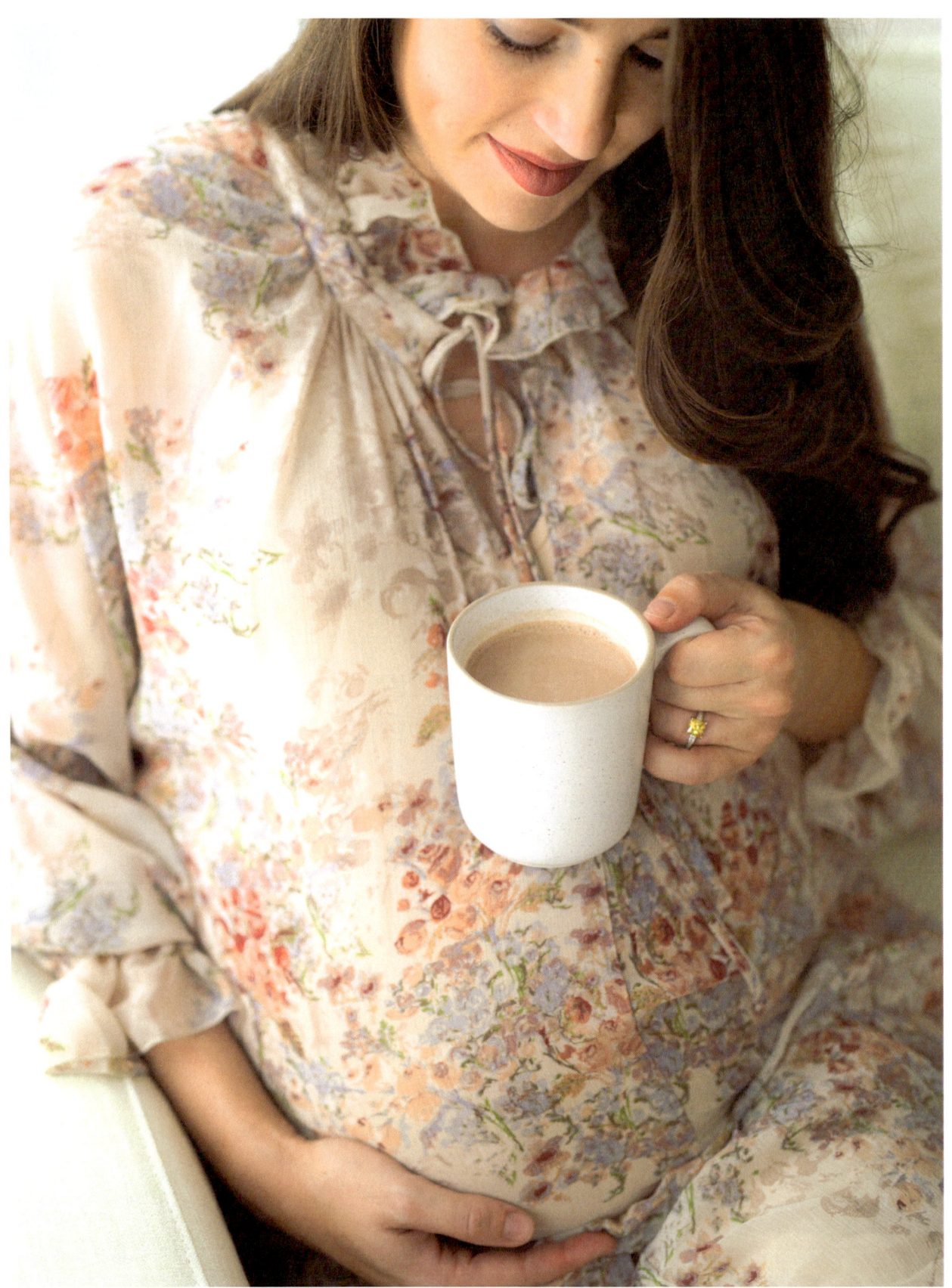

HOT CACAO

RELAXING AND MAGNESIUM-RICH

Put your feet up and prep for the big birthday event with this comforting hot chocolate drink. Magnesium is essential in pregnancy. It aids digestion, helps with late-pregnancy insomnia, relieves aches and muscle spasms, and helps calm an excited mind. This warm, rich, and delicious bevvy is great for an afternoon rest or part of your bedtime ritual.

INGREDIENTS | SERVES 1

60 grams cacao paste (2 ounces)
120 grams cacao butter (4 ounces)
1 teaspoon lucuma powder
3–4 tablespoons maple syrup
½ teaspoon vanilla extract
½ cup coconut cream
½ cup almond milk
1 tablespoon ashwagandha powder

DIRECTIONS

1. In a small saucepan, bring ¼ cup water to a boil. Place a small metal bowl over the top and add the cacao paste and cacao butter. Slowly melt the two together, stirring to incorporate.
2. Add the lucuma, maple syrup, and vanilla and stir to combine.
3. Carefully remove the bowl from the top of the saucepan, set aside, and empty the water from the saucepan.
4. Return the saucepan to the stove and add the coconut cream and almond milk, whisking to incorporate.
5. Bring to a low simmer and add the cacao mixture and ashwagandha. Stir to combine, and enjoy!

This magical hot chocolate is full of superfoods, however the ingredients may be hard to find at your typical grocery store. Source cacao butter, lucuma, and ashwagandha at whole-foods stores, natural markets, or online.

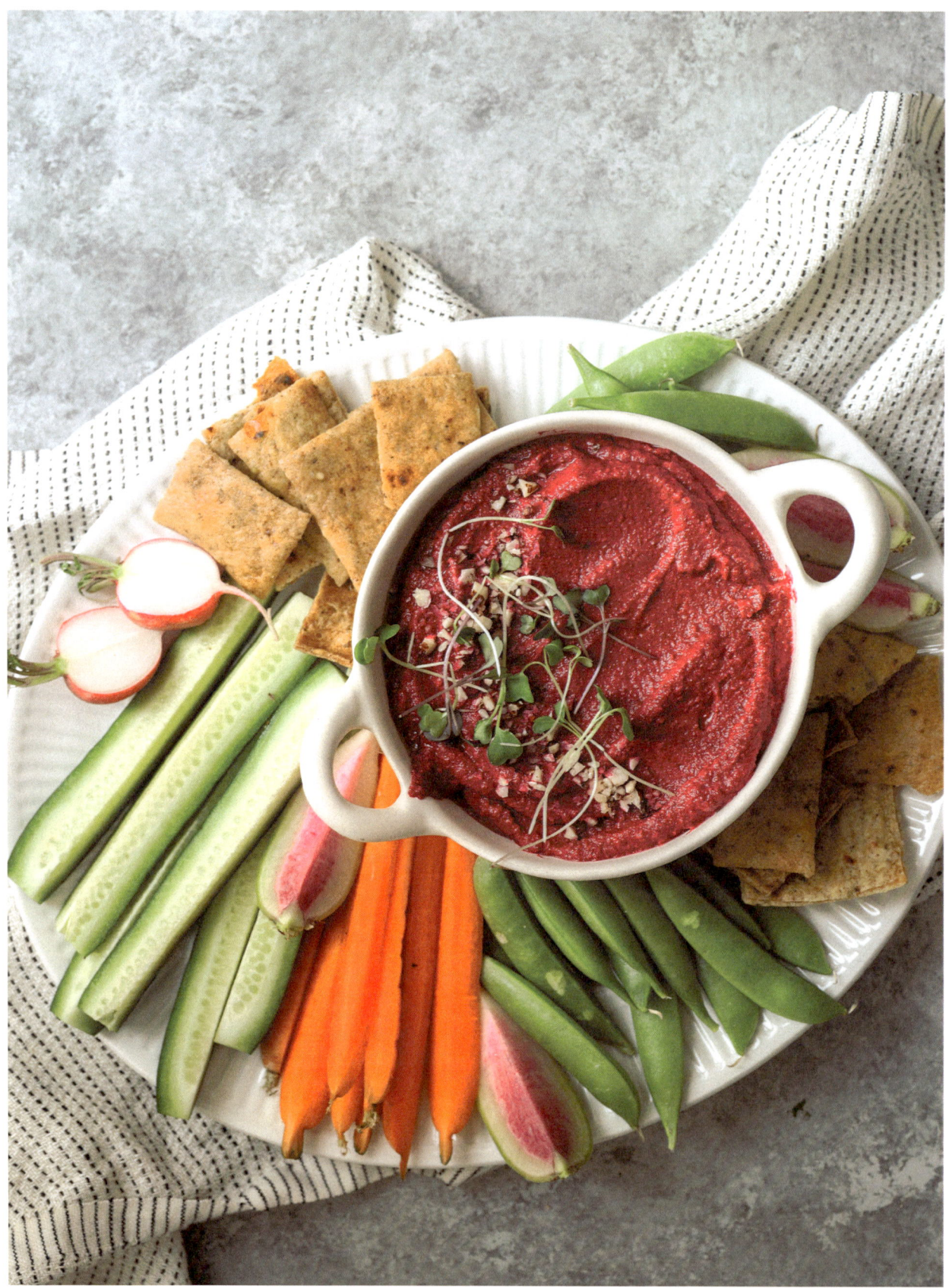

BEET DIP

WITH MINT AND LEMON

In the third trimester, 80 percent of a mother's iron stores are transferred to the baby in preparation for its life outside the womb. Beets are high in iron, but nonheme (vegetarian) sources are best absorbed when paired with vitamin C, as in this recipe. Enjoy this dip with your favourite crackers, with cucumber slices, or on a sandwich!

INGREDIENTS | YIELDS 1 ½ CUPS

- ½ cup raw, unsalted cashews
- 1 ½ cups chopped, cooked beets, divided
- ½ tablespoon minced garlic
- 2 ½ tablespoons lemon juice
- 3 tablespoons high-quality extra-virgin olive oil
- 1 teaspoon pasteurized honey
- ½ teaspoon sea salt
- 2 ½ tablespoons mint chiffonade
- 1 teaspoon lemon zest, for garnish (optional)

DIRECTIONS

1. Place the cashews in a bowl and cover with fresh water. Place in the fridge overnight.
2. The next day, drain and rinse the cashews.
3. In a food processor, pulse ½ cup of the beets until minced or shredded. Remove from the food processor and set aside.
4. In the food processor, combine the cashews, garlic, lemon juice, extra-virgin olive oil, honey, and salt. Pulse until the cashews have broken down into tiny pieces and are well combined.
5. Add the last cup of beets to the food processor and purée until smooth.
6. Transfer to a bowl and stir in the shredded beets and fresh mint. Garnish with the lemon zest.

I baked 6 medium beets at 425° F in parchment paper for 1 hour. (Total cooking time will depend on the size of your beets.) I then peeled the beets and chopped them. If you have leftover beets or can buy precooked organic beets, they will work perfectly!

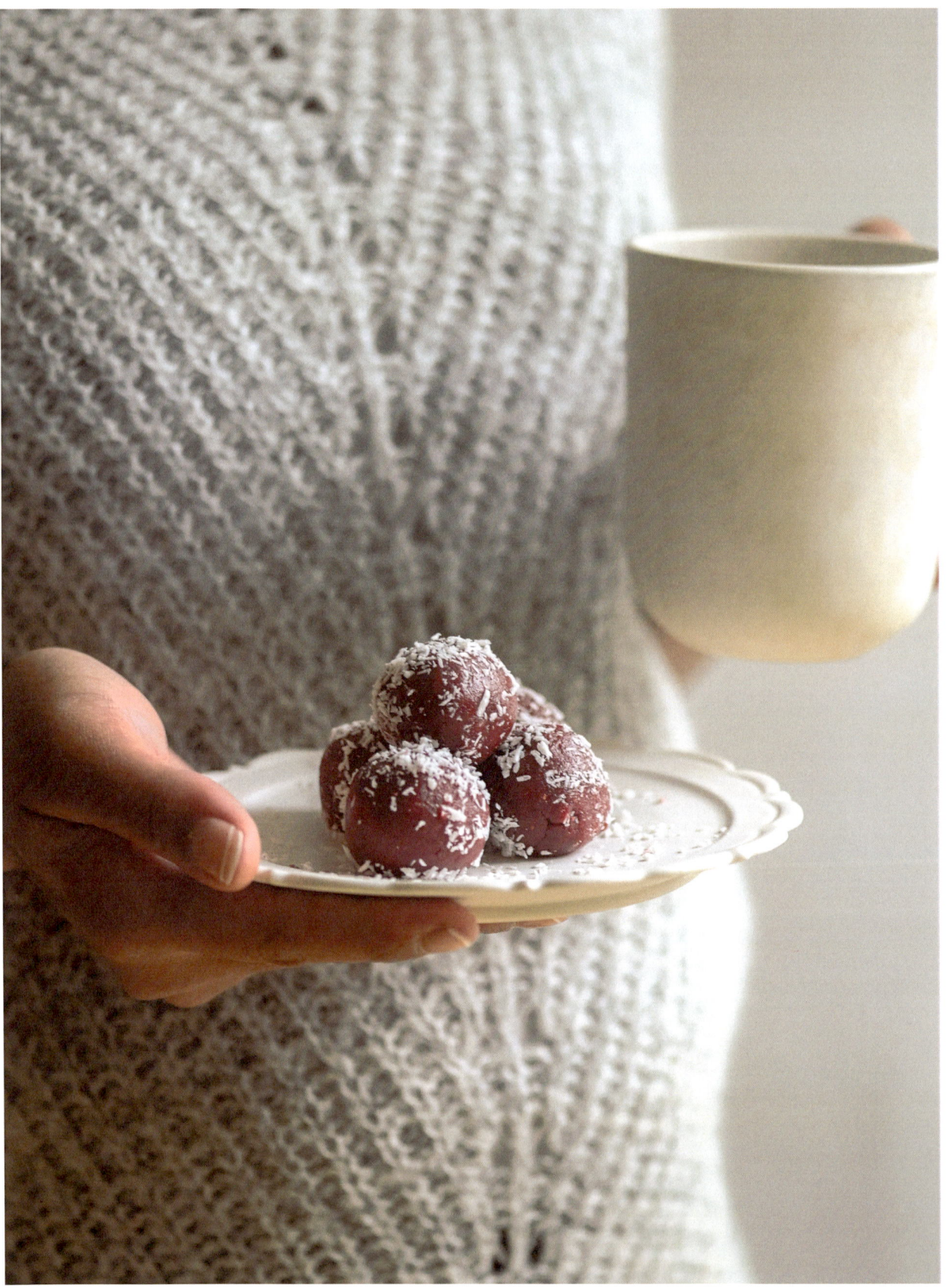

RED RASPBERRY BITES

DR. CARRIE'S "RIPE AND READY" SNACKS

Red raspberry leaf is one of Dr. Carrie's favourite botanicals for labour preparation, so roll up a double dose of these yummy snacks and share them with all your pregnant friends! Red raspberry leaf has been shown to tone and strengthen the uterine muscles when taken throughout the third trimester. In the last stretch of pregnancy, you really can't go wrong with these sweet, uterus-toning snacks.

INGREDIENTS | YIELDS 15 BALLS

18 organic red raspberry leaf tea bags, divided

1 ½ cups raw, unsalted cashews

4–5 dates, pits removed

½ cup almond butter

½ cup dried goji berries or dried blueberries

2 teaspoons vanilla extract

¼ cup unsweetened shredded coconut

DIRECTIONS

1. Place the cashews and 3 tea bags in a large bowl or glass jar.
2. Boil 1 cup of water and pour over the cashews and tea bags. Let them steep for 30 minutes.
3. Transfer the cashews and ⅓ cup of the tea to a food processor. Discard the tea bags and discard the extra tea.
4. Add the dates, almond butter, goji berries, and vanilla extract to the food processor. Pulse until everything is chunky and combined.
5. Cut open the 15 red raspberry leaf tea bags. Pour the loose-leaf tea into the food processor. (If you have loose leaf tea, use 3 tablespoons.)
6. Add the coconut and blend in the food processor until the mixture becomes thick and sticky.
7. Scoop a tablespoon of the mixture and roll it into a ball between your palms. Repeat with the remaining mixture.
8. Line up the balls on a baking sheet and place in the refrigerator to chill for at least an hour, or overnight if possible.
9. Store the Raspberry Bites in an airtight container in the refrigerator or freezer for up to 2 weeks.

The prescription: Enjoy 2 yummy "ripe and ready snacks" mid-afternoon with a steaming cup of red raspberry leaf tea. For an added benefit, combine with 5 minutes of deep-belly breathing as your hands cradle your precious babe. Visualize their perfect face, breathe deep, and ground yourself in your innate maternal strength.

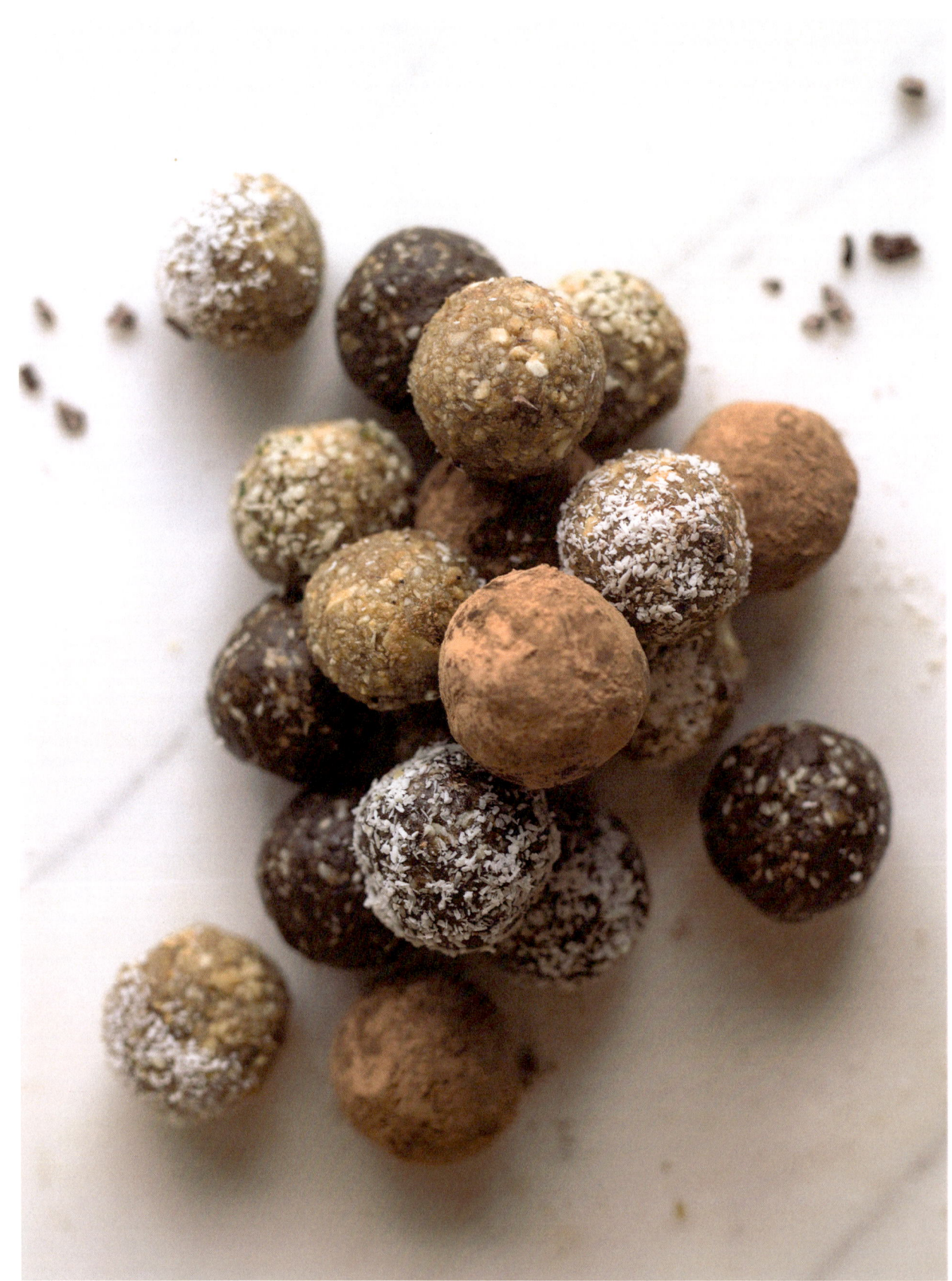

BLISS BALLS

WITH BANANA, WALNUT, AND FIGS

Leg cramps, Braxton Hicks, pelvic floor spasms (lightening crotch pelvis, anyone?) ... Mamas, we are going through it by the end of pregnancy! Packing magnesium- and calcium-rich meals and snacks will help ease cramping and spasms and help you feel your best in the last weeks of your pregnancy. Do your future self a huge favour—double this recipe and freeze half for easy postpartum snacks!

INGREDIENTS | YIELDS 20 BALLS

½ cup banana, tightly packed
½ cup plus 1 tablespoon walnuts
¾ cup almonds
3 tablespoons pumpkin seeds
12 dried figs or dates
6 medjool dates, pits removed
¼ cup plus 2 tablespoons almond butter
½ teaspoon vanilla extract
2 tablespoons vegan vanilla protein powder
1 ½ tablespoons chocolate chips (optional)
¼ cup hemp hearts, shredded coconut, cacao powder or crushed dried banana chips for dusting

DIRECTIONS

1. Blend the banana in a food processor. Once smooth, transfer to a medium bowl.
2. Add the walnuts, almonds, pumpkin seeds, figs and dates to the food processor. Pulse until they resemble crumbles.
3. Add the almond butter, vanilla extract, and protein powder. Pulse until well combined.
4. Transfer the mixture to the bowl with the banana and stir to combine. Add chocolate chips if desired and stir again.
5. Take about 1 tablespoon of the mixture and roll it into a ball in your hand; repeat with the remaining mixture.
6. Roll each ball in hemp hearts, coconut, cacao powder, or crushed banana chips.
7. Keep in the fridge for up to 2 weeks, or freeze for future use.

Magnesium is best absorbed through the skin, so try a magnesium-rich Epsom salt bath followed by an application of magnesium lotion or gel. Finish with a banana walnut bliss ball and an electrolyte drink high in salt and magnesium.

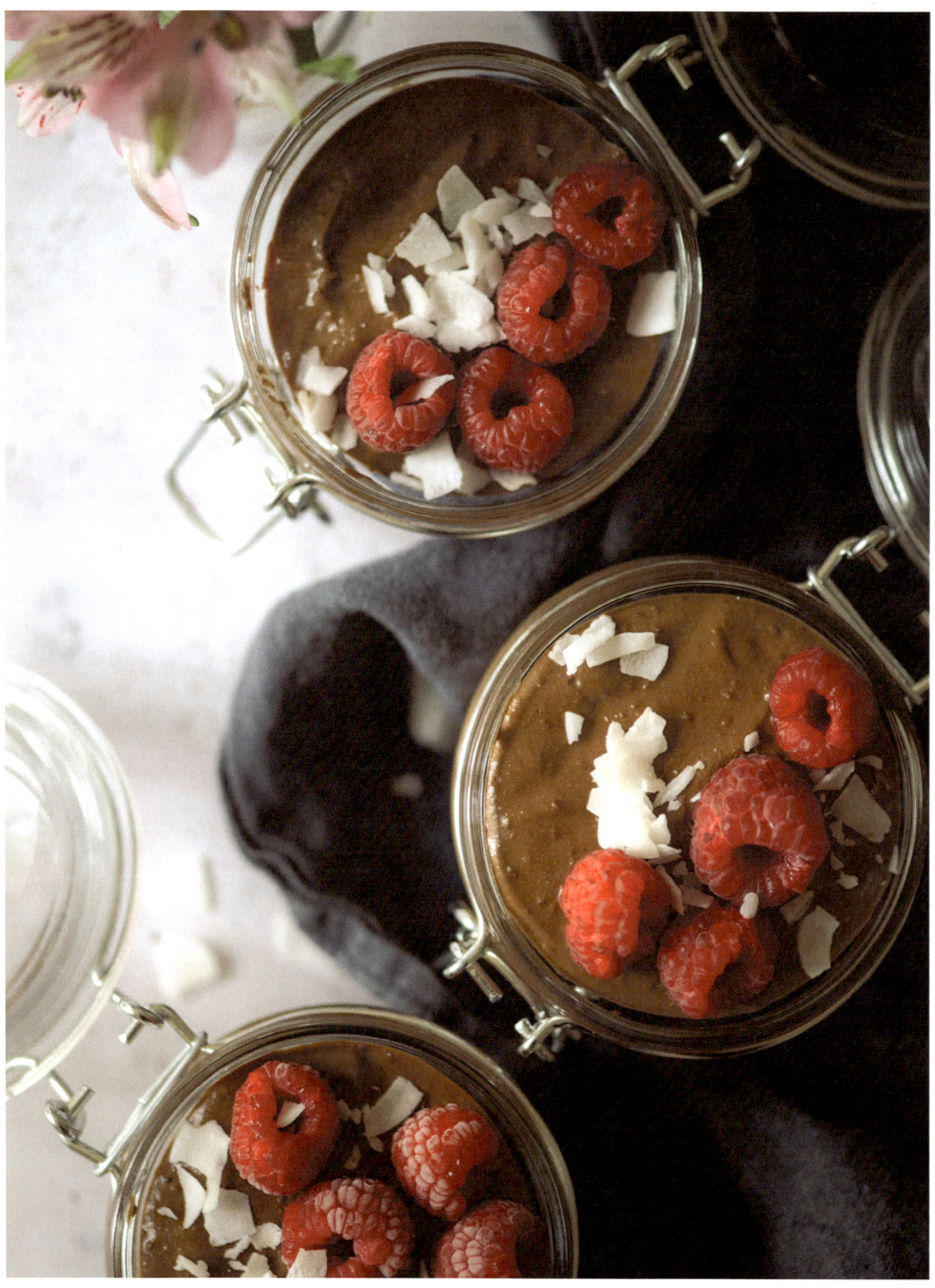

LABOUR PREP CHOCOLATE PUDDING

WITH DATES, AVOCADO, AND CHIA SEEDS

Dates are the number-one food to eat daily in the third trimester. Pregnant mommas who eat 4–6 dates a day in the third trimester experience higher rates of spontaneous labour, easier cervical dilation, and shorter initial labour times. Sign us up! These chocolatey pudding cups pack all the amazing benefits of dates as well as protein and fibre. Make a huge batch and enjoy daily along with your red raspberry leaf tea!

INGREDIENTS | YIELDS 2 CUPS

- 2 tablespoons chia seeds
- ½ cup light coconut milk
- 12 dates, pits removed
- 4 ½ tablespoons cacao powder
- 1 avocado, pit removed
- 2 tablespoons nut butter
- ⅛ teaspoon sea salt
- ½–1 tablespoon maple syrup (optional)
- 1/2 cup raspberries, optional

DIRECTIONS

1. Add the chia seeds to a food processor and pour the coconut milk over top. Stir to combine and let the chia seeds sit with the milk for 20 minutes. Do not turn on the food processor yet!
2. If your dates are hard, place them in a separate bowl and cover them with boiling water. Let them soften while the chia seeds are sitting.
3. After the chia seeds have sat for 20 minutes, drain the dates and add them to the food processor. Purée the chia seeds and dates until smooth.
4. Add the cacao powder, avocado flesh, nut butter, and salt. Pulse again until everything is fully combined.
5. Taste and add maple syrup if desired. Purée again until smooth and transfer to little glass jars. Enjoy with a few fresh raspberries if you desire!

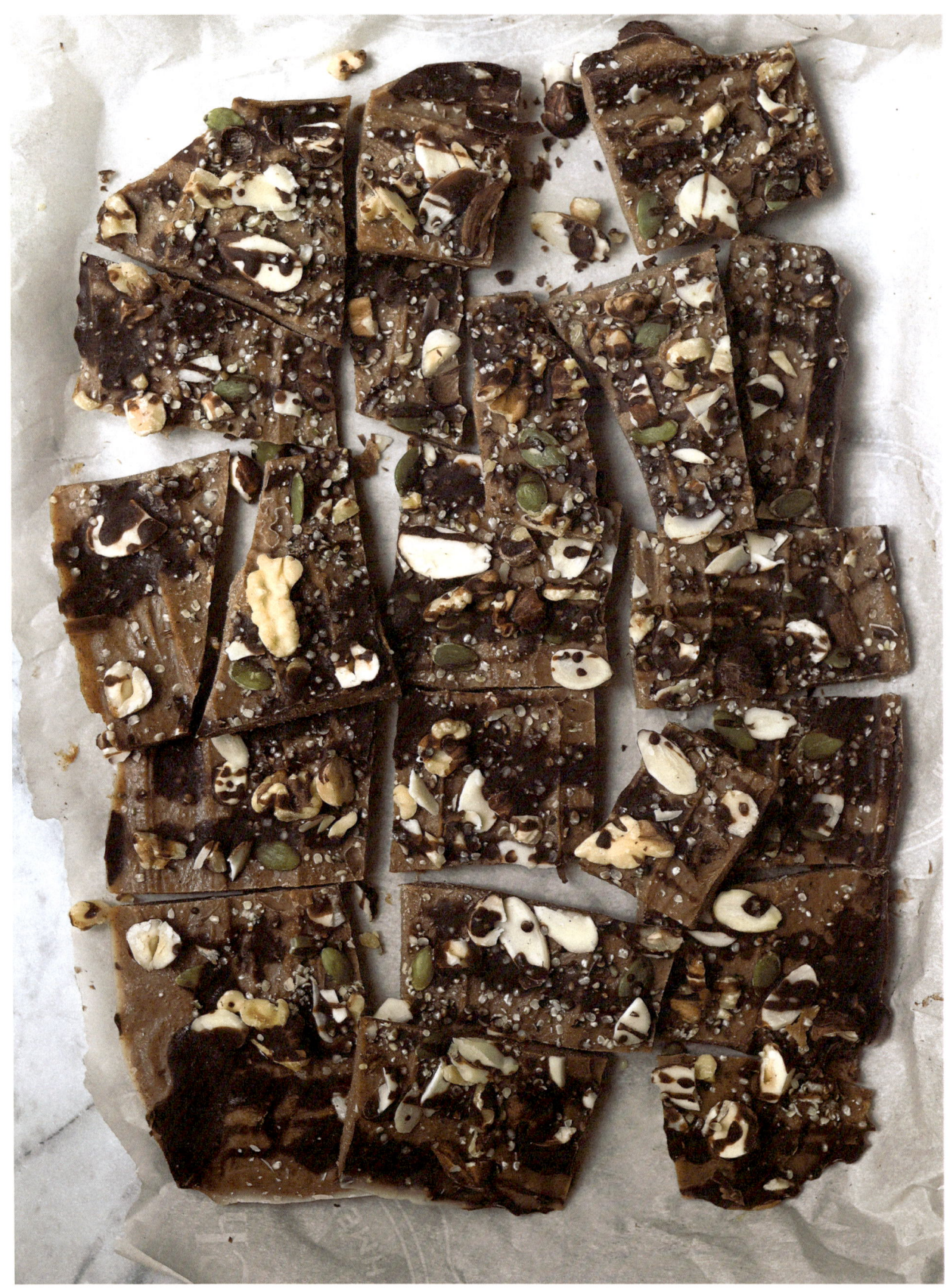

CHOCOLATE BRITTLE

WITH PEANUT BUTTER AND CINNAMON

One of the biggest regrets many seasoned mamas share is that they focused too much on childbirth and didn't spend more time preparing and thinking about the postpartum adventure. We share this sentiment to encourage mamas to visualize and prepare for those first weeks and months after baby arrives.

So, while you munch on this decadent combination of chocolate and peanut butter, meditate on some of these big questions:

1. How do you plan to feed your baby? Do you have breastfeeding support or a backup plan should your first choice not work?
2. Who is your support system? Ask for help from parents, in-laws, friends.
3. What do you think you will need from your support system?
4. How do you plan to nourish, feed, and hydrate yourself?
5. What are your and your partner's expectations regarding the postpartum division of labour?
6. How will you seek help on the days when you are low on energy or experiencing the "baby blues"?
7. Will you need a postpartum doula or nanny?

INGREDIENTS

1 cup peanut butter (or any nut butters you have on hand)

3 tablespoons coconut oil, divided

¼ cup maple syrup

½ cup chopped walnuts

¼ cup chopped Brazil nuts

¼ cup almond slices

½ cup pumpkin seeds

¼ cup sunflower seeds

¼ cup dark chocolate chips or vegan carob chips

1 teaspoon cinnamon

¼ teaspoon sea salt

Optional superfood add-ins: 1–2 tablespoons collagen, spirulina, or Dandy Blend

DIRECTIONS

1. Line a cookie sheet with parchment paper. Set aside.
2. In a small saucepan over low heat, gently heat the peanut butter, 2 tablespoons of the coconut oil, and the maple syrup, stirring to combine until everything is melted together and fully incorporated.
3. Stir in the chopped nuts, sliced almonds, and seeds.
4. Spread the mixture over the lined cookie sheet. Set aside.
5. In a small saucepan, bring ¼ cup water to a boil. Place a small metal bowl over the top and add the chocolate chips and 1 tablespoon of the coconut oil. Slowly melt together the chocolate chips and oil, stirring to incorporate. Remove the mixture from the heat, and stir in the cinnamon, salt, and any of the superfoods you want to add.
6. With a spoon, drizzle the chocolate mixture over the peanut brittle.
7. Freeze the brittle for at least an hour, and enjoy straight from the freezer!

Adding cinnamon is a great way to help balance blood sugar levels and slow the absorption of sugars.

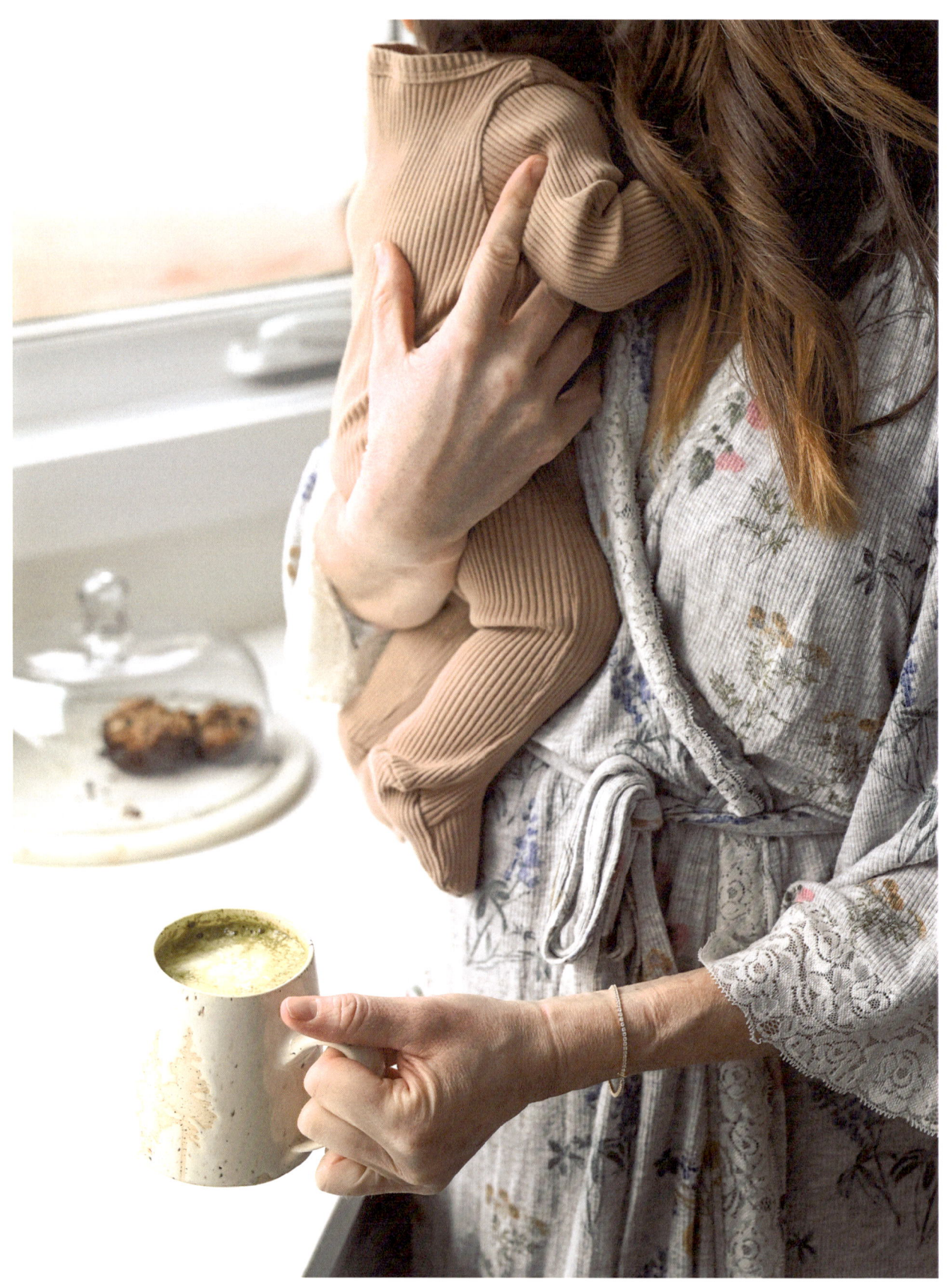

FOURTH TRIMESTER

CONGRATULATIONS, MAMA. WE ARE SO PROUD OF YOU!

Birth is a physically, emotionally, and spiritually intense experience, but all your hard work has been worth it. Here you are with your gorgeous prize. Now we begin to integrate ourselves as mothers and nourish this sacred mother–baby dyad. The fourth trimester is here, and no other time is so beautiful and yet so wild: a complete one-eighty from the way life used to be.

We often channel all our efforts into taking care of this precious, tiny being. However, this is one of the most important times to nourish Mama with increased focus and care. We want you to thrive after baby arrives, honouring your own birth into motherhood. You are your baby's everything. See your importance through their eyes, and nourish yourself like the goddess you are.

Most parents don't realize that if they're breastfeeding, they actually need more calories in the fourth trimester than they did at the end of their pregnancy. Feed this inevitable need by adding more food to your diet. Pop some snacks beside your breastfeeding station and munch away. Ask friends and family to help prepare some of the postpartum recipes here in exchange for baby cuddles. An extra 500 calories daily is often enough for Mama and babe during these exciting and exhausting months.

If you are breastfeeding, a further nutrient depletion can occur if you don't consume enough vitamins, minerals, and essential macronutrients. Postpartum eating revolves around comforting, warming, nourishing foods that replenish what is missing, preventing further deficiencies, and supporting lactation.

Nutritionally, in this "trimester" we will be balancing hormones, supporting milk supply, rebuilding blood, providing gentle energy, supporting the nervous system and immune system, and replenishing fluids lost during birth and breastfeeding. Warming and grounding foods like root vegetables, bone broth, organ meats, and spices like cinnamon, ginger, and turmeric are therapeutic during this time. Just like in previous chapters, every recipe here has been thoughtfully developed to provide your postpartum healing journey with everything it needs. Most recipes are freezable for future use, easy to digest, and easy enough for a loved one to make for you!

The first forty days after birth are intense and awe-inspiring. They should be honoured as a chapter for healing and recovery, and for building deep love and affection with babe. The baby will continue to wake and grow, and mamas will feel stronger in their bodies as months progress, but it is essential to remember that we are forever postpartum. Take this time to rest, nourish, and fall in love with your bright baby—and with yourself.

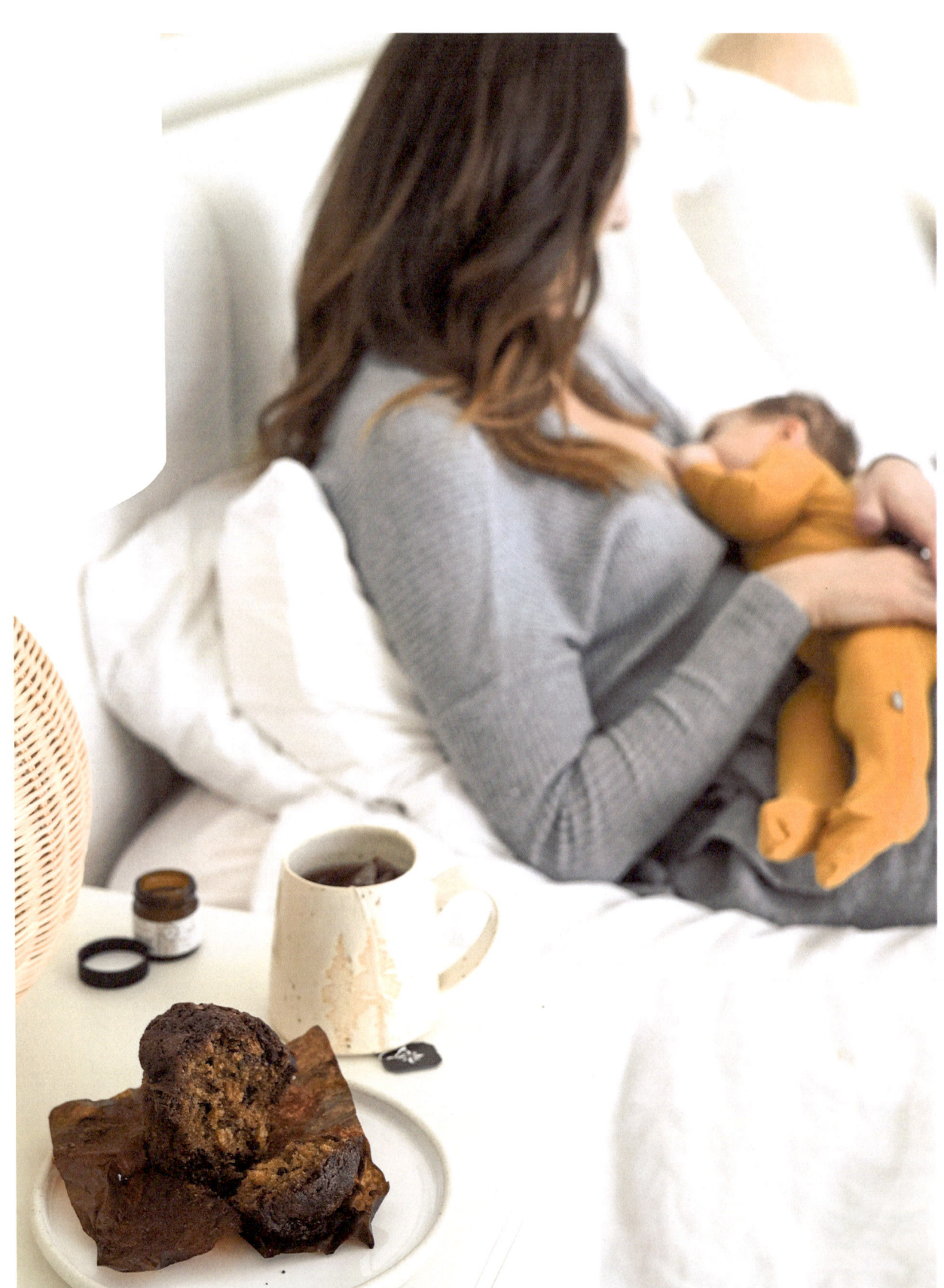

FOURTH TRIMESTER

TABLE OF CONTENTS

BREAKFAST
Post-Birth Healing Broth 145
Coconut Cardamon Millet Pudding with Spiced Pears and Pomegranate Molasses 147
Mini Frittatas with Asparagus and Roasted Tomatoes 149
Ayurvedic Kitchari Stew with Mung Beans, Cauliflower, and Spices 151
Blueberry Lemon Doughnuts with Citrus Glaze 153

LUNCH & DINNERS
Postpartum Nourish Bowl with Root Vegetables and Tahini Dressing 155
Creamy Wild Rice Soup with Cremini Mushrooms and Kale 157
Soothing Miso Ramen with Bone Broth and a Jammy Egg 159
Yam and Ginger Soup with Lentils and Greens 161
Roasted Salmon & Bok Choy with Coconut Lemongrass Broth 163
Root Vegetable Soup with Tomato, Mirin, and Roasted Garlic 165
Venison Meatballs with Ancestral Blend, Garlic, and Parsley 167
Ginger Turmeric Chicken Soup with Apricots and Chickpeas 169
Elk Larb Gai with Mango Avocado Salad 171

SNACKS AND SWEETS
Peanut Butter Cookies with Chocolate, Oats, and Fenugreek 173
Vanilla Coconut Custard with Honey-Stewed Rhubarb and Pistachios 175
No-Bake Granola Bars with Goji Berries, Dates, and Cranberries 177
Lactation & Immunity Smoothie with Berries, Moringa, and Camu-Camu 179
Beet & Apple Bundt Cakes with Cinnamon-Sugar Glaze 181
Spiced Muffins with Parsnips and Carrots 183

TEAS & ELIXIRS
Postpartum Healing Tea 185
Relaxing Reishi Rose Elixir 187
Energizing Matcha Latte 189
Grounding Coconut Chai 191

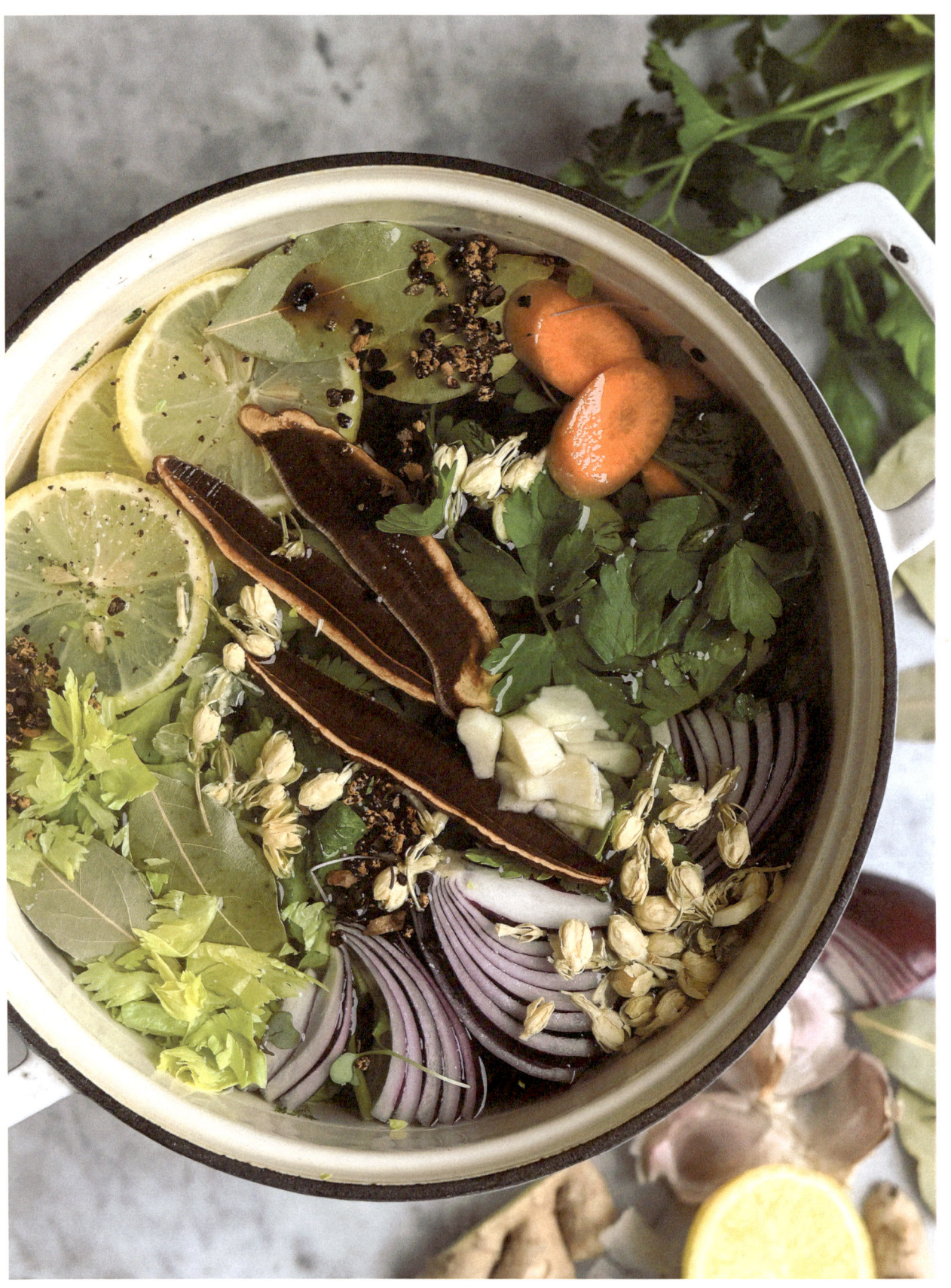

POST-BIRTH HEALING BROTH

After Anise's 3 births, bone broth was the first thing she sipped on, and for good reason! Nutrient needs are higher postpartum than they are during pregnancy, especially for mothers who breastfeed. Bone broth replenishes nutrients passed to baby during pregnancy, supports maternal bone density, and is full of electrolytes for ample hydration during recovery and breastfeeding. Properly made bone broth also contains the necessary glycine to support tissue growth and recovery after giving birth. This broth isn't made to be robust in flavour but to be a gentle, nourishing, and grounding mix of broth and spices to warm the body and soul after birth.

Give this transition—from pregnancy to delivery to early nurturing—the honour and respect it deserves by allowing yourself the time and space to heal fully. We invite you to welcome this warming broth as an essential staple of your post-birth healing plan.

INGREDIENTS | YIELDS 3 CUPS

4 dried allspice berries
1 teaspoon thinly sliced ginger
1 cinnamon stick
Mesh spice bag or cheesecloth
675 ml / 24 oz bone broth (beef or chicken)
¼ teaspoon sea salt
2 dried reishi mushroom slices

DIRECTIONS

1. Place the allspice, ginger, and cinnamon in the mesh bag or cheesecloth. If using cheesecloth, tie it into a bag with a piece of twine.
2. Place the bone broth and the spice pouch in a medium saucepan. Add the salt. Bring to a gentle simmer, cover, reduce the heat to very low, and cook for 10 minutes.
3. Remove the broth from the heat, add the reishi slices if using and let it sit, covered, for 20 minutes.
4. Remove the spice pouch and reishi slices and pour the broth into a large mason jar. Allow it to cool completely on the counter before putting the lid on and moving it to the freezer or fridge.
5. Make and freeze it a few weeks before your due date so it's ready to go when you begin labour. You can take it to the hospital in a thermos or warm it on your stovetop during a home birth.

Try to find a bone broth made with organic, free range bones. Typically ones in the freezer section in grocery stores are better quality than ones in the aisle. You can also make your own with leftover bones, apple cider vinegar, an array of aromatics, and patience!

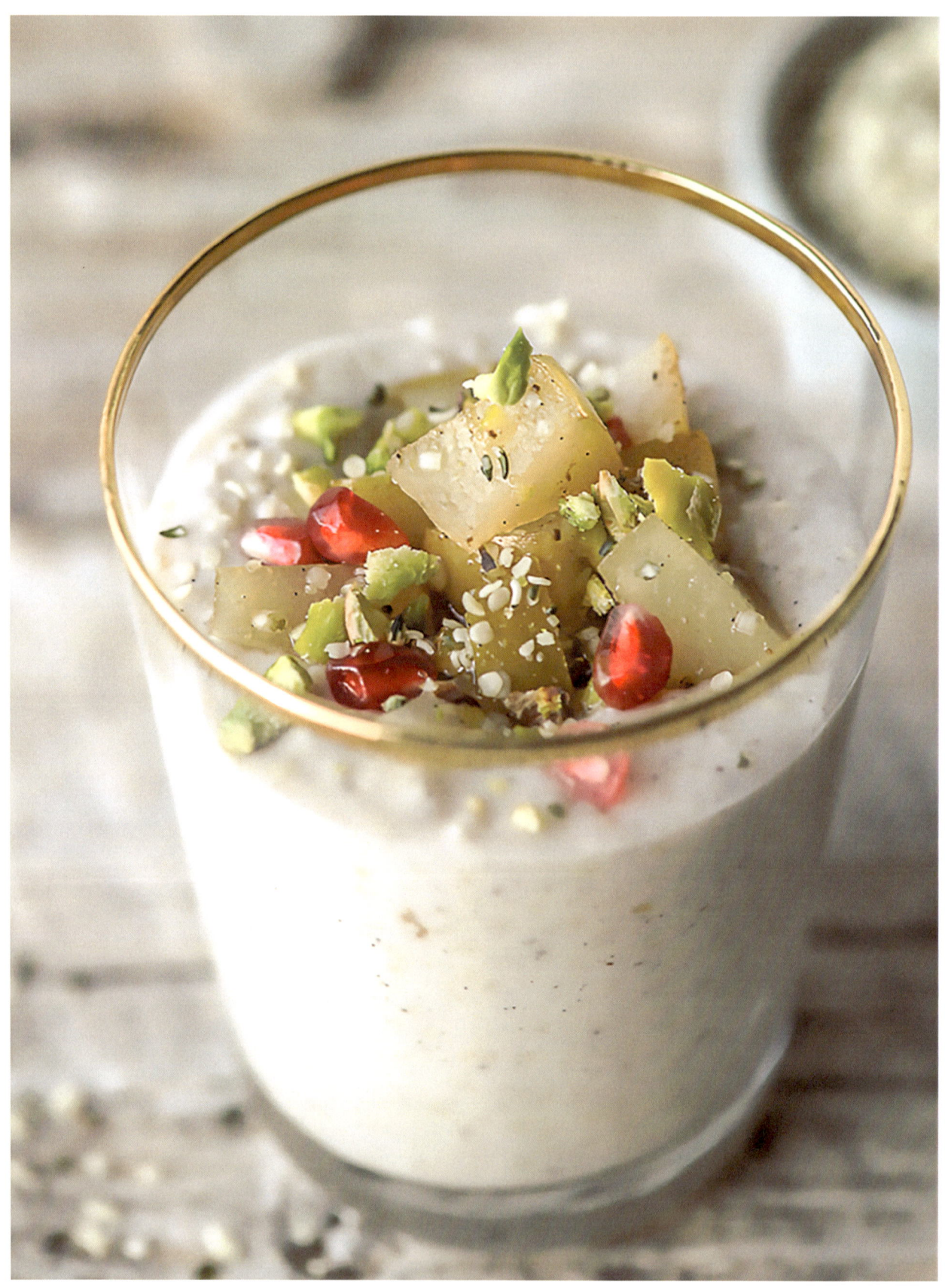

COCONUT CARDAMON MILLET PUDDING

WITH SPICED PEARS AND POMEGRANATE MOLASSES

The fourth trimester is a time to rest, snuggle, and bond with your sweet baby. After babe arrives, we crave warm, nutrient-dense, and easily digestible foods like this millet pudding. This nourishing breakfast is inspired by Anise's travels through Bali. "Bubur Injin" is traditionally made with black rice, but here she switches it up with millet. An Instant Pot will yield perfectly creamy pudding without much effort, while the stovetop variation requires a bit more care. Curl up on the couch with your newborn and a warm bowl of this millet pudding—preferably made by someone else!

INGREDIENTS | SERVES 2

Millet pudding:
½ cup millet
2 ¾ cups light coconut milk
½ cup full-fat coconut milk (if using an Instant Pot) or 4 cups full-fat coconut milk (if using a stovetop)
3 tablespoons maple syrup
1 teaspoon ground cardamom
1 teaspoon vanilla extract or paste

Pears:
1 pear, diced or sliced
1 (½ inch) piece ginger, sliced
3 ½ tablespoons honey or maple syrup
1 (2 inch) piece orange peel
Juice from ½ an orange
1 star anise

Pomegranate molasses:
½ cup pomegranate juice
2 tablespoons pasteurized honey or maple syrup

Optional:
Hemp hearts to garnish
Pomegranate seeds to garnish
Pistachios or walnuts to garnish

DIRECTIONS

1. Thoroughly wash and rinse the millet in a sieve under running water.

2. Stovetop variation: In a medium saucepan, bring the millet, 4 cups full-fat coconut milk, maple syrup, cardamom, and vanilla to a simmer. Cover the saucepan and simmer on low for 30 minutes, stirring frequently towards the end so it doesn't stick. If necessary, add additional coconut milk a little at a time to avoid burning. It should have a consistency similar to porridge when it's finished.

3. Instant Pot variation: combine 2 ¾ cups light coconut milk, ½ cup full-fat coconut milk, millet, maple syrup, cardamom, and vanilla in the Instant Pot. Seal the pot, and set it for 13 mins on manual then natural release for 8 minutes. Carefully open the lid.

4. While the millet is cooking, prepare the pears. In a medium saucepan, combine 2 cups of water with the pears, ginger, honey or maple syrup, orange peel, orange juice, and star anise. Bring to a simmer and poach the pears for 15 minutes or until they are fork-tender. Remove the pears from the saucepan and set aside.

5. To make the pomegranate molasses, add the pomegranate juice and additional 2 tablespoons of maple syrup to the pear-poaching liquid. Simmer, uncovered, for about 15 minutes until the liquid reduces to a syrup. Remove the aromatics and set aside the pomegranate molasses.

6. Divide the millet between 2 bowls and top with the pears, hemp hearts, pomegranate seeds, and pistachios or walnuts. Drizzle with the spiced pomegranate molasses.

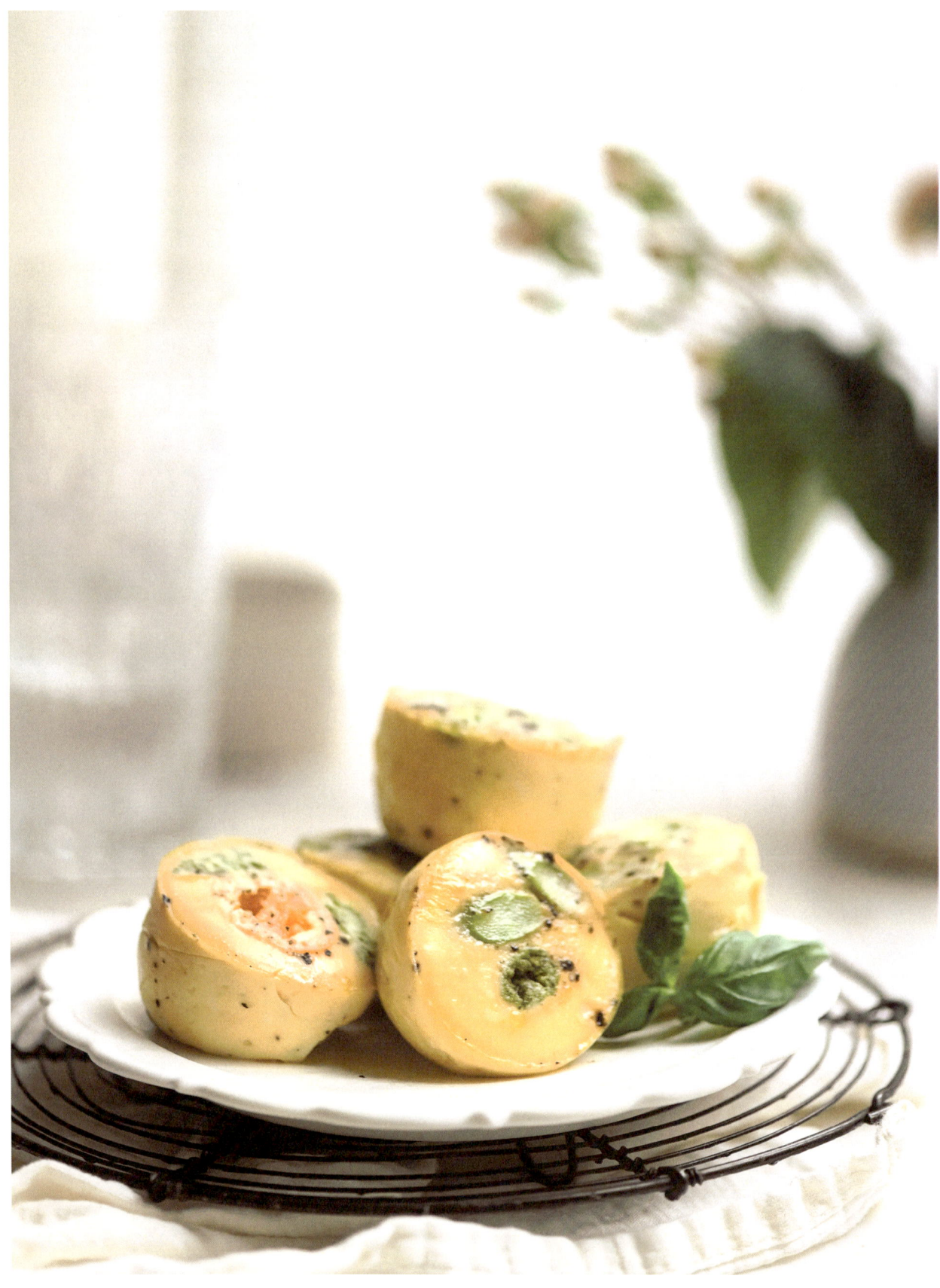

MINI FRITTATAS

WITH ASPARAGUS AND ROASTED TOMATOES

Frittatas are known as the leftover king: they bring new life to whatever is in the fridge at the end of the week. Eggs are an ideal fourth-trimester food. Choline, present in the egg yolk, is an essential nutrient during the postpartum period—our need for it actually increases during lactation. It is essential for Mama's mental health and baby's brain and memory development. These choline-packed mini frittatas are a great make-ahead breakfast or snack for the whole family. They can also be made in an instant pot for a quick and easy sous-vide version.

INGREDIENTS | YIELDS 24

1 cup cashew cream (*directions to the right*), organic cream, or full-fat organic goat milk

16 cherry tomatoes, quartered

20 small asparagus spears, ends trimmed, cut on the bias into 1-inch pieces

1 ½ teaspoons sea salt, divided

¾ teaspoon freshly cracked pepper, divided

1 tablespoon extra-virgin olive oil

16 free range, organic eggs

3 tablespoons finely chopped fresh basil

½ cup pesto (optional)

This is just one of many combinations you can try. We also like:

- *Leftover roasted sweet potatoes, roasted fennel, and bison sausage*
- *Caramelized mushrooms, greens, and goat cheese*
- *Parma ham, Parmesan, and peas*
- *Leftover roasted broccoli and cheese*

DIRECTIONS | PREHEAT OVEN TO 400° F

1. If you are making the cashew cream: Place 1 cup raw cashews in a medium bowl and cover with boiling water. Chill in the refrigerator for 6–8 hours or overnight. Drain the cashews and add to a high-speed blender. Add ½ cup plus 2 tablespoons filtered water and purée until smooth. Set aside. (You will need only 1 cup of cashew cream for this recipe.)

2. Lay the cherry tomatoes and asparagus onto a parchment paper–lined baking sheet, and toss with ½ teaspoon salt, ¼ teaspoon pepper, and 1 tablespoon of extra-virgin olive oil. Roast at 400°F for 10 minutes while you prepare the eggs.

3. In a bowl, beat the eggs with with 1 cup of cashew cream, milk or cream, 1 teaspoon salt, and ½ teaspoon pepper until light and fluffy. Set aside.

4. Remove the asparagus and tomatoes from the oven. Toss them with the basil and set aside.

5. Turn the oven down to 375°.

6. Pour the egg mixture into a silicone muffin mould, filling each mould halfway. Add a few pieces of asparagus, basil, and a couple tomatoes to each mini frittata. Swirl about a ¼ teaspoon of pesto, if using, into each frittata. Cover the mould tightly with parchment paper (preferred) or aluminum foil.

7. Bake the mini frittatas at 375° for 10–12 minutes until all the eggs have set and the centres barely jiggle.

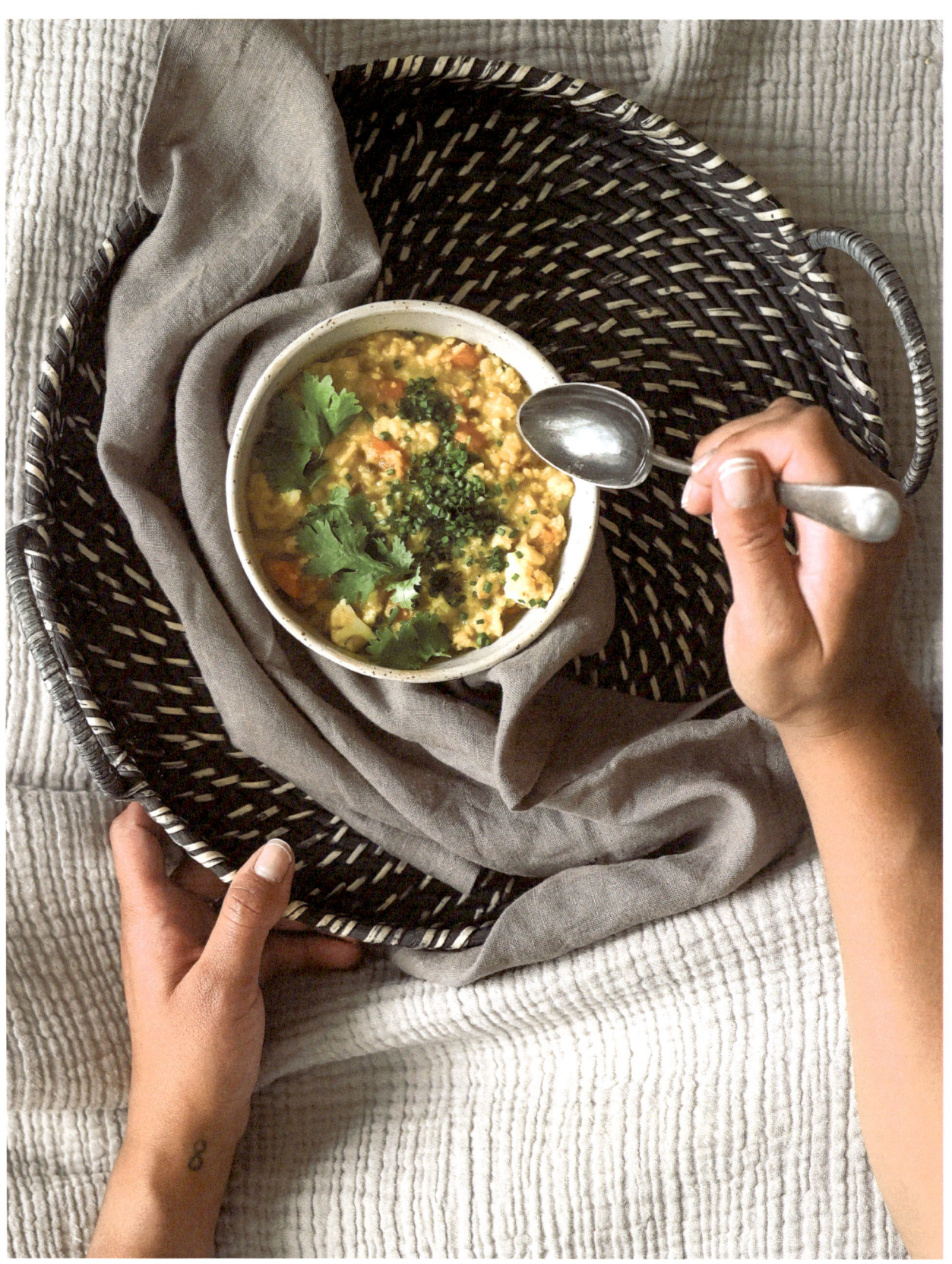

AYURVEDIC KITCHARI STEW

WITH MUNG BEANS, CAULIFLOWER, AND SPICES

You were up throughout the night and then again at 4 a.m. A cold smoothie won't cut it for breakfast. During those postpartum days, you need hearty, warm, pre-made, calorie-rich goodness to start the day. Kitchari is a healing, Ayurvedic, porridge-like dish that is particularly nourishing and easy to digest. Turmeric and ginger are anti-inflammatory with robust antioxidants: perfect as the postpartum body resets after birth. Have someone make this the night before and you're set for breakfast, or a midnight snack, throughout the week.

INGREDIENTS | SERVES 4

1 cup brown basmati rice
1 teaspoon sea salt, divided
2 tablespoons ghee
1 teaspoon cumin seeds
1 teaspoon fenugreek seeds
½ cup minced shallots
1 cup finely diced carrots
1 bay leaf
½ teaspoon ground ginger
¼ teaspoon ground turmeric
1 cup finely chopped cauliflower
1 ½ cups split mung beans
4 ½ cups bone broth or vegetable stock
Freshly cracked pepper
Fresh cilantro and/or chives to garnish

DIRECTIONS

1. Soak the rice in pure, filtered water overnight if possible. If you forget, rinse the rice thoroughly for 3–4 minutes in a fine mesh sieve as you rub it between your hands. In a medium saucepan, add 2 cups filtered water, ½ teaspoon salt, and rice and bring to a boil. Cover, reduce heat to low, and simmer for 22–25 minutes. Towards the end, check that it doesn't need more water; if it does, add the water quickly so as not to release too much steam. Remove the rice from the heat and let it sit, covered, for 10 minutes. (This can also be done in an Instant Pot.)

2. Prepare the kitchari: In a large Dutch oven or saucepan, melt the ghee over low heat. Add the cumin seeds and fenugreek seeds and cook for 1–2 minutes. They should sizzle and become fragrant but not burn.

3. Add the shallots and carrots and cook for 3–4 minutes until vegetables are softened.

4. Add the bay leaf, ginger, turmeric, ¼ teaspoon salt, cauliflower, and mung beans and stir to coat. Toast for about 1 minute until fragrant.

5. Add the broth or stock, another ¼ teaspoon of salt, and a few cracks of pepper, and bring everything to a low simmer. Turn the heat down to medium-low, cover, and let the kitchari simmer for 35–40 mins until the mung beans are cooked through and soft.

6. Serve with the basmati rice and fresh cilantro and chives. Store in the fridge up to 5 days.

Soaking grains, beans, and legumes overnight makes them easier to digest and removes phytic acid, a compound that hinders nutrient absorption.

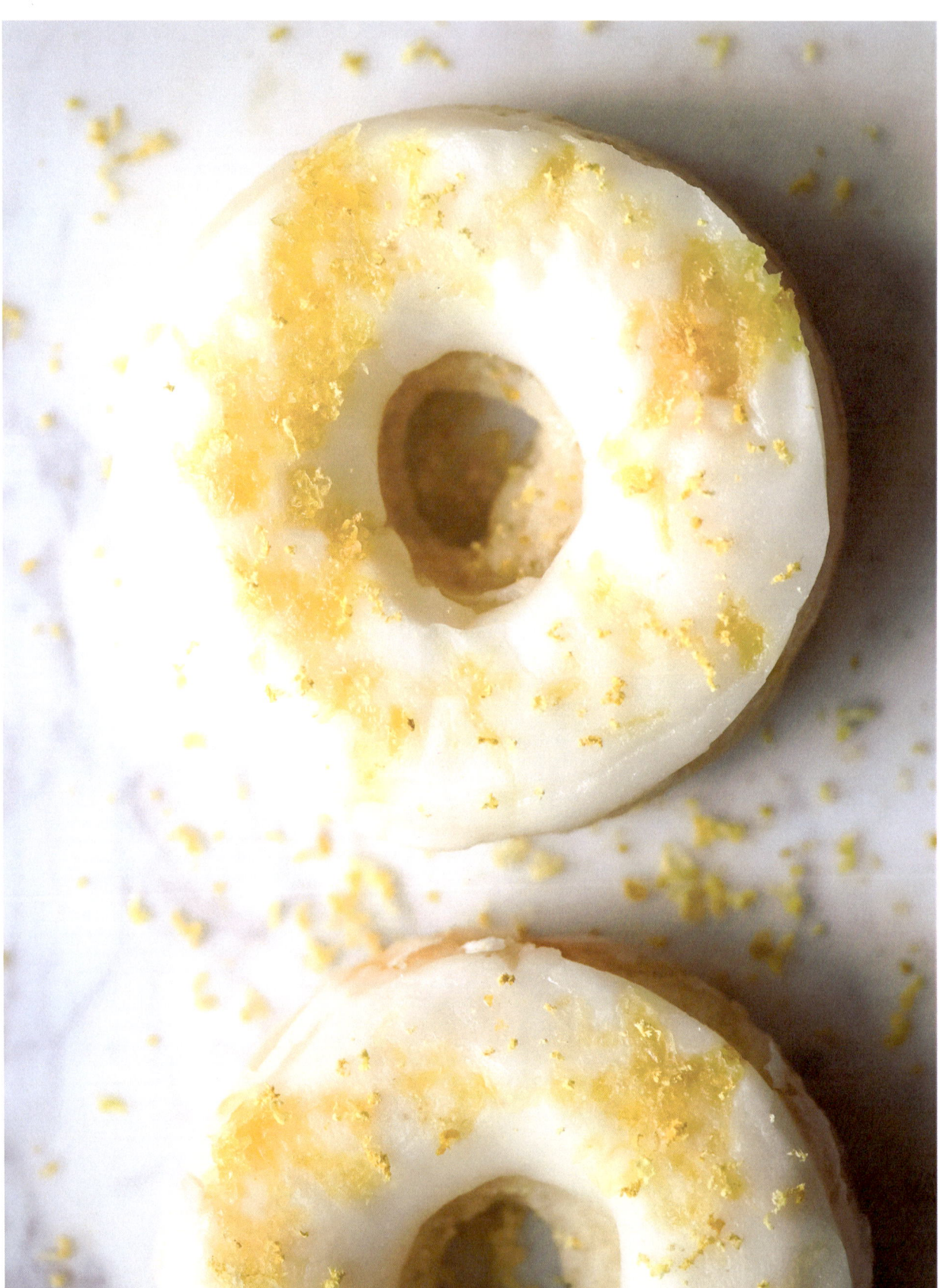

BLUEBERRY LEMON DOUGHNUTS

WITH CITRUS GLAZE

Meet your new favourite make-ahead breakfast! Almond flour and coconut flour are two of Anise's favourite flours to work with: nutrient dense, grain free, and high in healthy fats, they are a staple in her pantry. Combined with natural sugars, eggs, and antioxidant-rich blueberries, this is a breakfast or snack you will come back to again and again!

INGREDIENTS | YIELDS 12

Doughnuts:

1 ½ cups almond flour, spooned and levelled

½ cup coconut flour, spooned and levelled

2 tablespoons arrowroot starch or additional almond flour

1 teaspoon baking soda

¼ teaspoon sea salt

4 free range, organic eggs

½ cup maple syrup

Zest of 2 lemons

3 tablespoons freshly squeezed lemon juice

1 teaspoon vanilla extract

¼ cup coconut oil, melted and cooled

Avocado oil to grease the pans

½ cup fresh blueberries

Citrus Glaze (optional):

1 cup organic powdered sugar

2 tablespoons fresh lemon, grapefruit or orange juice

DIRECTIONS | PREHEAT OVEN TO 350° F

1. In a medium bowl, combine the almond flour, coconut flour, arrowroot starch, baking soda, and salt and mix thoroughly, breaking up any clumps.

2. In a large bowl, combine the eggs, maple syrup, lemon juice, lemon zest, and vanilla. Whisk to combine. Add the cooled coconut oil, very slowly if it is still a bit warm. Stir or whisk as you are pouring in the coconut oil.

3. Pour the dry ingredients into the wet ingredients and stir gently to combine. Set aside for at least 5 minutes so the coconut flour can fully absorb the liquid.

4. Prepare a silicone doughnut mold: place a few drops of avocado oil into each doughnut mould and rub it around the sides of the mould with a pastry brush or your fingers.

5. Pour in the mixture until each doughnut mould is about ¾ full.

6. Place 4–5 blueberries into each mould and press them down into the batter. (I like to separate them this way instead of pouring them into the batter so you don't get clumps of berries which make the doughnuts mushy and hard to remove from the moulds.)

7. Bake at 350° for 20–22 mins or until a toothpick inserted in a doughnut comes out clean.

8. While the doughnuts bake, prepare the glaze: in a small bowl, combine the powdered sugar and fruit juice. Stir to combine. Set aside.

9. Remove the doughnuts from the oven and let them cool completely before removing them from the moulds.

10. Drizzle with the citrus glaze if desired.

11. Place in an airtight container for 5–7 days

You can use this recipe in any silicone mould, such as a muffin tray, mini-muffin tray, or mini Bundt pan.

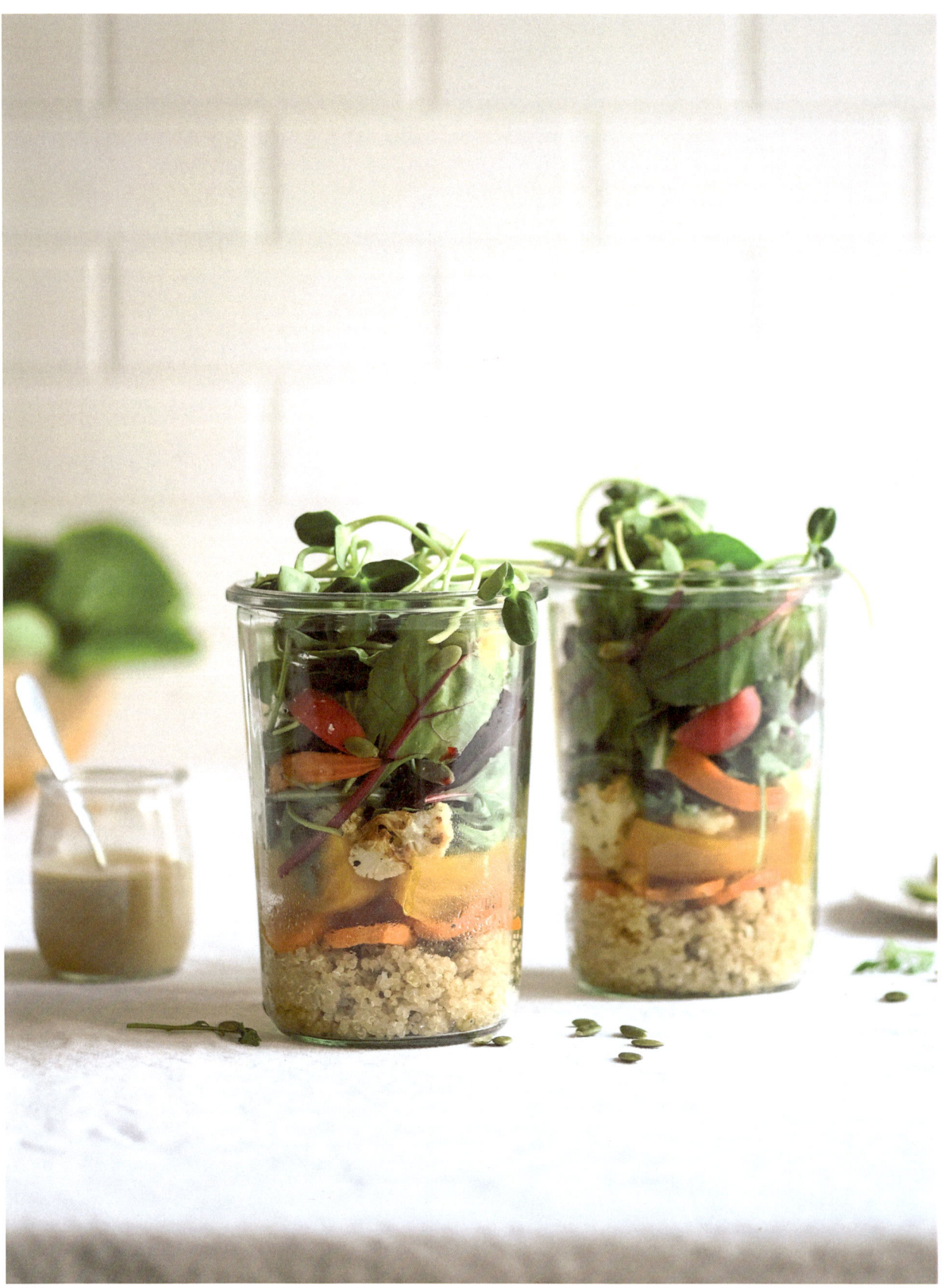

POSTPARTUM NOURISH BOWL

WITH ROOT VEGETABLES AND TAHINI DRESSING

Grain bowls, Buddha bowls, yoga bowls … Whatever you want to call them, they are nourishing, all-in-one, whole-food bowls that can be a saviour on busy postpartum days. Fenugreek is a botanical galactogogue, or milk-boosting ingredient, that has been used therapeutically for thousands of years. It is a hearty seed full of protein and vitamin C, and it boasts anti-inflammatory properties as well. Have someone roast the vegetables and make the dressing for you, and precook your grains and/or protein ahead of time. Store servings in individual glass containers to eat throughout the week. Meals between breastfeeding and napping just got a whole lot easier!

INGREDIENTS | SERVES 4

1 ½ cups quinoa
1 ⅛ teaspoons sea salt, divided
1 cup peeled and chopped beets (1 inch chunks)
1 cup chopped carrots
1 cup chopped sweet potatoes
1 cup chopped cauliflower
2 ½ tablespoons coconut oil, divided
Freshly cracked pepper
½ teaspoon ground cumin
4 tablespoons pumpkin seeds
2 avocados
2 cups mixed greens
Fresh parsley, cilantro, or mint to garnish

Tahini fenugreek dressing:
½ cup tahini
¼ cup plus 1 tablespoon lemon juice
2 teaspoons Dijon mustard
4 teaspoons maple syrup
¼ teaspoon sea salt
6 tablespoons water
¼ teaspoon red pepper flakes
¼ teaspoon fenugreek powder or 1 fenugreek capsule (optional, to support milk production)

DIRECTIONS | PREHEAT OVEN TO 425° F

1. Thoroughly rinse quinoa in a fine mesh sieve under running water for 2–3 minutes. In a medium saucepan, bring 3 cups water and ½ teaspoon sea salt to a boil. Add the quinoa. Cover, reduce heat to low, and simmer for 15 minutes. Remove from the heat and let the quinoa stand for 5 minutes, covered. Fluff with a fork and set aside. (This can also be done in an Instant Pot.)

2. Line a rimmed baking sheet with parchment paper and set aside.

3. In a medium bowl, toss the beets, carrots, and sweet potatoes with 2 tablespoons oil, ½ teaspoon salt, and a few cracks of pepper. Place on the baking sheet in a single layer.

4. In the same bowl, add the cauliflower, ½ tablespoon oil, ⅛ teaspoon salt, and cumin, and toss to coat. Set aside.

5. Transfer the tray to the oven and roast the beets, carrots, and sweet potatoes at 425° for 20 minutes.

6. Add the cauliflower to the baking sheet and continue roasting for another 20 minutes or until all vegetables are fork-tender. Remove the vegetables from the oven and set aside.

7. While the vegetables roast, prepare the dressing: In a medium metal bowl, vigorously whisk together all the dressing ingredients. (Add more water if you want it a bit thinner.) Pour the dressing into a glass jar with a tight-fitting lid; can be stored in the fridge up to 10 days.

8. If you are pre-portioning meals, place ½ cup cooked quinoa into each of four glass containers, and top each with ¼ of the root vegetables, 1 tablespoon of pumpkin seeds, and ½ cup fresh greens. When you are ready to serve, top each serving with ½ an avocado, sliced and sprinkled with salt, fresh herbs, and ¼ of the dressing.

If your vegetables are organic, save time and leave the peel on for added nutrition!

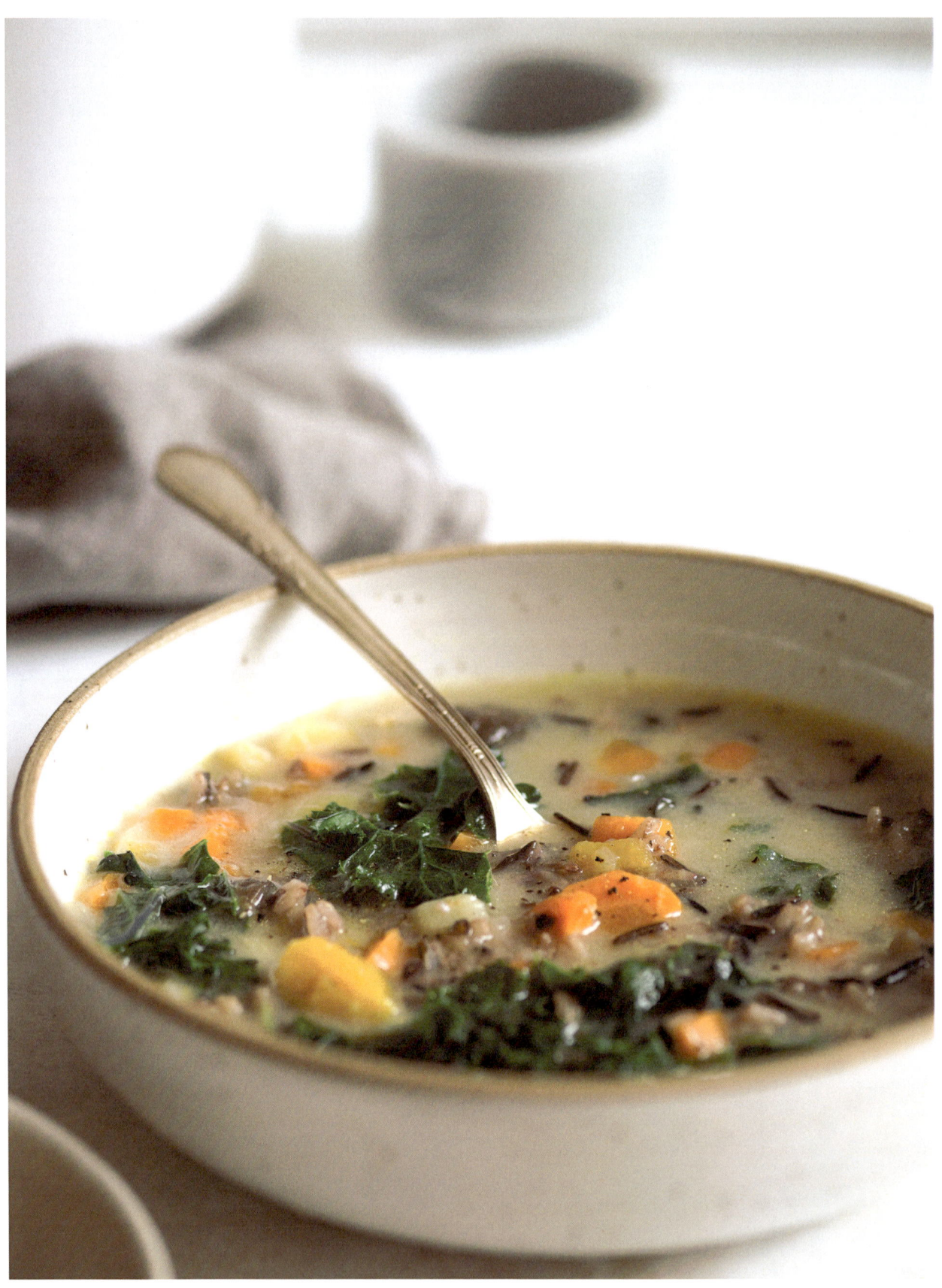

CREAMY WILD RICE SOUP

WITH CREMINI MUSHROOMS AND KALE

The third day postpartum is infamous for being emotionally, mentally, and physically challenging. Your milk supply is ramping up, birth adrenaline is wearing off, and there is massive shift in hormones. Mamas can often feel overwhelmed, weepy, and nervous. It's a perfect time to accept help from the community. Ask an auntie, grandma, or best friend to drop a warm pot of this creamy soup at the front door, and take the extra time to sit in the sunshine with a good book.

You got this, Mama.

INGREDIENTS | SERVES 4-6

Cashew Cream:
1 cup cashews
¼ teaspoon sea salt

Soup:
4 tablespoons ghee, butter, or coconut oil, divided
1 large onion, diced
3 large carrots, diced
3 large celery stalks, diced
½ plus ⅛ teaspoon sea salt
Freshly cracked pepper
450 grams cremini mushrooms, wiped clean, quartered (16 ounces)
¼ cup white wine
5 cups chicken bone broth
½ cup wild rice
2 teaspoons poultry seasoning
4 thyme sprigs
1 rosemary sprig
2 bay leaves
1 bunch kale or any greens, chopped

DIRECTIONS

1. Place the cashews in a medium bowl and add boiling water to cover. Chill in the fridge for 6–8 hours or overnight.

2. In a large Dutch oven or stockpot, melt 2 tablespoons of ghee over medium heat. Add the onions, carrots, and celery, sprinkle with ¼ teaspoon of salt, and sauté until the onions are soft, about 5 minutes.

3. Add the mushrooms and the remaining 2 tablespoons of ghee or oil. Sprinkle with ¼ teaspoon of salt and freshly cracked pepper. Continue to sauté over medium heat until the mushrooms are soft, about 5 minutes, stirring occasionally.

4. Add the white wine, stir, and deglaze the pan for about 2 minutes. Add the bone broth, rice, poultry seasoning, thyme, rosemary, and bay leaves. Turn the heat to medium-low, cover, and simmer until the rice is tender, about 40 minutes.

5. While the soup cooks, make the cashew cream: drain and rinse the soaked cashews. Add cashews to a high-speed blender. Add ½ cup plus 2 tablespoons of filtered water and ¼ teaspoon salt. Purée until smooth. Set aside.

6. Remove the thyme sprigs, rosemary stalk, and bay leaves from the broth.

7. Add in the chopped greens, ⅛ teaspoon salt and simmer for 2–3 minutes until soft. Stir in the cashew cream to thicken. Taste and season with more salt and pepper if necessary.

You can also cook this in an Instant Pot: Add everything except the cashews and greens to the inner pot. Set your Instant Pot to manual: high for 25 minutes and let it natural release for 10 minutes. Add the greens after the rice has cooked through, and simmer until the greens are tender. Add the cashew cream and stir to combine.

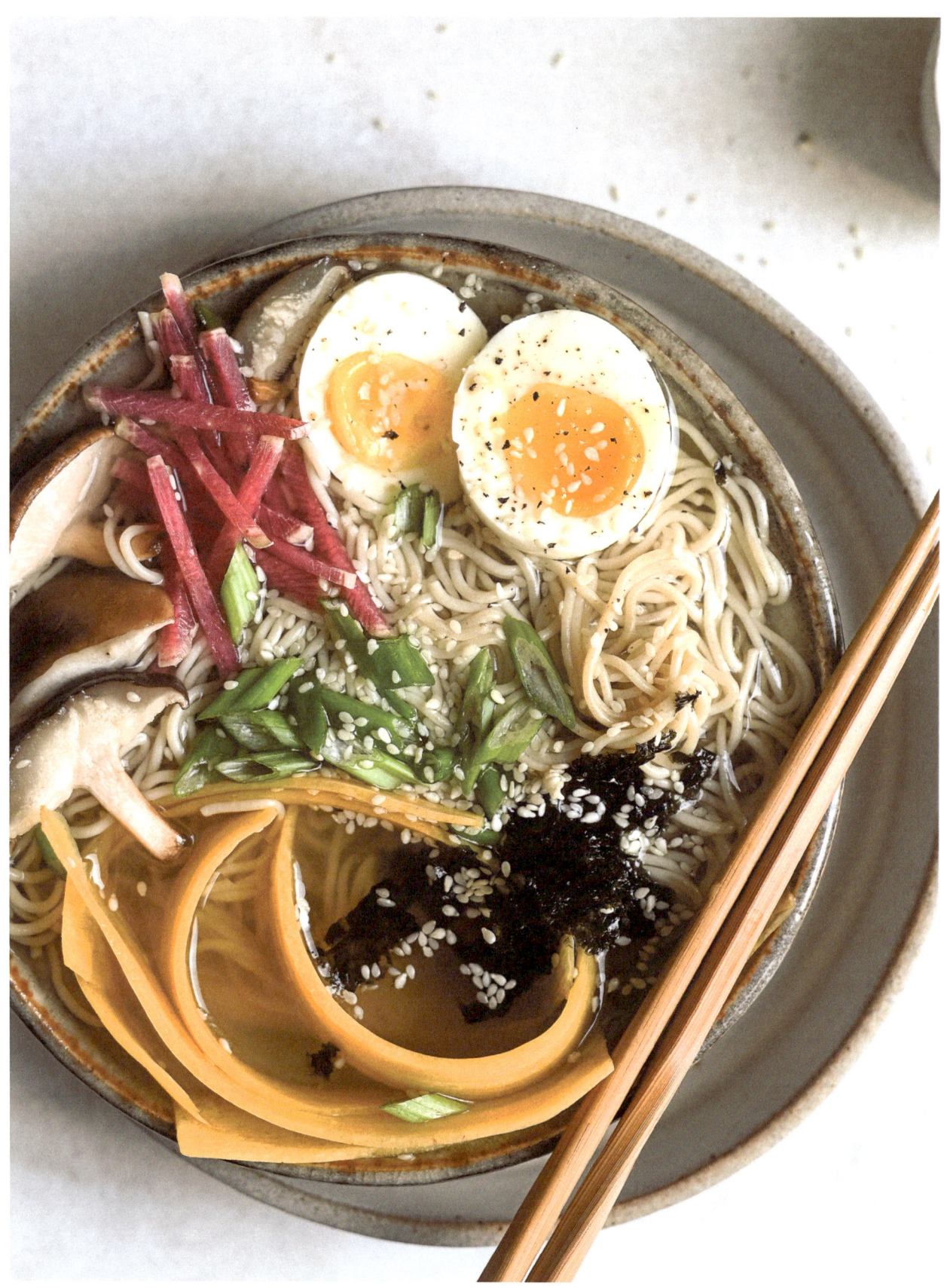

SOOTHING MISO RAMEN

WITH BONE BROTH AND A JAMMY EGG

This soothing bone broth ramen is the perfect support for fourth-trimester healing and recovery. Nutrition needs are even higher postpartum than in the final months of pregnancy, and substituting bone broth for regular stock in your soups will give your meals greater nutrition. Bone broth is full of protein, collagen, and electrolytes (magnesium, phosphorus, potassium, calcium, and sodium): a bonus for mamas who feel like they can never quench their thirst while breastfeeding. Add in an egg, seaweed, and miso, and you have a stellar postpartum lunch.

INGREDIENTS | SERVES 4

- 5 cups bone broth (chicken or bison)
- 2 tablespoons tamari
- 1 cup sliced shiitake mushrooms, wiped clean with a paper towel
- ¾ cup sliced carrots, cut on the bias
- 4 free range, organic eggs
- 2 packets whole-grain ramen noodles
- 3 ½ tablespoons red or genmai miso (but white miso works well too)
- 3 teaspoons sesame oil
- 2 green onions, thinly sliced on the bias
- 2 tablespoons sesame seeds, divided
- 1 seaweed sheet, shredded
- Chili oil or chili paste (optional)
- 2 watermelon radish, cut julienne, to garnish

DIRECTIONS

1. In large saucepan or Dutch oven, combine the bone broth and tamari. Bring to a low simmer and add mushrooms and carrots. Cover and simmer over medium-low heat for 10–12 minutes until carrots are fork-tender.
2. While the broth simmers, make the boiled eggs: Fill a medium saucepan with enough water to cover 4 eggs, and bring to a simmer. Carefully place the eggs in the boiling water with a slotted spoon, cover, turn the heat to low, and simmer for 7 ½ minutes.
3. Prepare a bowl with ice water and set aside.
4. When the eggs are finished cooking, remove them from the boiling water with a slotted spoon and transfer to the ice bath. Set aside.
5. While the broth continues to simmer, bring a medium saucepan of salted water to a boil and cook the noodles per package instructions. Drain and set aside.
6. Remove the broth from the heat and whisk in the miso.
7. Peel the eggs, cut each in half, and set aside.
8. Divide the noodles among 4 bowls and ladle over the broth.
9. Drizzle ¾ teaspoon sesame oil into each bowl. Top with sliced green onions, sesame seeds, seaweed, and 2 halves of a jammy egg. Drizzle over a bit of chili oil or chili paste if you desire!

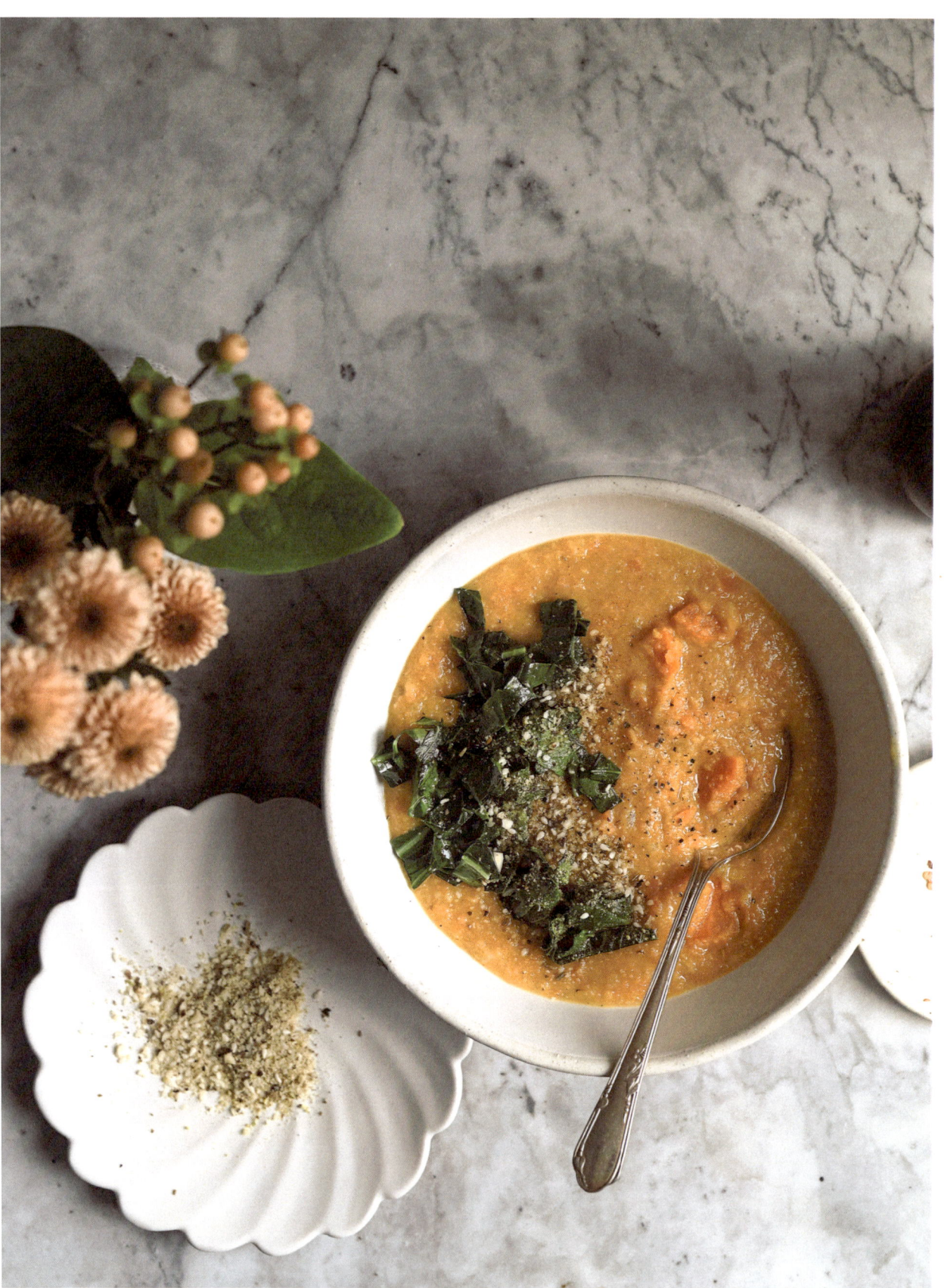

YAM AND GINGER SOUP

WITH LENTILS AND GREENS

Your body will do everything it can to give your baby the best start possible. Breastfeeding increases your nutrient requirements, and if your body can't get enough from your diet, it will take from your maternal stores. This yam and lentil soup is nutrient dense and will increase your stores of thiamine and vitamin A. Let's ensure that while you are giving your baby that liquid gold, you aren't leaving yourself depleted and exhausted.

INGREDIENTS | SERVES 4-6

- 2 tablespoons ghee
- 1 medium onion, diced
- 1 ½ teaspoons sea salt, divided
- 1 tablespoon freshly minced garlic
- 5 teaspoons minced or grated fresh ginger, divided
- ½ teaspoon ground cumin
- 5 cups bone broth
- 1 cube vegetable or chicken bouillon
- 1 cup diced carrots
- 4 cups diced yam (1–1 ½ inch cubes)
- ¾ cup dried red lentils
- ¼ cup almond butter
- ¼ teaspoon red pepper flakes
- 1 bunch collard greens, washed and stems removed

DIRECTIONS

1. In a large Dutch oven or stockpot, melt the ghee over medium-low heat. Add the onions and ¼ teaspoon of salt and sauté for 3–4 minutes, stirring frequently, until the onions soften.

2. Add the garlic, 3 teaspoons of ginger, and cumin, and sauté for another 1–2 minutes until fragrant. Stir frequently to avoid burning.

3. Add the bone broth, bouillon cube, carrots, yams, lentils, and ½ teaspoon of salt. Mix well to break down and incorporate the bouillon cube. Bring to a simmer, cover, and continue to simmer on low for 12 minutes, or until the yams are soft.

4. In a small bowl, combine the almond butter and a bit of the hot soup broth. Mix vigorously to thin it out, adding more broth if necessary. Add the almond butter mixture, the last 2 teaspoons of freshly grated ginger, ¾ teaspoon of salt, and the red pepper flakes to the soup, and stir to combine.

5. Using an immersion or high-powered blender, blend about half the soup, leaving behind some chunks to preserve texture.

6. Layer the collard greens in a pile and roll tightly. Cut the roll into strips. Add the collard greens to the soup and gently simmer for 2–3 minutes until the greens have softened.

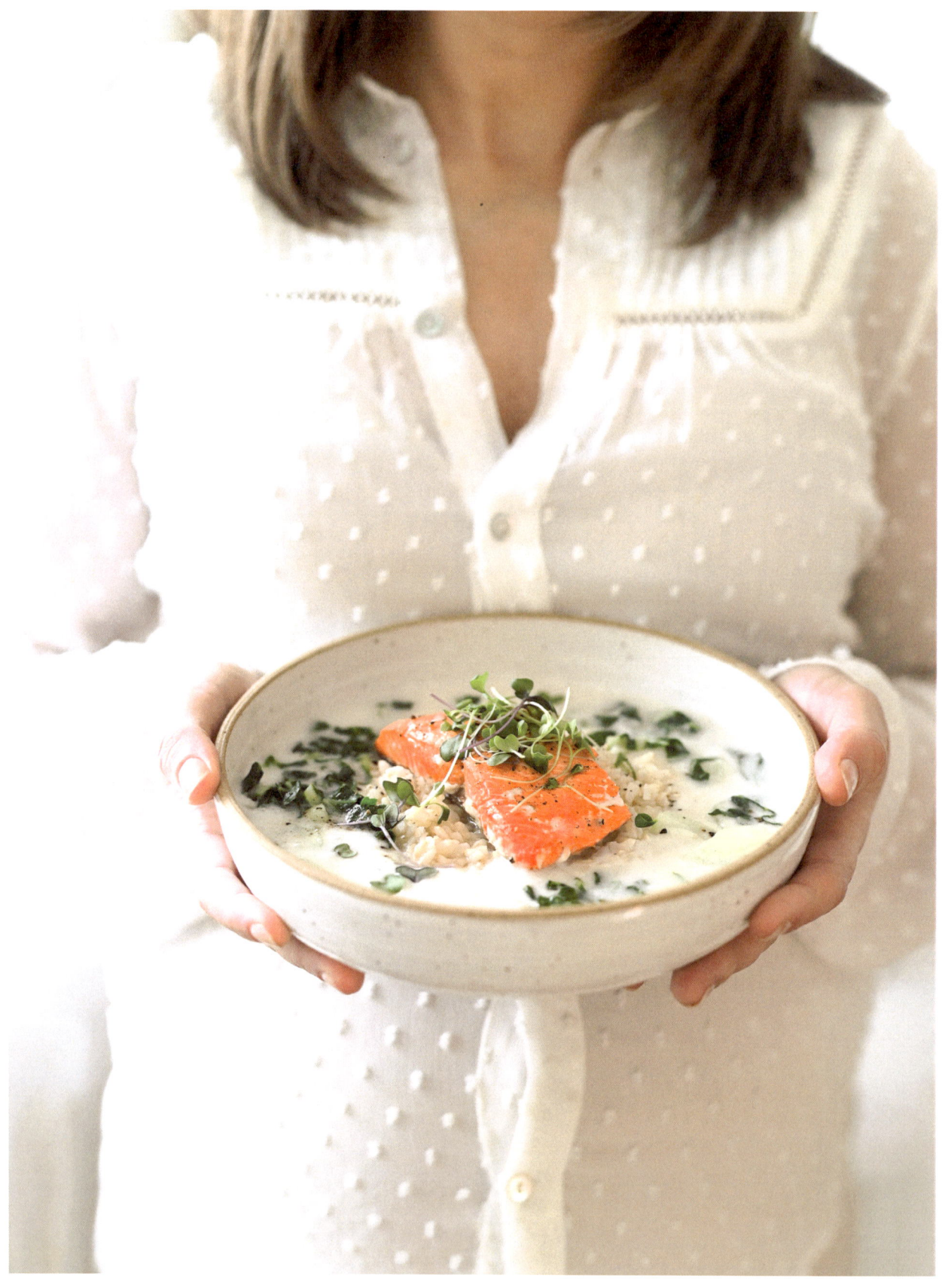

ROASTED SALMON & BOK CHOY

WITH COCONUT LEMONGRASS BROTH

Fish oil is essential for both mom and babe during the postpartum period, and wild salmon is a tasty source of omega-3 DHA. Not only does this essential fatty acid support Mama's mental health, but it also aids the newborn's brain and eye development. When we eat fatty fish or supplement our diet with a high-quality fish oil, we see a dramatic increase in DHA in the breast milk too.

INGREDIENTS | SERVES 2

Coconut lemongrass broth:
1 tablespoon extra-virgin olive oil
1 ½ tablespoons freshly minced garlic
2 tablespoons freshly minced ginger
2 teaspoons lemongrass paste
1 cup chicken bone broth
1 (400-ml) can light coconut milk (14 ounces)
½ teaspoon sea salt
1 (6–7 inch) lemongrass stalk, smashed open
2 tablespoons white or shiro miso
1 tablespoon lemon juice

Salmon and bok choy:
340 grams salmon fillets (12 ounces)
2 tablespoons avocado or coconut oil
½ teaspoon sea salt
Freshly cracked pepper
½ lemon
1 head bok choy

Brown rice or brown-rice pad Thai noodles, to serve

DIRECTIONS

1. In a medium pot, add the olive oil, garlic, ginger, and lemongrass paste. Sauté over low heat for 2 minutes until fragrant, stirring frequently so it doesn't burn.

2. Add the broth, coconut milk, salt, and smashed lemongrass stalk. Bring to a simmer over medium heat, cover, reduce to low heat and simmer for 15 minutes.

3. While the broth cooks, prepare the salmon: In a large frying pan or cast-iron skillet, heat avocado or coconut oil over medium heat. Season the salmon fillets with ½ teaspoon salt, freshly cracked pepper, and a squeeze of the half lemon. Place the fillets skin side down in the hot oil and cover. Cook over medium heat for 6 minutes until the skin is crispy. Flip, cover, and cook for another 4–6 minutes, depending on the thickness of the salmon and your preference.

4. While the salmon cooks, rinse the bok choy and chop into small pieces.

5. When the salmon is done, remove from the pan and set aside.

6. Once the broth is done, add the bok choy; let it simmer for 2–3 minutes until soft.

7. In a separate small dish, whisk the miso into a little of the broth until thoroughly dissolved. Remove the broth from the heat, add the miso mixture and lemon juice, and season with more salt to taste.

8. Place a scoop of brown rice in a bowl, ladle in the broth with the bok choy, and top with a piece of salmon.

This recipe is also great with white fish or shrimp poached right in the broth!

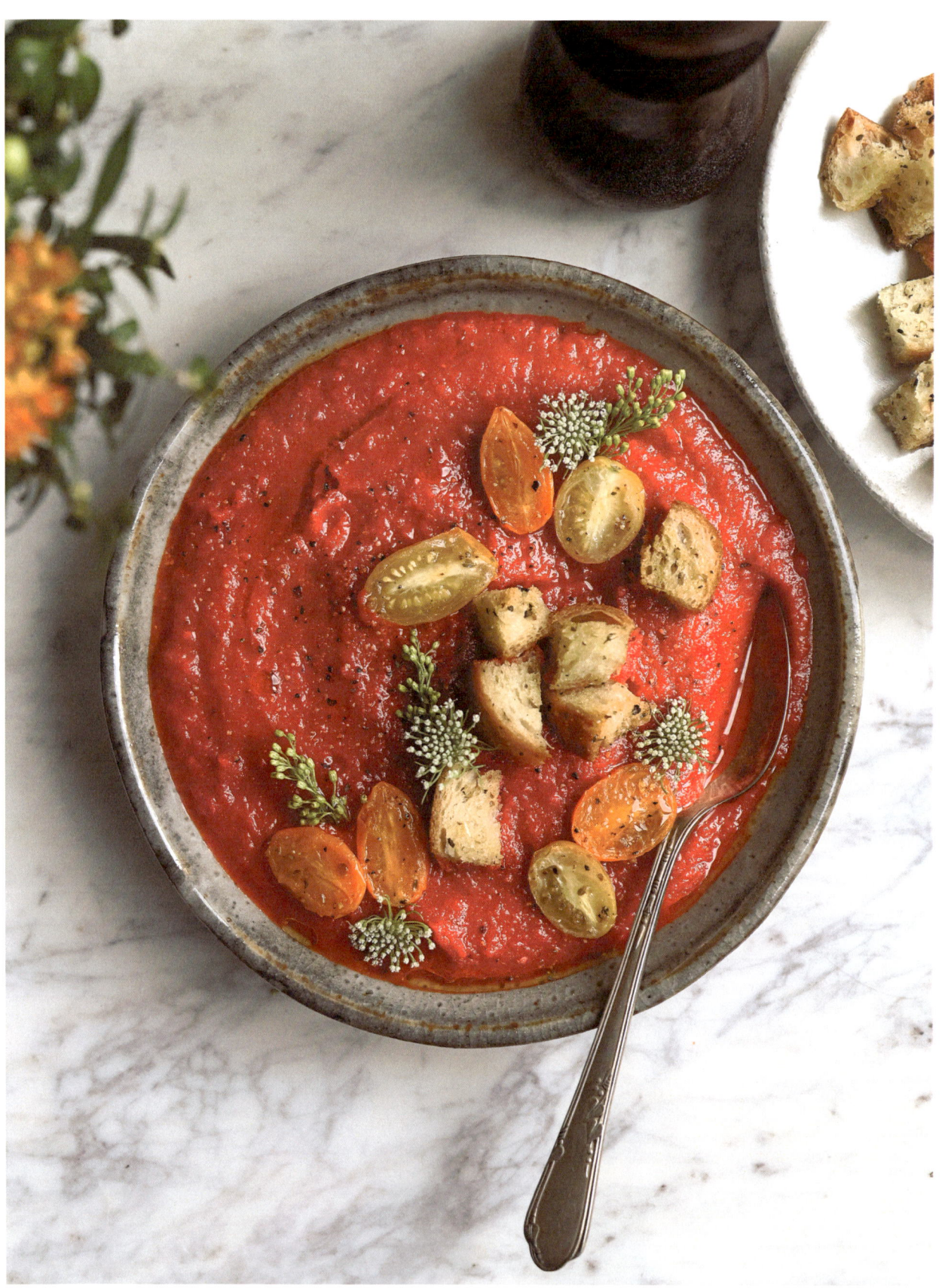

ROOT VEGETABLE SOUP

WITH TOMATO, MIRIN, AND ROASTED GARLIC

Warming, grounding, and therapeutic, root vegetables are a pillar of a healing postpartum diet. This versatile soup can be eaten with warm sourdough and butter, over spaghetti squash or gnocchi, as a dip for fried polenta sticks, or even as a pizza sauce. Blending makes this soup more easily digestible, and it's a fabulously sneaky way to ramp up the vegetable intake of postpartum parents and baby's older siblings.

INGREDIENTS | SERVES 4-6

1 cup peeled, roughly chopped rutabagas (½ inch cubes)

1 cup roughly chopped sweet potatoes

1 cup roughly chopped carrots

¾ cup peeled, roughly chopped beets

¾ cup peeled, roughly chopped turnips

26 cocktail tomatoes (about 680 grams or 1 ½ pounds)

3 tablespoons plus ¼ cup extra-virgin olive oil, divided

¾ teaspoon sea salt, divided

Freshly cracked pepper

1 whole garlic bulb

3 tablespoons mirin

1 ½ cups bone broth or vegetable stock

¼ teaspoon red pepper flakes

2 tablespoons white or shiro miso

1 cup sourdough croutons to garnish (optional)

DIRECTIONS | PREHEAT OVEN TO 425° F

1. This recipe works best with a deep, ovenproof skillet or frying pan that you can move from oven to stove. Place your pan on the counter.
2. Layer your chopped vegetables in the bottom of the pan. Lay the cocktail tomatoes on top.
3. Drizzle 3 tablespoons of extra-virgin olive oil over the vegetables and sprinkle with ½ teaspoon of sea salt and a few cracks of black pepper. Toss the vegetables with your hands, ensuring that the tomatoes end up on top of the pile.
4. Cut off the top the bulb of garlic so the cloves are exposed. Make a little hole in the centre of the vegetables and place the garlic bulb in the hole. Drizzle just enough olive oil over the garlic to wet the top.
5. Place the pan in the oven and roast the vegetables for 1 hour.
6. When the hour is up, carefully transfer the pan to the stove and turn on the burner to medium-low.
7. Remove the garlic bulb and place on a cutting board.
8. Add ¼ cup extra virgin olive oil, mirin, broth or stock, red pepper flakes, and ¼ teaspoon salt to the pan with the vegetables. Stir, and let everything simmer over low heat while you complete the remaining steps.
9. Squeeze the garlic cloves out of the bulb; discard the garlic skin and return the softened cloves to the pan.
10. In a small bowl, stir together 2 tablespoons of miso and 1 tablespoon of warm water until the miso is completely dissolved. Turn off the stove, remove the pan from the heat, and stir the miso into the vegetable and tomato mixture.
11. Using an immersion blender, blend the mixture until smooth. If you don't have an immersion blender, transfer the mixture to a high-speed blender and blend until the soup has reached a consistency you like. Add more stock if you like it thinner.

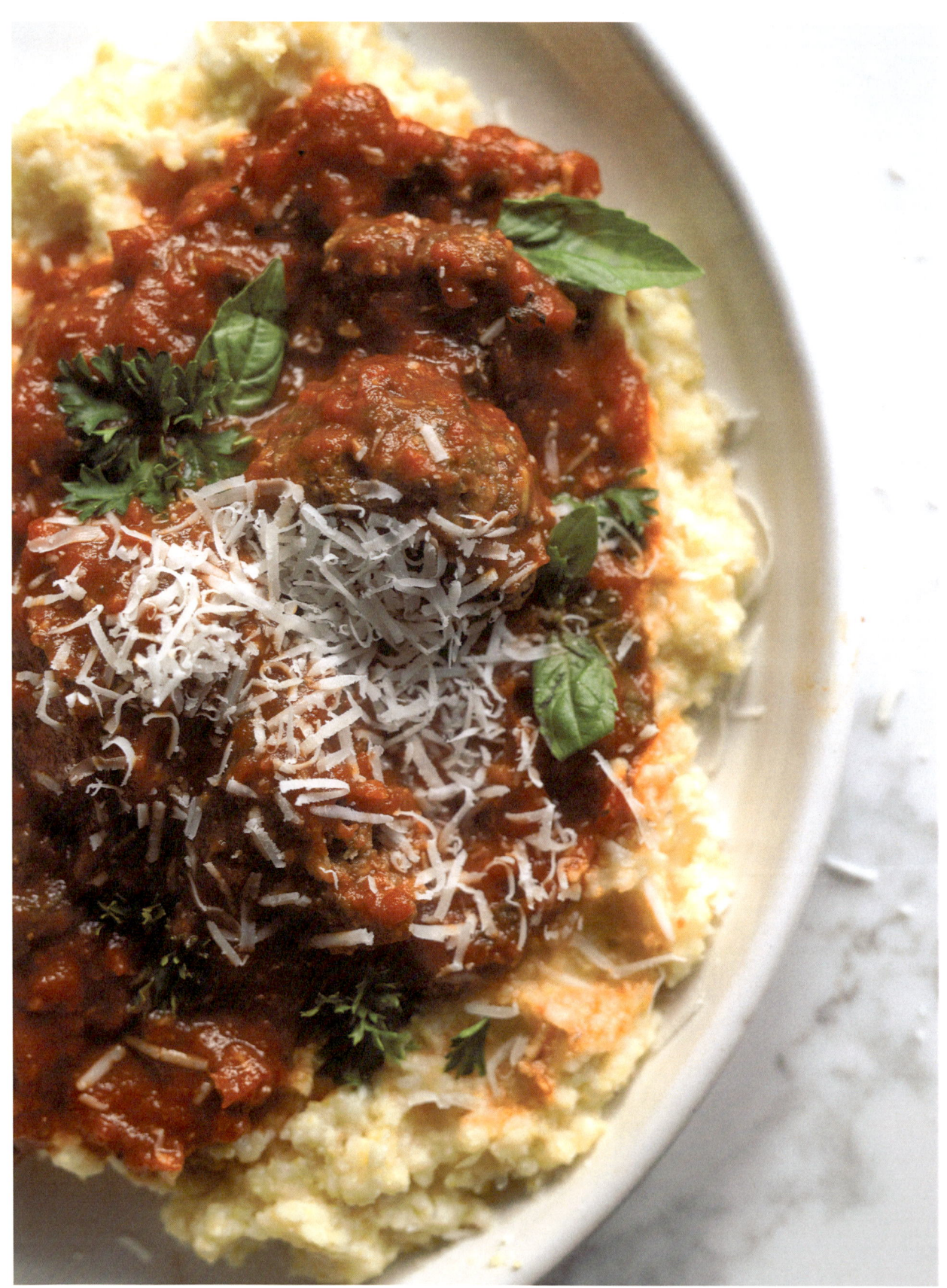

VENISON MEATBALLS

WITH ANCESTRAL BLEND, GARLIC, AND PARSLEY

In the last weeks of pregnancy, iron was transferred to the growing babe in preparation for their life outside the womb. After giving birth our iron levels also go down due to birth and postpartum blood loss. Building blood stores, with healthy iron levels, is important to ward off postpartum anemia and other unwanted symptoms. By choosing game meats that are blended with organ meats, we are providing our bodies with a boost of bioavailable iron, copper, selenium, vitamin A and B vitamins. If you are turned off from the smell and taste of organ meat, an ancestral blend (typically 10% organ meat, 90% ground meat) is a fantastic way to dip your toe in! Using it for a recipe like meatballs is an even further way to disguise the flavour. Look for organic, grass-fed and finished meat.

INGREDIENTS | SERVES 4-6

- 450 grams ground venison or ancestral blend (1 pound)
- 450 grams ground pork (1 pound)
- 2 free range, organic eggs, beaten
- 2 ½ tablespoons freshly minced garlic
- ½ cup chopped fresh parsley
- ½ cup almond flour
- 2 teaspoons salt
- 2 tablespoons avocado oil

DIRECTIONS

1. In a large bowl, use your hands to thoroughly combine all the meatball ingredients except for the avocado oil.
2. Take 2 tablespoons of the meat mixture and roll into a ball. Continue with the remainder of the mixture.
3. In a large skillet, warm 2 tablespoons of avocado oil over medium heat.
4. Add the meatballs and cook until browned on one side. Flip and continue cooking until most of the outside is browned.
5. Add the meatballs to a sauce of your choice (or the root vegetable soup on the previous page), cover, and simmer over medium-low until cooked through, about 10 minutes. Alternatively, you can transfer to the oven and continue cooking in the skillet or in a muffin tin.
6. Enjoy in meatball subs, on cauliflower pizza crusts, or over polenta, gnocchi, or pasta.

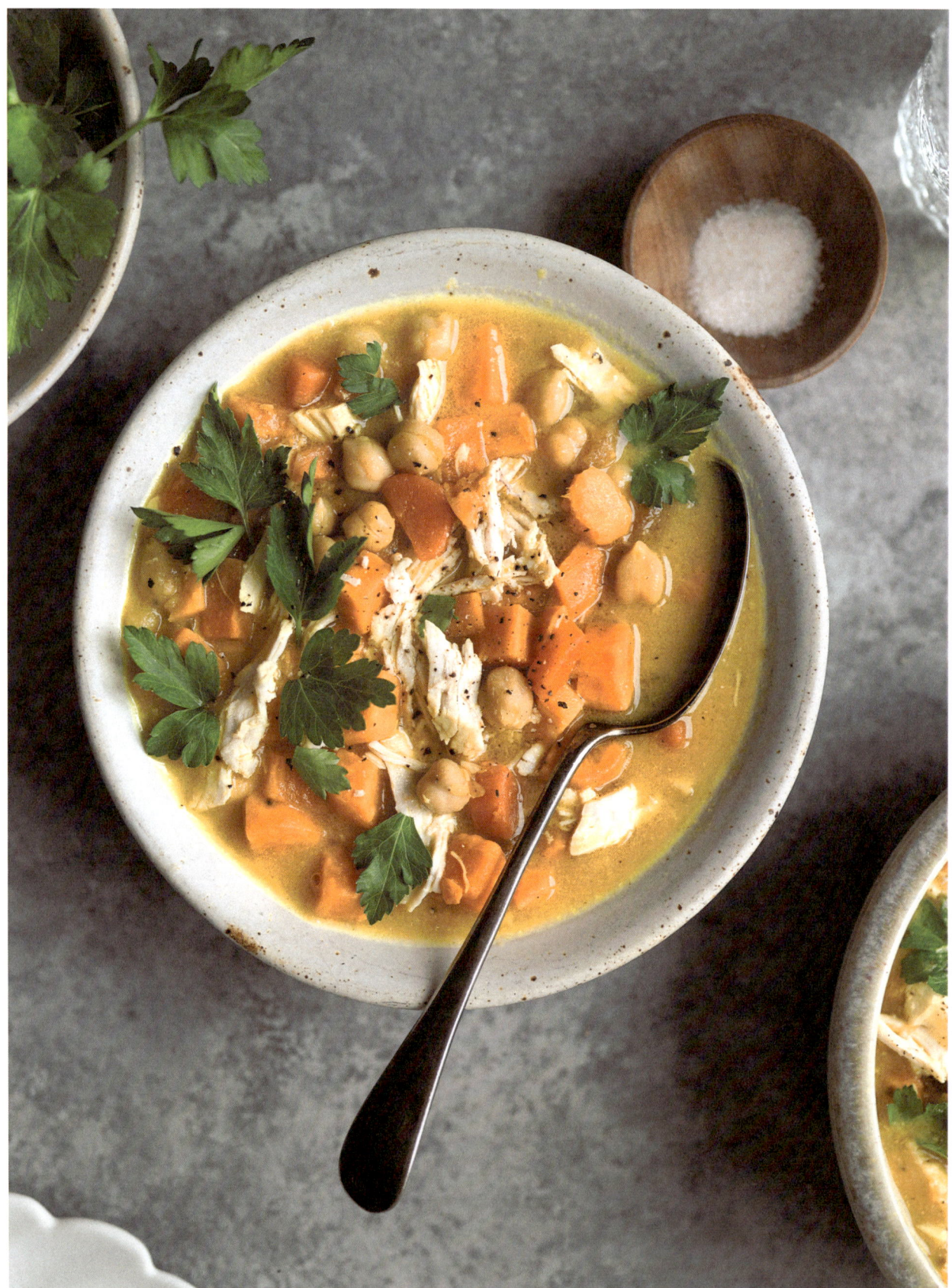

GINGER TURMERIC CHICKEN SOUP

WITH APRICOTS AND CHICKPEAS

Hair loss is a normal—but definitely bothersome—feature of the postpartum period that can begin 3 to 6 months after babe's arrival. Although this is a natural occurrence, nutritional deficiencies of iron, folic acid, zinc, biotin, and protein can all contribute to excessive hair loss. However, this soup is rich in all the above!

Use your meals as your medicine to feel energetic while worrying less about your luscious locks. Scoop up a big bowl of this flavourful soup, and don't forget to give yourself some unconditional self-love and grace as you navigate another postpartum change.

INGREDIENTS | SERVES 4-6

1 ½ tablespoons ghee or avocado oil

450 grams boneless, skinless chicken thighs, excess fat removed, resting at room temperature (1 pound)

1 ½ teaspoons sea salt

¼–½ teaspoon freshly cracked pepper

½ cup sliced yellow onions

1 cup chopped carrots

2 teaspoons ground ginger, divided

1 ½ tablespoons freshly minced garlic

5 cups chicken bone broth

¼ teaspoon turmeric powder

1 cup chopped sweet potatoes (½-inch cubes)

1 (398-ml) can chickpeas, drained and rinsed (14 ounces)

12 dried apricots, thinly sliced

1 can (400-ml) light coconut milk (14 ounces)

1 tablespoon freshly squeezed lemon juice

1 tablespoon freshly grated ginger

¼ cup chopped fresh parsley

DIRECTIONS

1. In a large Dutch oven, melt the ghee and avocado oil over medium-low heat.
2. Season the chicken thighs with ½ teaspoon salt and freshly cracked pepper on both sides.
3. Brown the chicken for 4 minutes, flip, and brown for another 5 minutes.
4. Add the onions, carrots, 1 teaspoon ground ginger, and ½ teaspoon of salt, and sauté for 3–4 minutes until the onions are translucent.
5. Add the garlic, stir, and sauté for 1 minute until fragrant.
6. Add the bone broth, the remaining 1 teaspoon of ground ginger, turmeric, sweet potatoes, chickpeas, and apricots. Simmer for 12–15 minutes until the sweet potatoes are fork-tender.
7. Remove chicken and set aside.
8. Add the coconut milk, lemon juice, fresh ginger, parsley and the last ½ teaspoon salt.
9. Simmer the soup on low heat while you shred the chicken.
10. Return the shredded chicken to the soup and stir to combine.

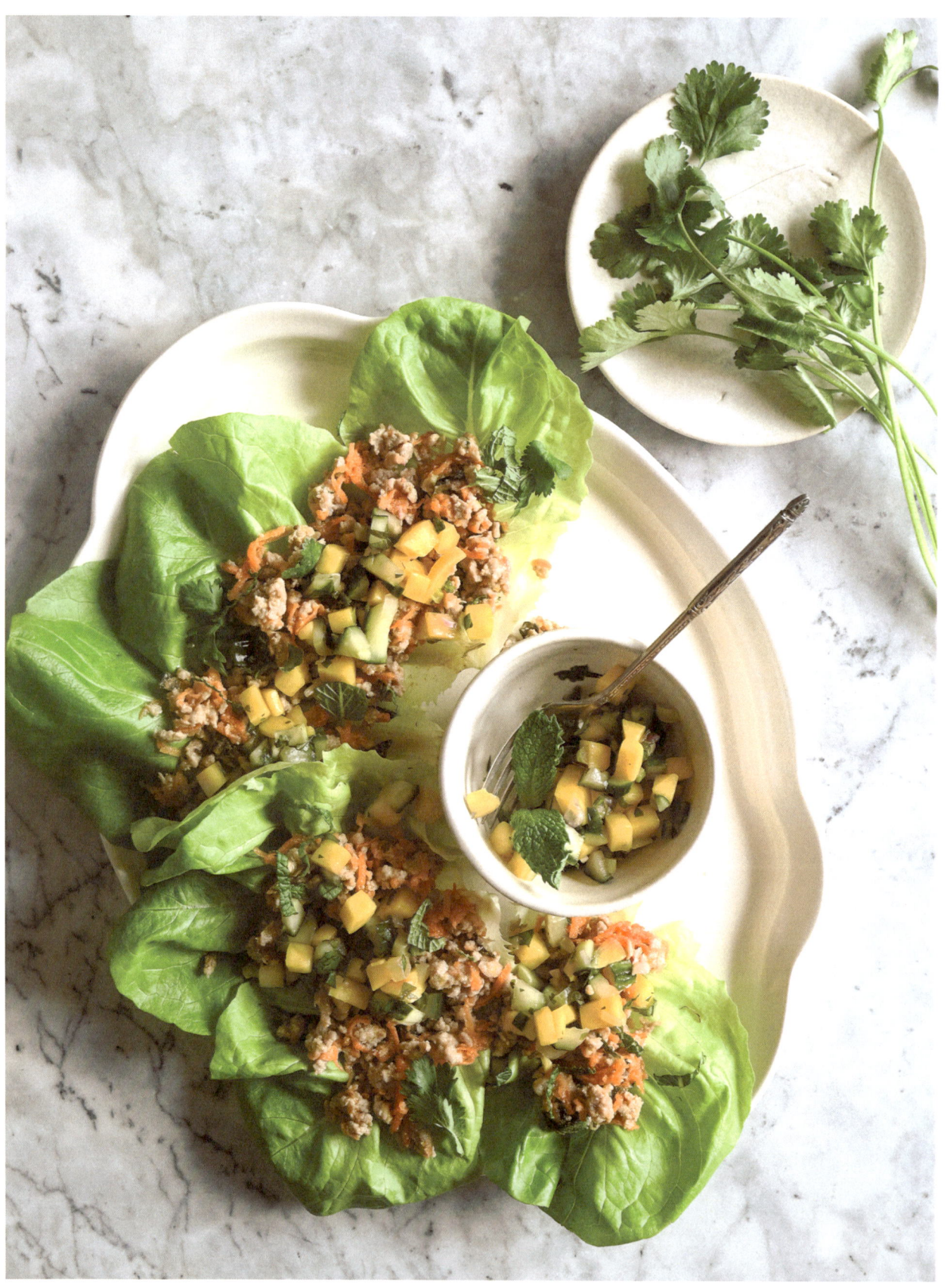

ELK LARB GAI

WITH MANGO AVOCADO SALAD

Childbirth, whether vaginal or Caesarean, normally involves the loss of half a litre to a full litre (or more) of blood. That is a lot! Postpartum is a time of red blood cell, iron, and B12 replenishment. Prioritize iron- and B12-rich foods—while continuing to take a prenatal vitamin. Choosing a ground meat blend that includes organ meat (typically called "ancestral blend") gives you a mighty dose of iron, vitamin A, choline, zinc, and vitamin B12, all essential for postpartum healing. Ask your local butcher or farmers' market meat shop if they carry ancestral blends.

Larb Gai, a traditional Thai dish, is typically made with ground chicken, mint, basil, and lime. We adore this dish on a hot day to help replenish blood and iron stores. We need all the energy we can get to keep up with our wee ones!

INGREDIENTS | SERVES 4

Mango avocado salad:
½ teaspoon pasteurized honey
1 tablespoon lime juice
¾ teaspoon lime zest
⅛ teaspoon sea salt
1 teaspoon minced jalapeño
½ cup diced mango
¼ cup diced cucumber
¼ cup diced avocado
1 ½ tablespoons chopped cilantro
½ tablespoon basil chiffonade

Dressing:
1 ½ tablespoons fish sauce
4 tablespoons lime juice
¾ tablespoon pasteurized honey
1 teaspoon lemongrass paste
¾ teaspoon roasted red chili paste

Larb gai:
1 ½ tablespoons ghee
675 grams ground elk, preferably with 10 percent organ meat, "ancestral blend" (1 ½ pounds)
¼ teaspoon sea salt
1 large shallot, thinly sliced
½ cup finely grated carrots
1 ½ tablespoons lime zest
2 tablespoons mint chiffonade
2 tablespoons basil chiffonade
2 tablespoons chopped cilantro
1 head butter leaf lettuce
¼ cup crushed peanuts, optional

DIRECTIONS

1. Prepare the mango avocado salad: In a large bowl, whisk together the honey, lime juice, lime zest, salt, and minced jalapeño. Add the mango, cucumber, avocado, cilantro, and basil. Gently stir ingredients together.

2. Prepare the dressing: In a bowl or jar, combine all the dressing ingredients and stir or shake to combine. Set aside.

3. Prepare the larb gai: Melt the ghee in a large frying pan over medium heat. Add the ground elk and ¼ teaspoon of salt. Cook over medium heat, breaking the meat into crumbles.

4. When the meat is almost cooked through, stir in the shallots and cook for another 2 minutes.

5. Transfer the meat to a medium bowl and add the shredded carrots and lime zest. Stir to combine. Drizzle over the dressing and toss with the fresh mint, basil, and cilantro. Taste and season with more salt if necessary.

6. Arrange butter lettuce leaves on a plate, and spoon the elk larb gai mixture into the lettuce cups. Top each with the crushed peanuts and the mango avocado salad.

This mango avocado salad is also a great topping for blackened fish!

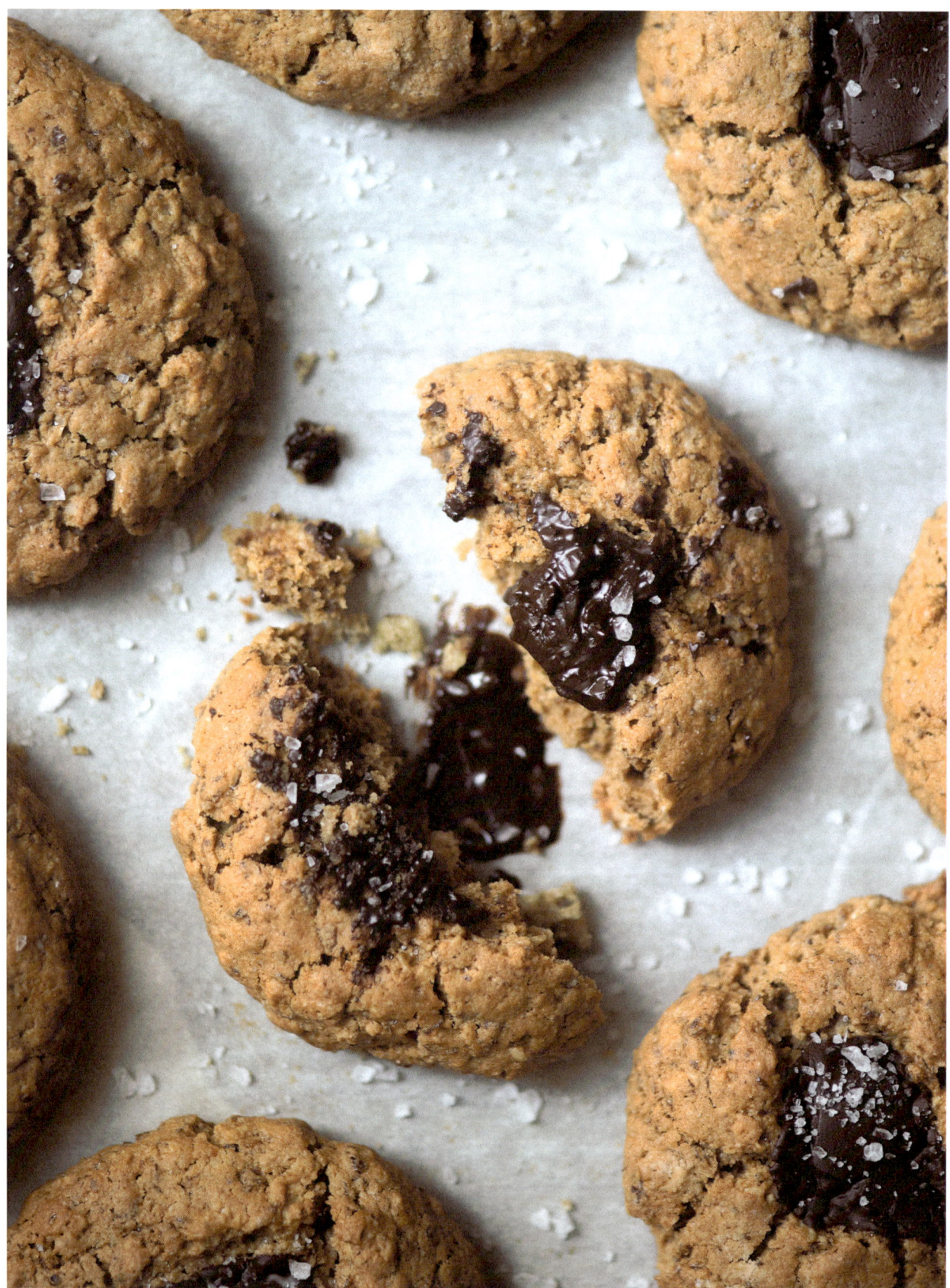

PEANUT BUTTER COOKIES

WITH CHOCOLATE, OATS, AND FENUGREEK

The journey to a healthy and happy breastfeeding relationship can be more challenging than we expected. Even after baby nails the latch, we often feel like we could be making more milk, despite a satisfied and growing babe. The synergy of oats, fenugreek, flax, wheat germ, and nutrient-dense ingredients in these cookies can give you a gentle boost and help maintain milk supply for hungry newborns.

Note to mamas: reach out for professional help if breastfeeding or chestfeeding is challenging. While cookies, teas, and tinctures may help milk production, there is nothing like support from lactation consultants, doctors, or other specialized health care providers. Be gentle and patient with yourself. Know that things will get better and that however you choose to feed your baby is completely acceptable and your choice!

INGREDIENTS | YIELDS 16

- 2 tablespoons milled flaxseed
- 1 cup oat flour
- ¼ cup almond flour
- ¼ cup wheat germ or almond flour
- 4 capsules fenugreek powder (optional for milk support)
- ½ teaspoon baking soda
- ¼ teaspoon sea salt
- ¼ cup grass-fed butter, soy-free vegan butter, or coconut oil
- ¼ cup plus 2 tablespoons organic, unsweetened, smooth peanut butter
- 1 egg yolk, free range, organic
- 1 teaspoon vanilla
- ½–¾ cup light brown sugar or coconut sugar
- 1 (110 grams) bar dark chocolate, broken into small chunks (4 ounces)

DIRECTIONS | PREHEAT OVEN TO 375° F

1. Line a baking sheet with parchment paper and set aside.
2. In a large bowl, combine the milled flaxseed and 4 tablespoons of water. Set aside.
3. In a medium bowl, combine oat flour, almond flour, wheat germ, the powder of 4 fenugreek capsules (if using), baking soda, and salt. Stir to combine and set aside.
4. In a small saucepan over very low heat, melt together the butter and peanut butter. Remove from the heat and set aside.
5. Add the egg yolk, vanilla, and sugar to the bowl with the flaxseed and water. Stir together until fully combined.
6. Slowly add the peanut butter mixture to the egg-and-sugar mixture, and stir to combine.
7. Gently fold the dry ingredients into the wet ingredients.
8. Place golf ball–sized balls of cookie dough about 3 inches apart on the parchment-lined baking sheet. Using three fingers, press down gently to slightly flatten each cookie. Place a chunk of chocolate in the middle of each one. Keep the remainder of the dough in the fridge while the first batch cooks.
9. Bake at 375° for 10 mins. Do not overbake! These will continue to cook and firm up as they cool.
10. Repeat with the remainder of the dough.
11. Store at room temperature for up to 5 days.

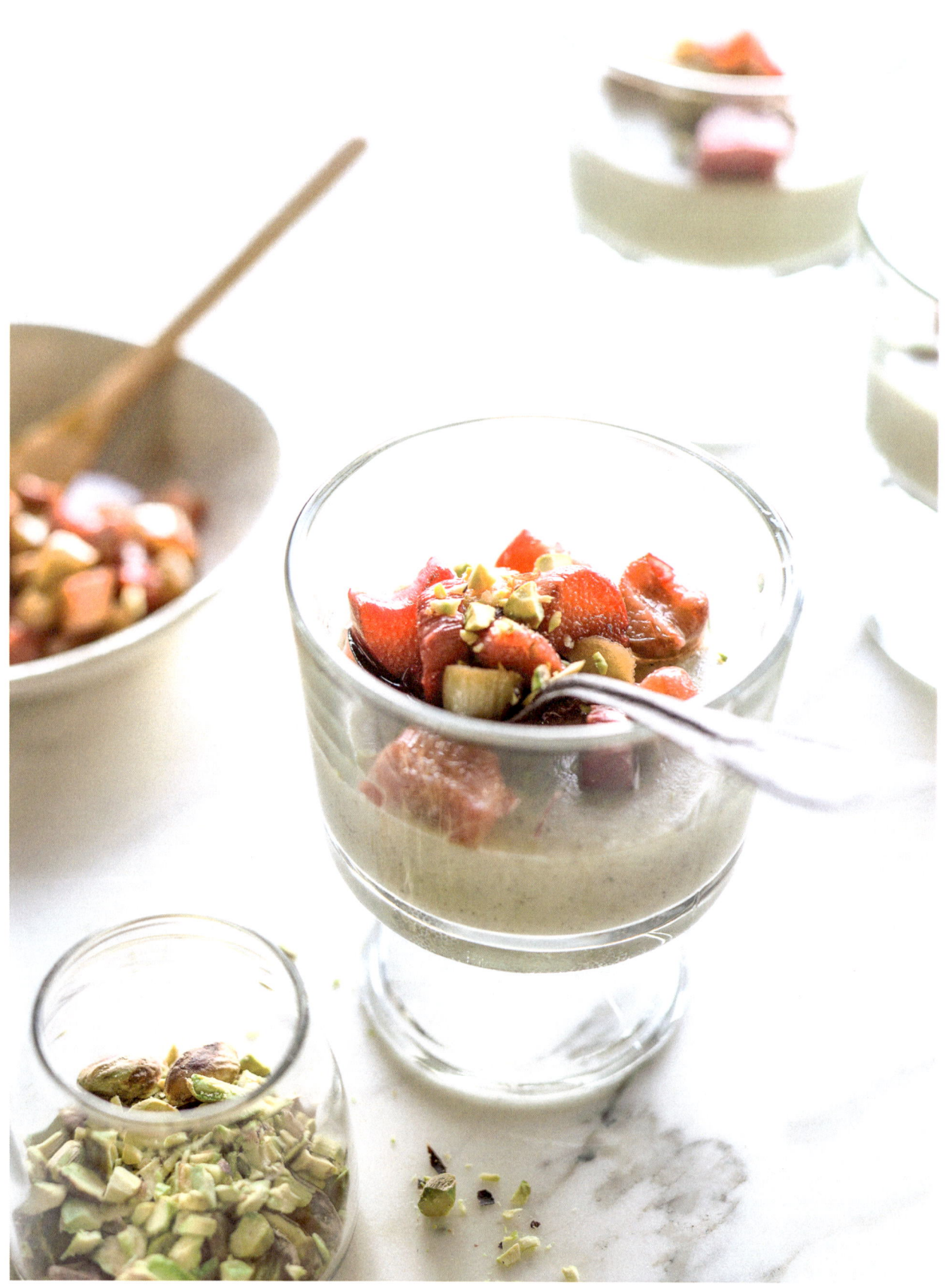

VANILLA COCONUT CUSTARD

WITH HONEY-STEWED RHUBARB AND PISTACHIOS

This custard is a fun and easy way to get more eggs into your diet. Eggs—full of protein, choline, vitamin D, iron, and DHA—and high-fat coconut milk are a postpartum match made in heaven.

INGREDIENTS | SERVES 4

Custard:

1 (400-ml) can full-fat coconut milk (14 ounces)

2 teaspoons vanilla extract

1–2 tablespoons pasteurized honey

4 large or 6 small egg yolks, free range, organic

⅓ cup organic cane sugar or coconut sugar*

3 tablespoons cornstarch or ¾ teaspoon agar powder**

¼ cup crushed pistachios

Rhubarb topping:

1 cup chopped rhubarb stalks

2 tablespoons water

1–2 tablespoons pasteurized honey

1 teaspoon orange zest or freshly grated ginger

* *Coconut sugar will turn the custard brown, whereas the cane sugar will keep it a cream colour.*

** *Cornstarch will yield a pudding-like consistency; agar powder will yield a gelatin-like consistency.*

DIRECTIONS

1. Combine the coconut milk, vanilla, and honey in a medium saucepan. Bring to a gentle simmer over low heat, whisk, then remove from the heat. Set aside.

2. In a large bowl, whisk together the egg yolks and sugar. Very, very slowly drizzle the warm milk into the egg mixture, whisking constantly. Return the coconut milk and egg mixture to the saucepan.

3. In a small dish, combine the cornstarch with 3 tablespoons of cold water (or combine the agar powder with 1 tablespoon of cold water). Stir.

4. Add the cornstarch or agar mixture to the saucepan with the coconut milk and bring to a gentle simmer over medium-low heat. Turn the heat to medium and cook, whisking frequently, until the mixture thickens, about 4–5 minutes.

5. Remove the mixture from the heat and pour into four small pudding containers. Let them cool at room temperature; once cooled, transfer them to the fridge to chill.

6. Prepare the rhubarb topping: In a small saucepan, stir together all the rhubarb ingredients. Simmer over low heat for 4–5 minutes until the rhubarb has softened. (I like mine "al dente," but if you want them broken down a bit more, continue cooking for another 3–4 minutes.)

7. Remove the rhubarb from the heat and layer it on top of each custard pot after the custard has set. Top each with 1 tablespoon of crushed pistachios

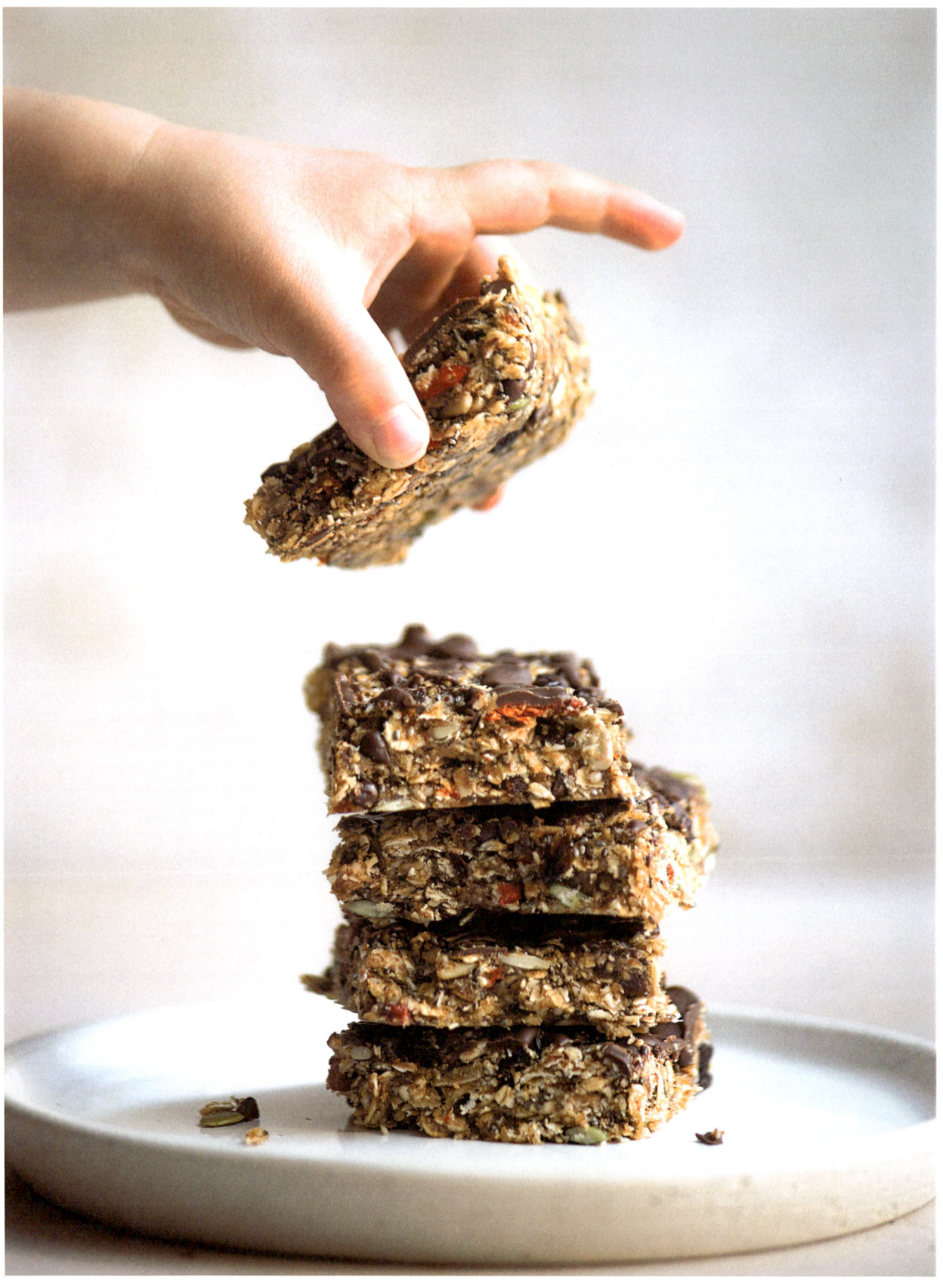

NO-BAKE GRANOLA BARS

WITH GOJI BERRIES, DATES, AND CRANBERRIES

These are perfect when you get the breastfeeding munchies or when you need a quick bite while preparing baby's bottle. Nuts and seeds have amazing amounts of zinc, magnesium, fat, and protein, all so supportive of hormone health and progesterone production. Postpartum is a time of functional progesterone deficiency, which can leave us feeling vulnerable to depression and postpartum mood disorders. Sometimes knowing why we are feeling "off" helps us normalize our feelings. Know that maternal mental health matters, and reach out for support if needed.

INGREDIENTS | YIELDS 16

2 cups dates, stems trimmed
1 cup rolled oats
½ cup nut butter or seed butter (or a combination)
¼ cup pumpkin seeds
¼ cup sunflower seeds
⅓ cup goji berries
3 tablespoons cranberries
2 tablespoons chia seeds
2 tablespoons hemp hearts
¼ cup shredded coconut
¼ cup dark chocolate chips
1 tablespoon coconut oil

DIRECTIONS

1. Line a 9-by-9-inch glass baking dish with parchment paper.
2. Place dates in a medium bowl and add hot water to cover. Soak the dates until soft. Drain, reserving a few tablespoons of the date water. Transfer the dates to a food processor and blend until smooth. If the mixture is still quite hard, add some of the hot date water and blend again until the dates become a sticky paste you can mould with your hands.
3. Transfer the date mixture to a bowl and add the remaining ingredients except the chocolate chips and coconut oil. Mix thoroughly with your hands until everything is well incorporated. Flatten the granola mixture into the parchment-lined dish.
4. Boil ¼ cup of water in a small saucepan and place a small metal bowl over top. Add the chocolate chips and coconut oil to the bowl. Over low heat, gently melt the chocolate and stir to combine with the coconut oil.
5. Drizzle the chocolate over the granola mixture and place in the fridge or freezer to harden before cutting.
6. Cut the hardened mixture into small squares or rectangles and store in the fridge for up to a week.

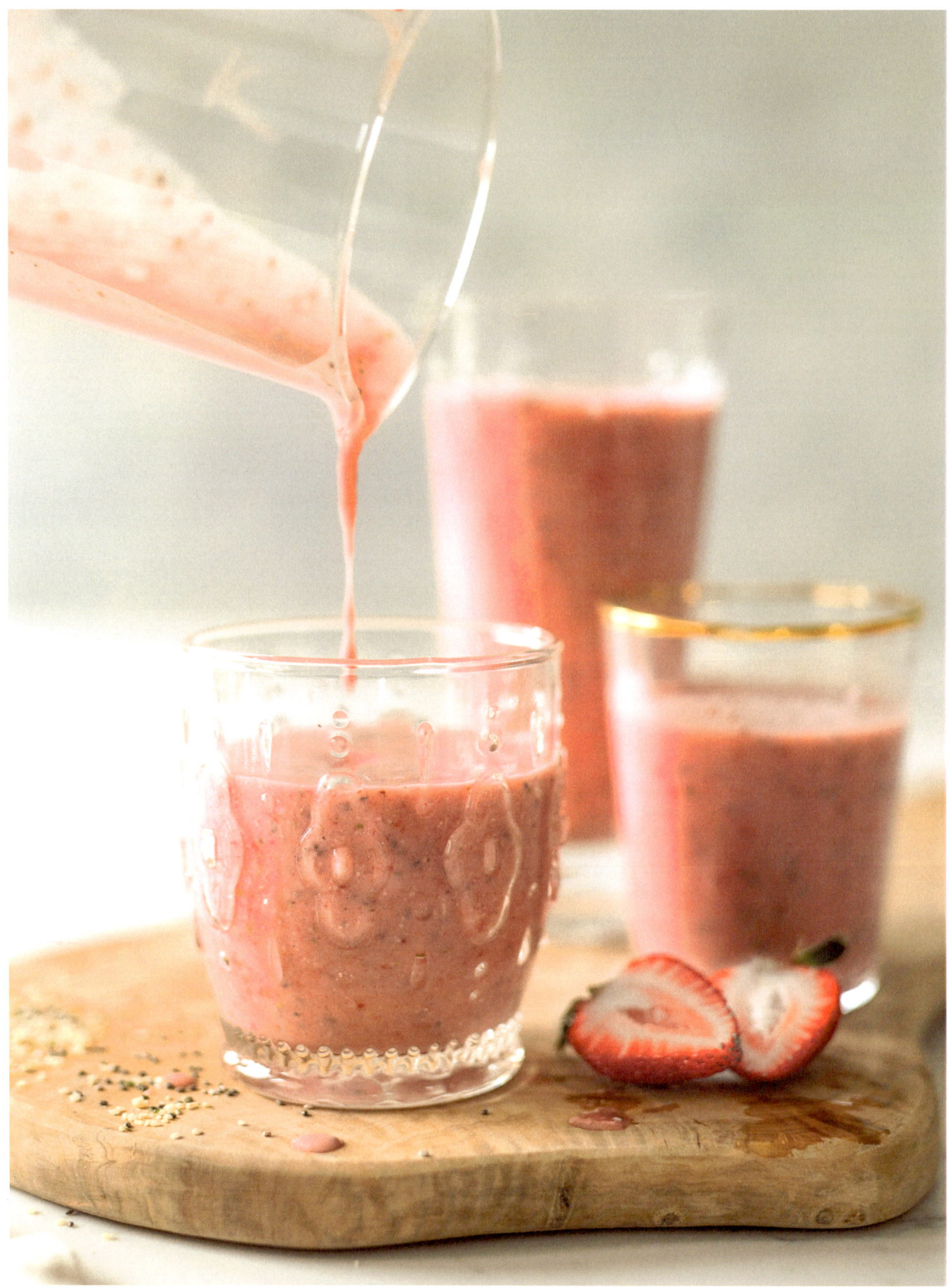

LACTATION & IMMUNITY SMOOTHIE

WITH BERRIES, MORINGA, AND CAMU-CAMU

This fourth trimester smoothie is an effective way to establish or increase breast milk production. One of the main reasons women stop breastfeeding sooner than they had hoped is because they worry they aren't making enough milk—even though this often isn't the case!

Brewer's yeast, flax, moringa, and oats are all galactagogues: botanical medicines that encourage the body's milk production. They also contain protein, iron, B vitamins, and trace minerals. Coconut water is a hydration bonus, and the fruit and camu camu support a healthy immune system.

INGREDIENTS | SERVES 2

½ cup coconut water or water kefir
½ cup fresh orange juice
¾ cup frozen strawberries
½ cup frozen raspberries
½ cup frozen dragon fruit
3 inches frozen banana
2 dates, pits removed
2 tablespoons milled flaxseed
4 tablespoons rolled oats
1 tablespoon brewer's yeast
1 tablespoon camu camu
1 tablespoon moringa
2 tablespoons collagen (optional for added protein)

DIRECTIONS

1. Combine all the ingredients in a blender, and blend on high until smooth. Enjoy!

While there is lots of advice out there for mamas worried about insufficient milk production, little is said about what to do if you're an over-producer of milk! Chat with your doctor, naturopath, or midwife if this is causing you problems like clogged ducts. However, mint tea can help calm milk production, and ingesting soy lecithin capsules, applying hot compresses, taking hot showers, and massaging the chest area can help manage clogged ducts. Make sure to get clog duct issues taken care of before they turn into mastitis.

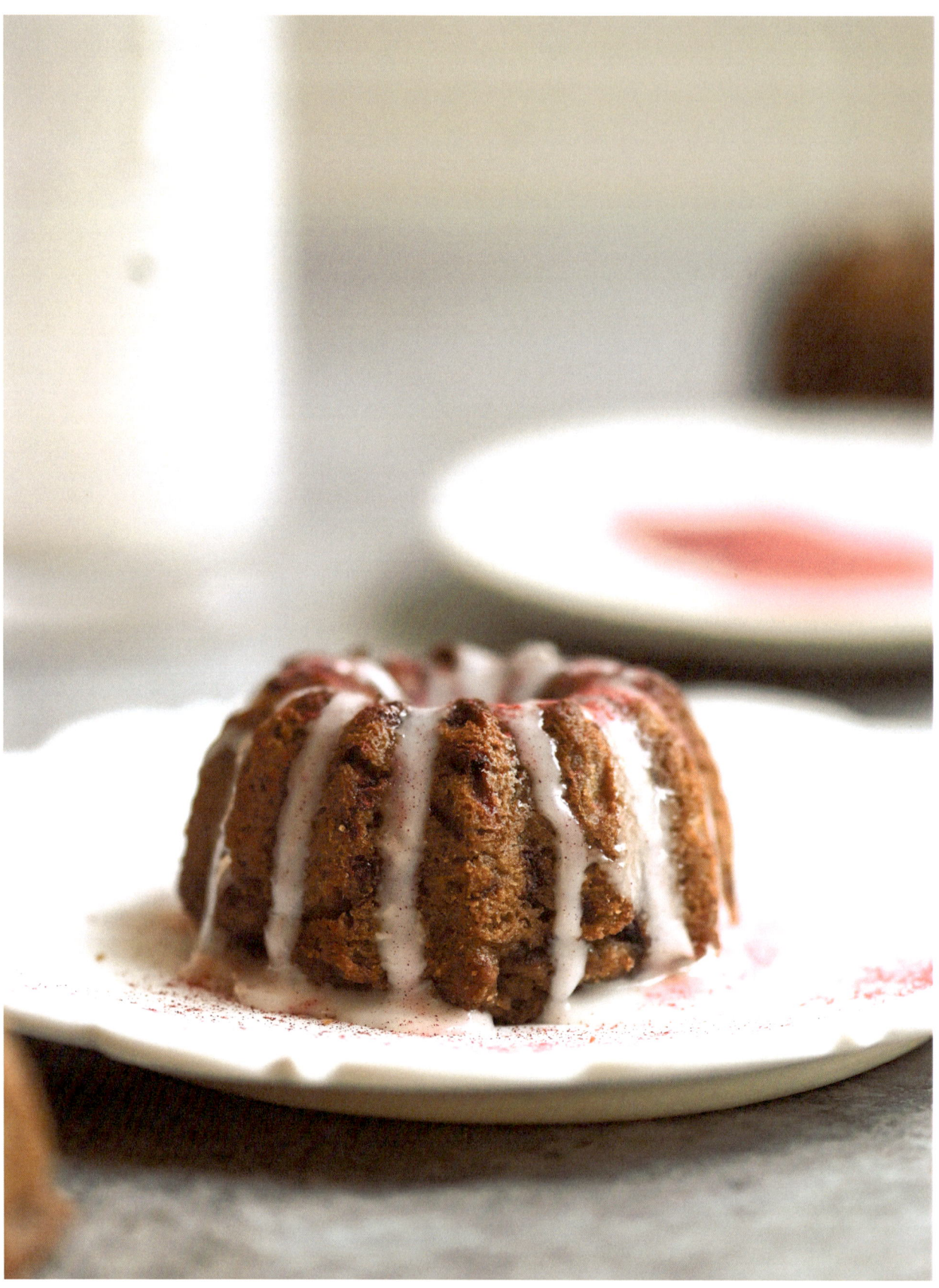

BEET & APPLE BUNDT CAKES

WITH CINNAMON-SUGAR GLAZE

These gluten-free, dairy-free, perfectly spiced cakes are sure to become a staple in your kitchen. Not all new parents need to restrict dairy or other foods in their diets, but many breastfed babes can in fact be sensitive to some foods through the breast milk. We kept this in mind while developing this beet and apple cake, which nonetheless delivers iron and a plethora of healthy fats.

INGREDIENTS | YIELDS 12 MINI BUNDT CAKES

1 cup oat flour, spooned and leveled
½ cup coconut flour, spooned and leveled
½ cup almond flour, spooned and leveled
¾ cup coconut sugar
2 teaspoons apple pie spice*
1 teaspoon baking soda
1 teaspoon baking powder
½ teaspoon sea salt
4 organic, free range eggs
1 ½ teaspoons vanilla extract or paste
¾ cup unsweetened applesauce
½ cup coconut oil, melted and cooled
Zest from 1 orange
1 cup shredded raw beets
½ cup crushed walnuts (optional)
¼ cup dried cherries (optional)

Cinnamon sugar glaze:
1 cup organic powdered sugar or coconut sugar
2 tablespoons apple juice
1 tablespoon cinnamon

* *If you can't find apple pie spice, make your own with a variety of warming spices like cinnamon, cardamom, ginger, and cloves.*

DIRECTIONS | PREHEAT OVEN TO 350° F

1. In a medium bowl, combine the oat flour, coconut flour, almond flour, coconut sugar, apple pie spice, baking soda, baking powder, and salt. Set aside.
2. In a large bowl, combine the eggs, vanilla, applesauce, coconut oil, and orange zest.
3. Gently add the dry ingredients to the wet ingredients and stir gently to combine. Let it sit for a couple of minutes so the coconut flour can absorb the wet ingredients. (It's like a sponge!)
4. Fold in the shredded beets and the walnuts or cherries, if using.
5. Spoon the mixture into a silicone mini Bundt pan, filling each one ¾ full.
6. Bake in the oven for 22 minutes.
7. While the cakes are baking, prepare the cinnamon sugar glaze: in a medium bowl, combine powdered sugar, apple juice, and cinnamon. Whisk until combined. If using coconut sugar, blend in a blender until very fine then add to a bowl with the apple juice and cinnamon. Set aside.
8. When the bundt cakes are done, remove them from the oven and let them cool. The presence of the coconut flour makes it imperative to cool the cake completely before removing from the pan! Drizzle each bundt cake with glaze and enjoy!

This recipe also works well in a loaf pan (baked for 50–55 mins) or a muffin tin.

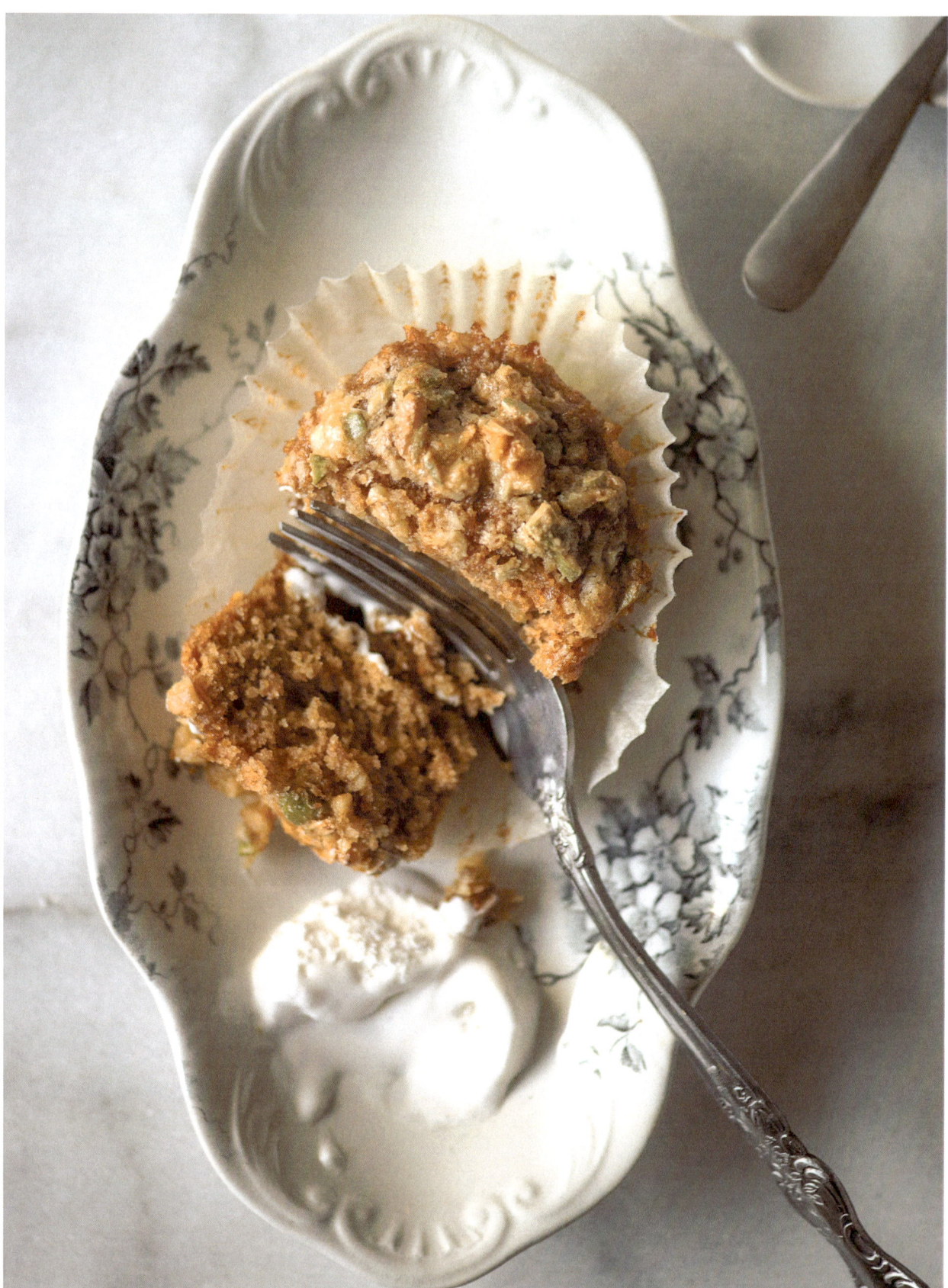

SPICED MUFFINS

WITH PARSNIPS AND CARROTS

It is better to eat nutritionally dense food frequently throughout the day instead of confining ourselves to mealtimes. Maintaining a consistent, elevated level of maternal vitamins, minerals, fats, and proteins in breast milk allows for baby's optimal growth and development.

Take a quick pic of this muffin recipe and send it off to a bestie or family member. Then soak in the nourishment and great company when they arrive with these grounding goodies!

INGREDIENTS | YIELDS 16 MUFFINS

1 cup almond flour
¾ cup oat flour
¼ cup arrowroot starch
¾ cup coconut sugar
2 teaspoons baking powder
1 ½ teaspoons warming spice blend like chai, pumpkin pie spice, or your own blend
½ teaspoon sea salt
3 free range, organic eggs
½ cup coconut oil, melted and cooled
¼ cup plus 2 tablespoons unsweetened applesauce
1 teaspoon vanilla extract
zest from ½ navel orange
1 cup grated parsnips
1 cup grated carrots

DIRECTIONS | PREHEAT OVEN TO 350° F

1. Line a muffin tin with liners or use a silicone muffin mould.
2. In a medium bowl, combine the almond flour, oat flour, arrowroot starch, coconut sugar, baking powder, spice blend, and salt. Stir to incorporate.
3. In a large bowl, stir together the eggs, coconut oil, applesauce, vanilla, and orange zest.
4. Pour the dry ingredients into the wet ingredients and stir to combine.
5. Fold in the grated parsnips and carrots.
6. Pour into muffin moulds. Bake for 15 minutes (for mini muffins) or 20 mins (for regular muffins).
7. Remove muffins from the oven and let them cool slightly in the tray before removing them to a rack.

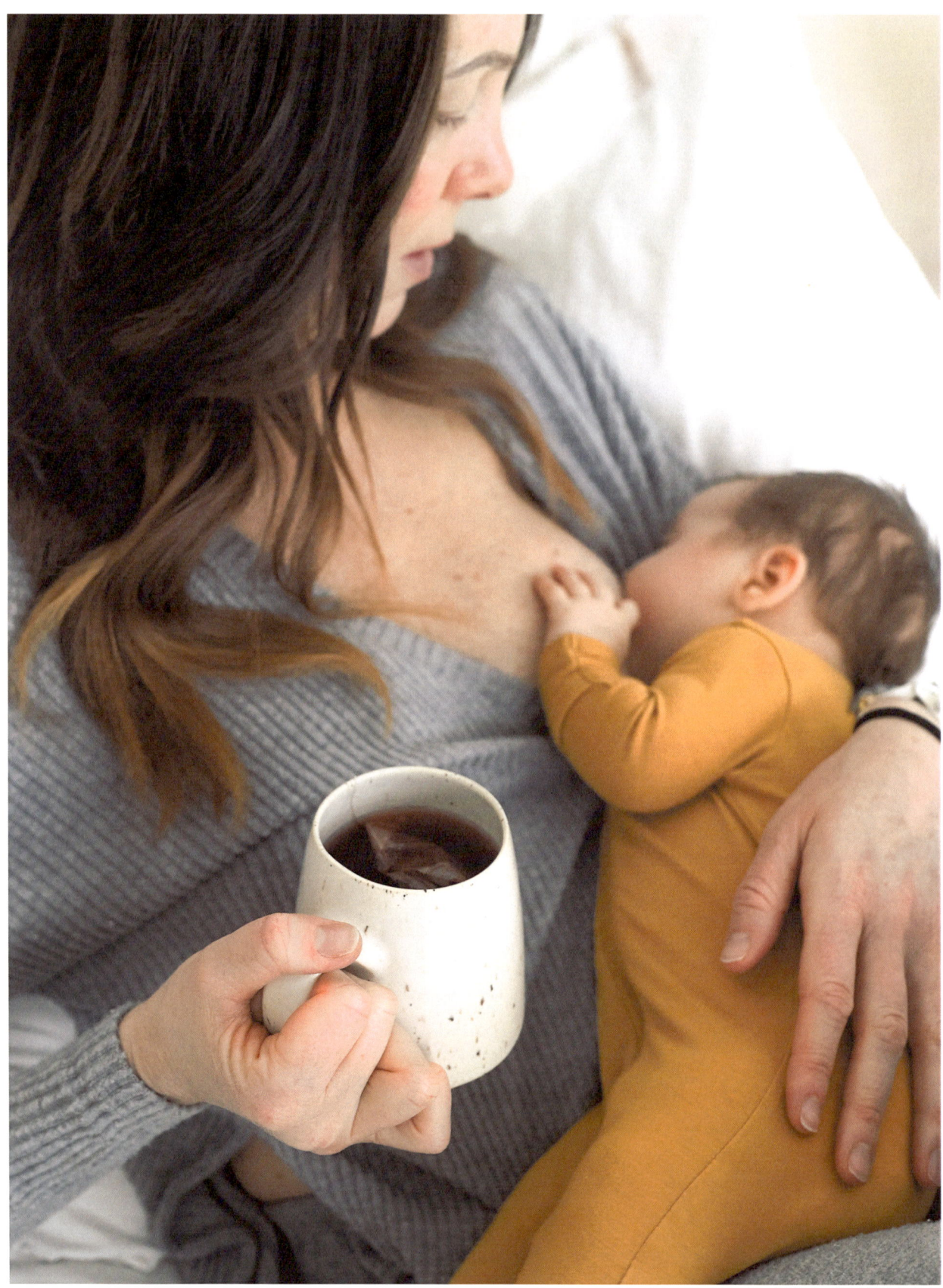

POSTPARTUM HEALING TEA

WITH STINGING NETTLE, LEMON BALM, AND OAT STRAW

Nettles really are magical; they offer a multivitamin-esque array of nutrients, decrease inflammation, and act as a diuretic to purge excess pregnancy fluids. Oat straw and lemon balm calm the mind, encourage relaxation, and help soothe the early postpartum "baby blues." Pour a warm cup, draw an Epsom salt and lavender bath, and soak your body and tender perineum, taking time to rest and heal like the goddess you are. This is the ultimate postpartum sip and soak!

INGREDIENTS | SERVES 1

½ teaspoon loose-leaf stinging nettle
½ teaspoon loose-leaf oat straw
½ teaspoon loose-leaf lemon balm
1 cranberry-pomegranate tea bag
1 cinnamon stick
¼–½ teaspoon honey

DIRECTIONS

1. Combine stinging nettle, oat straw, and lemon balm in a tea diffuser.
2. Place the tea diffuser in 1 cup of boiling water along with the pomegranate tea bag and cinnamon stick.
3. Let steep for 10 minutes.
4. Remove tea bag, diffuser, and cinnamon stick and add honey to taste.

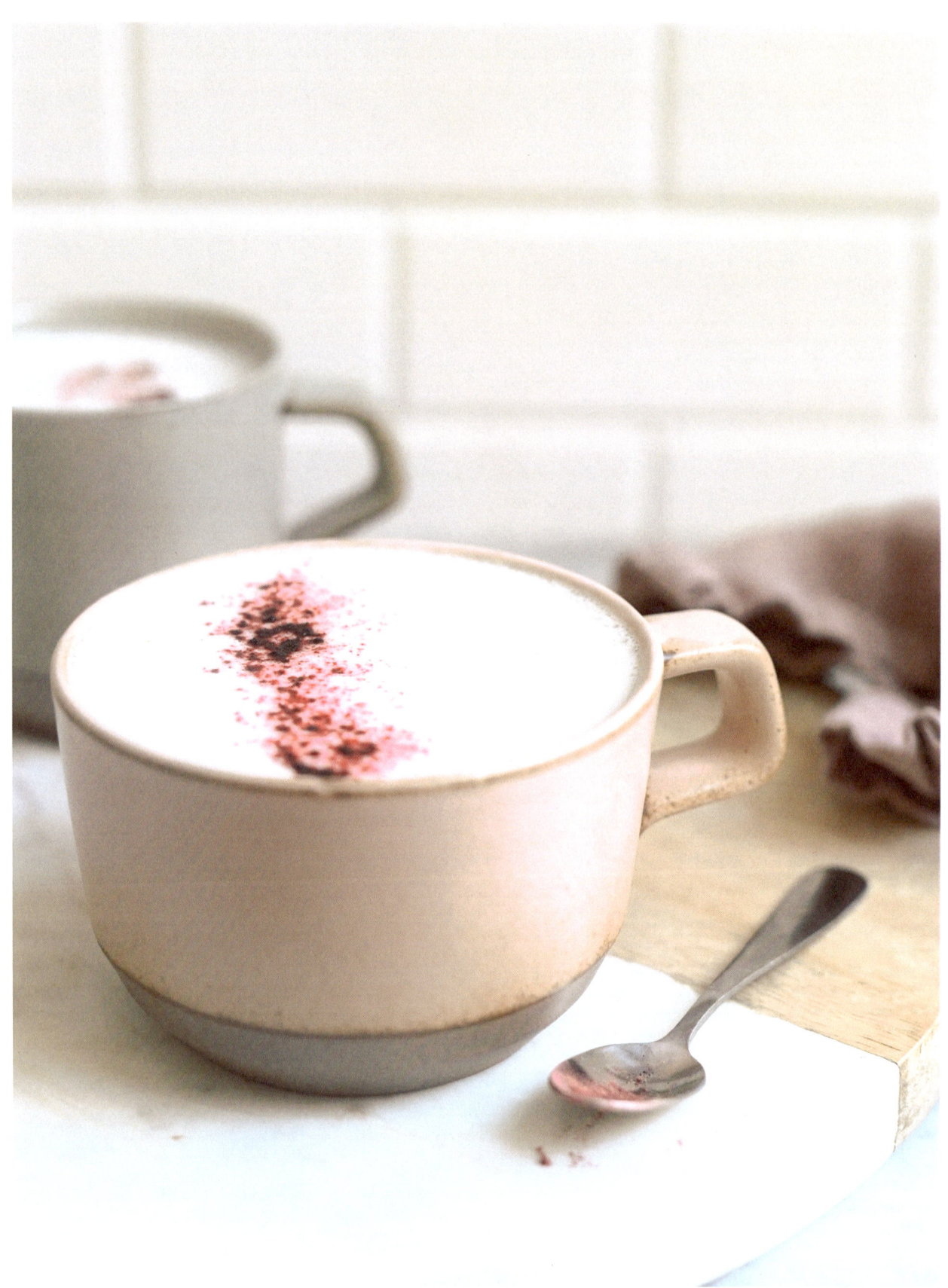

RELAXING REISHI ROSE ELIXIR

WITH REISHI, OAT STRAW, AND ASHWAGANDHA

Adaptogens, like reishi mushrooms and ashwagandha, are a must-have during the postpartum metamorphosis, allowing the body to adapt and heal from physical and mental stress. Adaptogens are able to settle down our nervous system if we are on overdrive, or give us a gentle pick-me-up if we need it. It's amazing how intuitive they are, working in accordance with our body's needs at any given moment. We invite you to sip on this gorgeous rose elixir (which tastes like Lindt white chocolate!) and remind yourself that you too are blooming and growing.

INGREDIENTS | SERVES 2

½ ounce dried reishi slices

1 tablespoon oat straw in a tea diffuser or tea bag

1 tablespoon cacao butter (or 5 round wafers)

2 tablespoons coconut butter

2 ½ tablespoons honey

¼ teaspoon ashwagandha powder

½ plus ⅛ teaspoon rose hydrosol

¼ teaspoon vanilla extract

Pinch salt

DIRECTIONS

1. In a small saucepan, bring 2 ½ cups filtered water to a simmer. Turn off the heat and add the dried reishi and oat straw tea bag.
2. Steep for 45–60 minutes.
3. Discard the mushrooms and tea bag and warm the tea on the stove over low heat.
4. Once warmed, transfer the tea to a high-speed blender and add cacao butter, coconut butter, honey, ashwagandha, rose hydrosol, vanilla, and salt. Blend on low until fully combined.
5. Pour into a mug and enjoy!.

The "five senses meditation" is one of Anise's favourite meditations to come into the present moment and calm a restless mind: name 5 things you see, 4 things you hear, 3 things you can feel, 2 things you smell, and 1 thing you taste. Take this elixir outside if possible, and sip while you are doing the meditation. (Hint: you can do this while baby-wearing if babe doesn't want to be put down!)

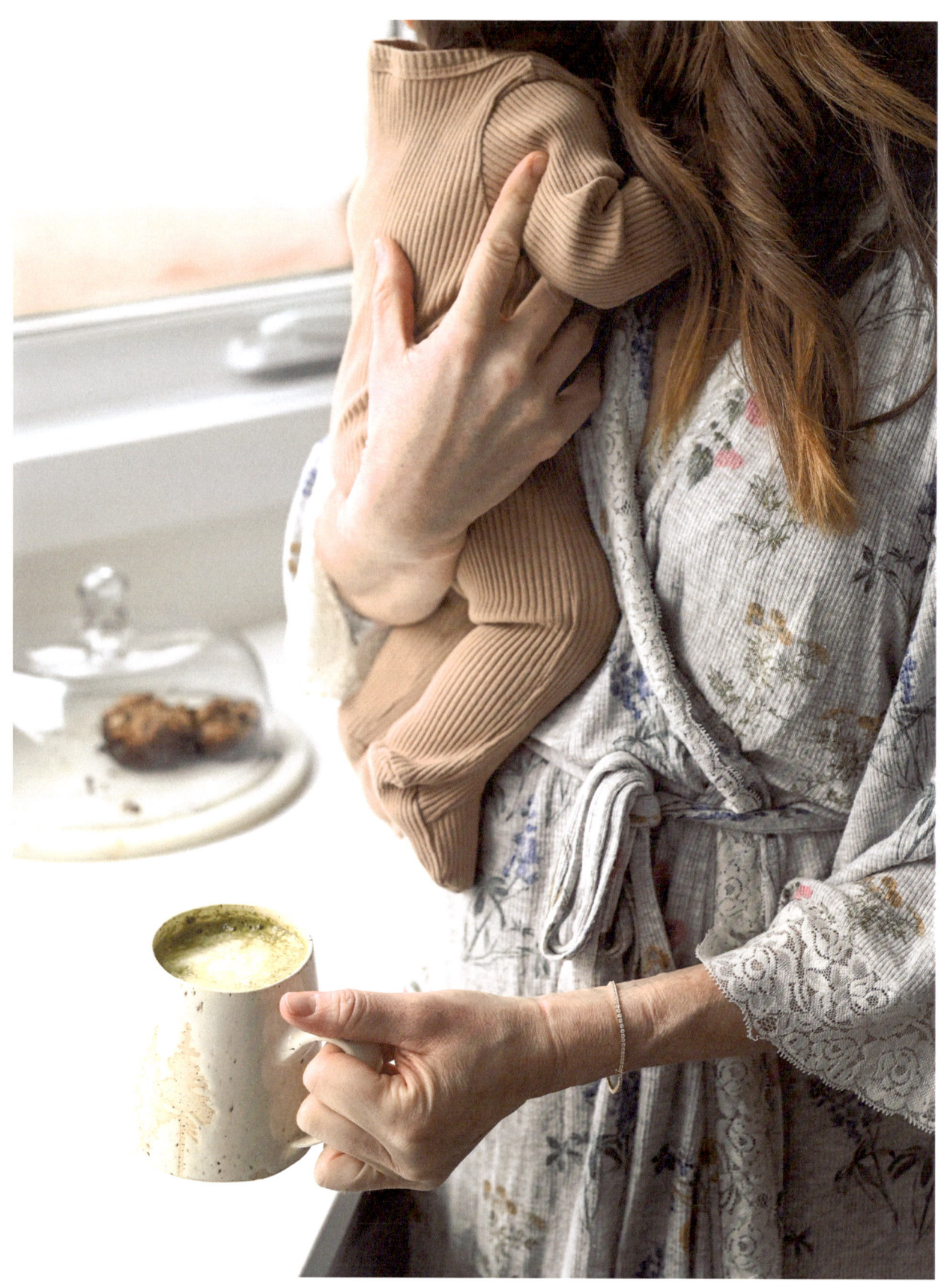

ENERGIZING MATCHA LATTE

WITH MORINGA AND COLLAGEN

Love and comfort sometimes come in a steamy mug, and that is welcome anytime of day! The powerful botanicals matcha and moringa boast both adaptogenic and lactation-boosting qualities. Matcha, a type of green tea, is known for providing gentle and steady energy, but it also supports our immunity. This decadent latte combines foundational plant medicine with energizing matcha for a deeply satisfying moment in your day.

INGREDIENTS | SERVES 2

1 cup light coconut milk
½ cup almond milk
1 ½ tablespoons honey
¼ teaspoon vanilla
Pinch salt
1 teaspoon matcha
½ teaspoon moringa
½ tablespoon collagen

DIRECTIONS

1. In a saucepan, bring the coconut milk and almond milk to a simmer over low heat.
2. Remove from the heat and stir in the honey, vanilla, and salt.
3. Whisk in the matcha, moringa, and collagen.
4. Pour into a mug and enjoy!

Daily affirmations, grounding breaths, and foundational nourishment can make all the difference in our postpartum experience. Choose one of the affirmations below to repeat throughout the day—or create your own.

"I am so grateful for my healing and will continue to love and nourish myself."

"I trust in the ways I choose to feed, support, nourish, and love my baby."

"I love and trust myself. I am recovering wonderfully and with grace."

"I am the best mom for my baby."

"My body is beautiful and has grown and nourished a baby. I am so thankful for this amazing body."

"I trust my intuition as a mother and whole person."

"Today is only a snippet of time; it will get better."

"I love myself and deserve support on all levels."

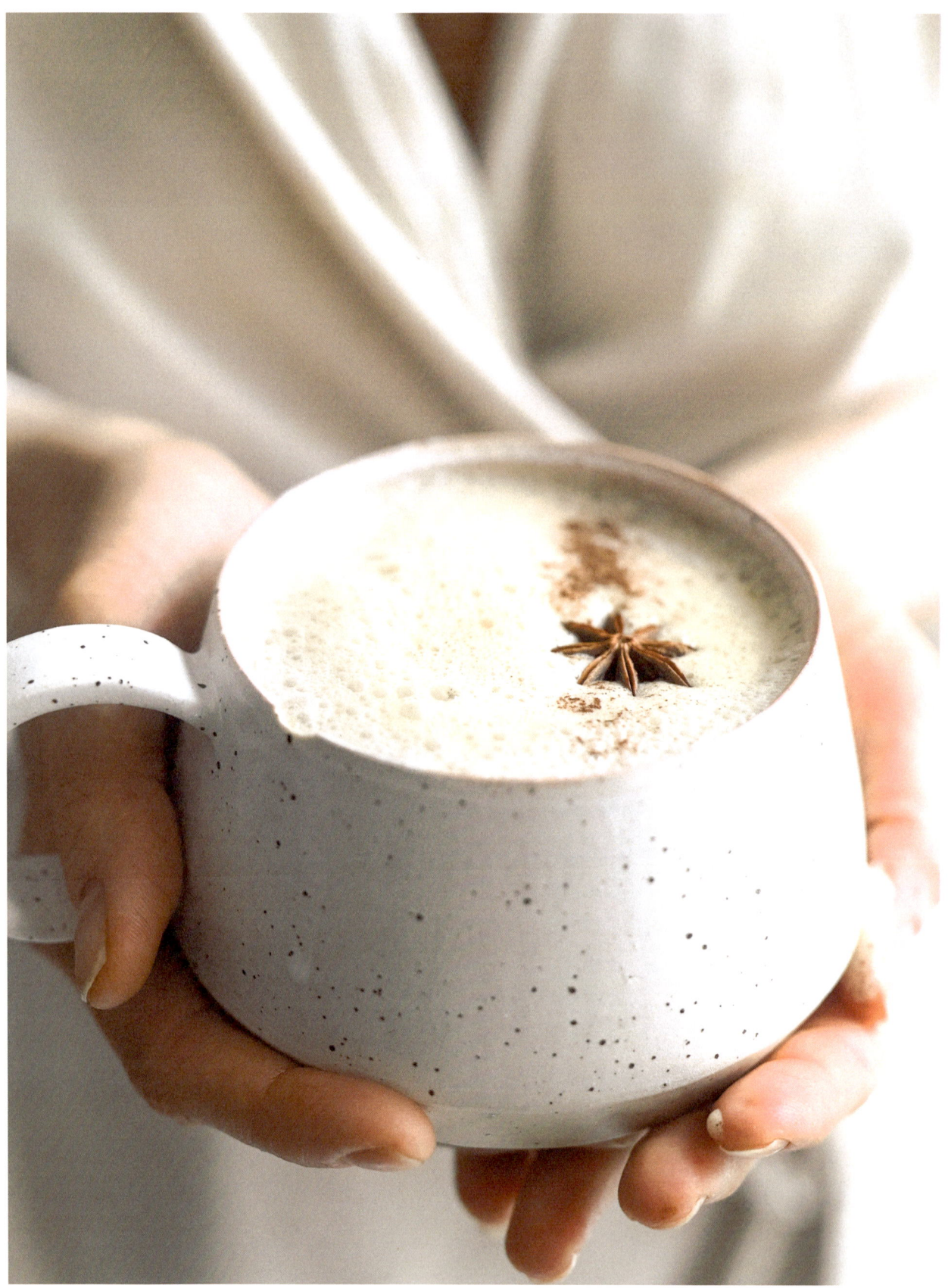

GROUNDING COCONUT CHAI

WITH HONEY AND VANILLA

Being a new mother can be one of the most amazing experiences. But perinatal mental health imbalances, including anxiety and depression, can make the postpartum journey extremely challenging. Our brains anatomically change during pregnancy, encouraging us to be more vigilant and alert. Add in feelings of overwhelm and isolation, changing relationships, and the responsibility of keeping a small human alive, and we can find ourselves at the end of our rope.

One way to stay present and grounded is to take this coconut chai outside, walk in the grass in your bare feet, take some deep breaths, and name 3 things you are grateful for. Here is your reminder to reach out to your mental health care provider, naturopathic doctor, medical doctor, health support team, or even a friend or partner for help if you are experiencing any postpartum depression or anxiety symptoms. Trust us—this is more common than you think! You are so loved, Mama, and you deserve all the support.

INGREDIENTS | SERVES 2

1 cup light coconut milk
½ cup almond milk
1 ¼ tablespoons pasteurized honey
½ teaspoon vanilla extract
Pinch of salt
1 ½ teaspoons stone-ground chai*

DIRECTIONS

1. In a small saucepan over low heat, or in a milk frother, warm the coconut milk and almond milk. Remove from the heat.
2. Stir in the honey, vanilla, and salt.
3. Whisk in the stone-ground chai until fully incorporated.
4. Pour into a mug and enjoy!

Stone-ground chai will give you a much richer flavour than a chai tea bag in water. You can try Chaiwala Original Chai and Genuine Tea Microground Chai.

ACKNOWLEDGEMENTS

To everyone who helped make this cookbook a reality....

To everyone that helped test recipes and gave your input, thank you for helping me fine tune every detail: Kristen Kitchen, Jessica Lindskog, Jess Kirby, Jill Galarneau, Philip Munson, James Munson, Dr Carrie Mitchell, and Shianna Pace.

To Amy Buchanan, what would I have done without my nanny for sweet Jones, taste-tester, cheerleader, prop assistant, constant supporter, and all around raddest chick to hang out with during the work days?!

To Laura Naaykens, Katrina Demers, Jacqueline Cuffie, Jill Galarneau and baby Louise: thank you for sharing such an intimate time with myself and my camera. You gave the photos such life and beauty.

Dr. Carrie Mitchell, thank you for your hard work to bring this cookbook to another level. What started out as a fun conversation in your office 8 years ago has turned into one of my most proud achievements.

To my editor and designer, Amanda Bidnall and Constance Mears: thank you for your patience and hard work. This was much harder than I anticipated but you held my hand along the way and were always there to answer questions. Just when I thought I *had* to be finished, it only took another 18 months!

To my family, thank you for your patience while I tested and re-tested all the recipes, the messy kitchen, the food photography items all over the dining room for years, and being extremely honest taste-testers. Thank you for your undying support and doing what was necessary to bring my ideas to fruition.

And last, thank you to my grandparents and parents: you taught me how to hold a knife, how to brunoise vegetables, how to make sausage rolls and whiskey chicken, and that a home-cooked meal is the ultimate expression of love.

ABOUT THE AUTHORS

Anise is a certified holistic nutritionist and mother of three living in Calgary, Alberta. When Anise moved to Canada in 2009, she developed a love for nutrition and was intrigued by the idea of food as medicine as well as the mind-body-soul connection. She graduated from the Canadian School of Natural Nutrition in 2014 and started Honoured Journey Prenatal Yoga Retreats, which specializes in yoga, empowerment and nourishment for the mama-to-be. She believes that choosing local, whole-food, in-season ingredients is a way to love ourselves and our family. You can find Anise blogging at Simply Sprouted or watch her culinary and family adventures @anisethorogood.

PHOTO: GENEVIEVE RENE

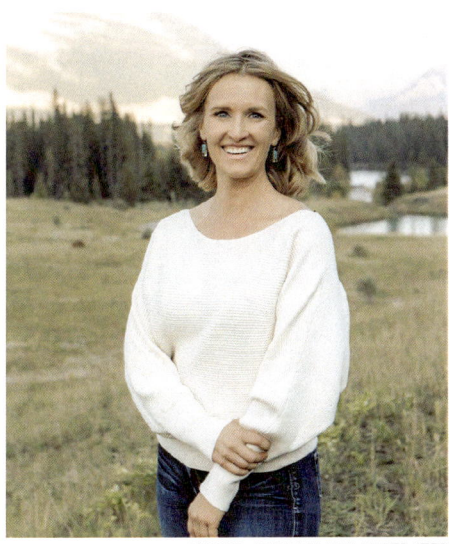

PHOTO: NATURALLY ILLUSTRATED

Anise has joined forces with Dr. Carrie Mitchell, mother of two and a perinatal-focused Naturopathic Doctor, to nourish the expectant mama in a way that is supported by science and years of clinical experience. Dr. Carrie is passionate about helping people thrive through the most transformative of times: fertility, pregnancy, postpartum and the young family years. She believes that how you feel during pregnancy, childbirth and postpartum can set the stage for a lifelong journey of health and vibrancy. Dr. Carrie can be found at Moss Postpartum House in Calgary, Alberta, or sneaking out for mountain adventures with her family.

INDEX

A

Adaptogens, 187
Affirmations, 189
Almond flour, 5, 11, 63, 89, 173, 181, 183
Almonds, 4, 15, 21, 37, 103, 135, 139
Aloe vera, 41
Ancestral blend, 9, 143, 167, 171
Anti-inflammatory, 7, 10, 89, 155
Antioxidants, 3, 6, 10, 35, 89, 105, 119, 127, 151
Anxiety, 95–96, 191
Apple cider vinegar, 6, 39, 73, 109, 119, 145
Apples, 6, 10, 99
Apricot, 55, 57, 103, 143, 169
Artichokes, 99, 113
Ashwagandha, 129, 187
Asparagus, 10, 27, 33, 143, 149
Avocado, 7, 11, 15, 19, 67, 69, 71, 73, 75, 105, 111, 115, 143, 153, 155, 171
Avocado and Corn Salsa, 99, 127
Avocado oil, 7, 63, 69, 71, 75, 79, 81, 127, 153, 167, 169
Avocado Toast, 15, 19
Ayurvedic, 143, 151

B

Baby blues, 139, 185
Banana bread, 45
Banana Carrot Bread with Cinnamon Pecans, 15
Bananas, 10, 45, 89, 105
Barbecue sauce, 35
Barley, 4
Basmati rice, 117, 151
Beet & Apple Bundt Cakes, 143, 181
Beet, Citrus & Lentil Salad, 109
Beet Dip, 99, 131
Beets, 45, 99, 109, 119, 131, 155, 165, 181
Beluga lentils, 117, 123
Berries, 6, 10, 17, 105, 133, 143, 145, 153, 177
Biotin, 4, 23, 43, 101, 169
Bison, 9, 15, 35, 99, 119, 149, 159

Bison Borscht, 99, 119
Black beans, 5, 127
Bliss Balls, 99, 135
Blood glucose levels/blood sugar, 5, 10, 19, 21, 47, 49, 59, 139
Blood loss, 167
Blood pressure, 51, 89, 95, 109
Blood volume, 51, 101
Blueberries, 55, 59, 133, 153
Blueberry Lemon Doughnuts, 143, 153
Bone broth, 67, 69, 123, 141, 161, 163, 165, 169
Brain development, 6
Brain health, 39
Braxton hicks, 135
Brazil nuts, 87, 139
Breastfeeding, 139, 141, 145, 155, 159, 173, 177, 179
Brewer's yeast, 179
Brittle, 99, 139
Broccoli, 55, 61, 67, 149
Brown basmati rice, 117, 151
Brown rice, 4–5, 10–11, 29, 33, 115, 163
Brown rice flour, 5, 11
Brownies, 55, 89
Brussels Sprout Hash, 15, 23
B12, 10, 13, 37, 79, 83, 85, 171
Bubur injin, 147
Buckwheat groats, 4, 49, 59
Butternut Squash Breakfast Buns, 55, 63

C

Cabbage, 25, 29, 81, 83, 99, 111, 119
Cacao butter, 129, 187
Cacao nibs, 17, 55, 93
Cacao powder, 47, 49, 57, 89, 135, 137
Cake, 11, 143, 181
Calcium, 6, 47, 61, 63, 71, 96, 135, 159
Camu camu, 87, 179
Camu-camu, 143
Cardamom, 17, 45, 49, 147, 181

Carrot Dip, 15, 43
Carrots, 43, 45, 55, 83, 115, 157, 159, 161, 165, 171, 183
Cashew cheese, 19, 69
Cashew cream, 27, 121, 149, 157
Cashews, 4, 37, 69, 117, 121, 133, 149, 157
Cassava flour, 5, 45
Cauliflower, 15, 31, 33, 35, 99, 115, 151, 155, 167
Cauliflower Carbonara, 15, 33
Cauliflower rice, 15, 31, 35, 115
Celery Root, 99, 121, 123
Cervical dilation, 137
Cervix, 6, 96
Chai, 143, 183, 191
Chanterelles, 55
Cheddar, 63, 71, 85
Cheese, 9, 11, 19, 27, 35, 63, 69, 71, 115, 149
Cherries, 181
Cherry tomatoes, 27, 39, 65, 77, 149
Chia, 4, 11, 15, 41, 47, 49, 99, 103, 105, 137, 177
Chia pudding, 15, 49
Chia seeds, 4, 41, 47, 49, 91, 99, 103, 137, 177
Chicken, 9, 15, 33, 37, 55, 143, 145, 157, 159, 169, 171
Chicken Souvlaki Salad, 55, 77
Chicken thighs, 37, 77, 117, 169
Chickpeas, 5, 113, 143, 169
Chimichurri, 55, 61
Chlorella and spirulina, 6
Chocolate, 15, 47, 93, 99, 129, 135, 173, 177, 187
Chocolate Avocado Brownies, 55, 89
Chocolate Brittle, 99, 139
Chocolate Hazelnut Chia Pudding, 15, 49
Chocolate Sesame Truffles, 15, 47
Choline, 9, 23, 39, 149, 171, 175
Chowder, 99, 121
Cilantro, 25, 101, 111, 117, 127, 155, 171
Cinnamon, 15, 17, 45, 57, 99, 143, 145, 181, 185
Citrus Avocado Crema, 15, 25
Coconut, 5–7, 11, 15, 37, 41, 45, 83, 119, 121, 123, 177, 179, 181, 189, 191
Coconut Cardamon Millet Pudding, 143, 147
Coconut flour, 5, 11, 45, 105, 153, 181

Coconut milk, 31, 49, 93, 103, 107, 117, 137, 175, 189, 191
Coconut oil, 7, 17, 21, 49, 57, 75, 79, 83, 85, 153, 155, 177, 181, 183
Coconut water, 41, 51, 97, 179
Coconut whip, 107
Collagen, 63, 81, 87, 93, 103, 159, 179, 189
Constipation, 5, 13, 41, 51, 95, 105
Cookies, 55, 57, 143, 173
Cramping, 135
Creamy Wild Rice Soup, 143, 157
Crumble, 49, 59, 135, 171
Custard, 143, 175

D

Dairy-Free Salmon Chowder, 99, 121
Dandelion Greens, 10, 55, 85
Dandy blend, 89, 139
Dark chocolate, 89, 93, 139, 173, 177
Dates, 6, 17, 47, 55, 77, 89, 96–97, 137, 143, 177, 179
Depression, 177, 191
DHA, 6, 9, 163, 175
Digestion, 5, 17, 21, 41, 51, 89, 129
Dip, 15, 37, 43, 55, 69, 131, 165, 167
Doughnuts, 143, 153
Dragon fruit, 179

E

Edamame, 55, 73, 111
Eggplant, 99, 123
Eggs, 9, 15, 23, 31, 61, 63, 89, 153, 159, 167, 175, 181, 183
Electrolytes, 97, 135, 145, 159
Elk, 9, 55, 79, 99, 123, 143, 171
Elk Larb Gai, 143, 171
Energizing Matcha Latte, 143, 189
Energy, 4–6, 10, 31, 37, 89, 95–97, 115, 117, 139, 141, 171, 189
Essential fatty acids, 4–6, 25, 39, 61, 75
Evening Primrose Oil, 96–97
Extra-virgin olive oil, 7, 27, 29, 31, 33, 127, 149, 163, 165
Eyes, 121, 141

F

Fatigue, 13, 41
Fenugreek, 143, 151, 155, 173
Fermented foods, 25, 83
Fibre, 4–6, 9–11, 13, 17, 33, 69, 95, 105, 123, 137
Figs, 10, 15, 35, 47, 99, 135
Flaxseed, 5, 7, 11, 27, 37, 39, 105, 107, 109, 173, 179
Folic acid, 4–5, 9–10, 13, 23, 31, 39, 85, 169
Food Sensitivities, 3
Fourth Trimester, 67, 93, 141, 153, 159, 161, 173, 175, 177, 187, 189, 191
Freezies, 55, 91
Fried rice, 99, 115
Frittata, 149
Frosting, 55, 89
Fruit Crisp, 55, 59

G

Galactagogues, 179
Game meat, 9, 35, 79, 123, 167
Ginger, 15, 17, 21, 75, 79, 99, 107, 111, 115, 151, 161, 163, 181
Ginger Carrot Sauce, 55, 79
Ginger Granola, 15, 21
Ginger Soy Sushi Bowl, 55, 73
Ginger Turmeric Chicken soup, 143, 169
Glucose tolerance test, 59
Glycine, 145
Goat milk, 61, 149
Gochujang, 19, 81
Goji Berries, 6, 133, 143, 177
Grain bowl, 155
Granola, 15, 17, 21, 87, 143, 177
Granola bars, 143, 177
Grass-fed butter, 6, 11, 17, 19, 45, 105, 117, 123, 173
Green peas, 5
Gremolata, 99, 109
Grilled Avocado, 55, 81
Grilled Lemon Halibut, 55, 75
Grounding Coconut Chai, 143, 191
Guava Kombucha Freezies, 55, 91
Gut Microbiome, 67, 83

H

Hair loss, 169
Halibut, 37, 55, 75
Hazelnut butter, 49
Hazelnut-Crusted Chicken, 15, 37
Healthy Fats, 11
  Avocados, 11
  Chia seed, 11
  Grass-fed butter, 11
  Oils, 11
Heart health, 19, 77, 89
Heartburn, 95, 111
Hemorrhoids, 95, 105
Hemp hearts, 5, 17, 19, 37, 47, 51, 87, 103, 105, 135, 147, 177
Hemp oil, 7
Hempseed oil, 27, 73, 77, 109
High blood pressure, 95, 109
Homeopathics, 97
Honey, 6, 29, 31, 41, 73, 111, 147, 171, 175, 185, 187, 189, 191
Honey mint yogourt, 31
Honey-Stewed Rhubarb, 143
Hormone health, 177
Hot Cacao, 99, 129
Hot chocolate, 129
Hydration, 41, 51, 145, 179

I

Ice cream, 59, 93
Immunity, 89, 143, 179, 189
Ina May Gaskin, 77
Instant pot, 109, 117, 119, 147, 149, 151, 155, 157
Iodine, 6, 73
Iron, 5–6, 9, 23, 25, 85, 89, 95–96, 105, 169, 171, 175, 179, 181
Iron transfer, 131, 167

J

Jalapeños, 25, 117
Jam, 55, 57, 63, 65

K

Karma cooking, 45
Kidney beans, 5
Kimchi, 15, 19, 25, 55, 71, 83
Kimchi Quesadilla, 55, 71
Kitchari, 143, 151
Kiwi, 87, 99, 103
Kohlrabi, 55, 81
Kombucha, 25, 55, 67, 91, 99, 125

L

Labour-Aid, 97
Labour induction, 96
Labour Prep, 96, 99, 137
Labour Prep Chocolate Pudding, 99, 137
Lactation, 141, 143, 149, 173, 179, 189
Lactation & Immunity Smoothie, 143, 179
Leg cramps, 135
Lemon, 6, 10, 15, 19, 69, 75, 77, 83, 85, 97, 121, 131, 143, 169, 185
Lemon Balm, 185
Lemon Broccoli Soup, 55, 67
Lemongrass paste, 29, 163, 171
Lentil and Spinach Dal, 15, 31
Lentils, 5, 9, 31, 55, 67, 99, 117, 123, 143, 161
Lettuce wraps, 29, 171
Listeriosis, 73
Low mercury fish, 75
Lucuma powder, 129

M

Macadamia nuts, 103
Magnesium, 4–5, 13, 17, 33, 53, 63, 105, 109, 129, 135, 159, 177
Make ahead, 149, 153
Mango, 55, 73, 87, 99, 111, 127, 143, 171
Mango Avocado Salad, 143, 171
Maple syrup, 6, 17, 21, 45, 47, 103, 105, 111, 129, 147, 153, 155
Mastitis, 179
Matcha, 93, 143, 189
Meditation, 95, 187
Mediterranean Quinoa Salad, 99, 113

Mental health, 5, 31, 149, 163, 177, 191
Mercury, 9, 11, 75, 105
Microbiome, 67, 83
Milk supply, 141, 157, 173
Millet, 4, 10, 143, 147
Minerals, 3–4, 6, 9–10, 57, 96–97, 119, 179, 183
Mini Frittatas, 143, 149
Mint, 15, 27, 29, 31, 51, 109, 111, 113, 125, 155, 171, 179
Mint chocolate, 55, 93
Mint Chocolate Nice Cream, 55, 93
Miso, 15, 37, 55, 67, 75, 81, 143, 163, 165
Miso Lemon Collard Greens, 15, 37
Mojito, 99, 125
Monounsaturated fats, 4, 19
Moringa, 143, 179, 189
Morning sickness, 19
Muesli, 55, 57, 99, 103
Muesli Cookies, 55, 57
Muffins, 11, 45, 143, 183
Mulligatawny, 99, 117
Muscle spasms, 129
Mushrooms, 23, 69, 71, 75, 115, 123, 149, 157, 159, 187

N

Natural Sweeteners, 6
    Coconut sugar, 6
    Dates, 6
    Honey, 6
    Maple syrup, 6
Nausea, 4, 10, 13, 21, 41, 51, 53
Nettles, 185
Neural tube, 9, 31
Niçoise Salad, 15, 39
No-Bake Granola Bars, 143, 177
Non-toxic cookware, 105
Nutritional yeast, 33, 83

O

Oat flour, 5, 11, 45, 105, 173, 181, 183
Oat straw, 185, 187
Oats, 4, 10, 15, 17, 21, 37, 47, 57, 59, 177, 179
Oleic acid, 11, 77
Olives, 39, 55, 77

Omega 3 essential fatty acids, 4–5, 11, 13, 25, 75, 79, 121
Organ meat, 9, 141, 167, 171
Organic dairy, 9

P
Pancakes, 99, 105
Papaya, 87, 99, 103
Parsnips, 45, 121, 123, 143, 183
Pasta, 10, 27, 33, 55, 69, 167
Peanut butter, 99, 139, 143, 173
Peanut Butter Cookies, 143, 173
Pears, 10, 59, 143, 147
Perineal Massage, 97
Perineum, 185
Pesto, 15, 27, 149
PFAS, 105
Phyllo, 55, 85
Phyllo dough, 85
Pie, 59, 99, 107, 123, 181, 183
Pistachios, 4, 113, 143, 147, 175
Pizza, 15, 35, 165, 167
Poached Eggs, 15, 23
Poached Salmon, 15
Polyunsaturated fats, 7, 93
Pomegranate, 10, 105, 143, 147, 185
Postpartum, 5, 9, 95–97, 115, 143, 165, 171, 175, 177, 185, 187, 189, 191
    Postpartum anemia, 167
    Postpartum depression, 191
    Postpartum Healing Tea, 143, 185
    Postpartum health, 9, 123
    Postpartum Nourish Bowl, 143, 155
    Postpartum prep, 131, 167
Potatoes, 15, 23, 39, 55, 83, 99, 119, 155, 165, 169
Prebiotics, 33, 39, 71, 113
Preeclampsia, 67, 95, 109
Pregnancy Whole Foods 101, 3
Probiotics, 25, 67, 71, 91
Progesterone, 9, 177
Protein powder, 47, 135
Pumpkin Caramel Smoothie, 99, 107
Pumpkin pie, 107, 183
Pumpkin purée, 69, 107
Pumpkin seeds, 4, 17, 21, 27, 45, 47, 49, 135, 139, 155, 177
Pumpkin smoothie, 107
Pumpkin Truffle Pasta, 55, 69

Q
Quinoa, 4, 10, 15, 27, 77, 99, 103, 111, 113, 155
Quinoa flakes, 103

R
Ramen, 143, 159
Raspberries, 15, 49, 55, 87, 89, 91, 137, 179
Raw balls, 133
Raw fish, 73
Recovery, 141, 145, 159
Red harissa, 81
Red Raspberry Bites, 99, 133
Red raspberry leaf, 96, 99, 125, 133, 137
Red Raspberry Leaf Mojito, 99, 125
Red raspberry leaf tea, 96, 125, 133, 137
Reishi, 143, 145, 187
Relaxation, 185
Relaxin, 63
Relaxing Reishi Rose Elixir, 143, 187
Rice bowl, 73, 163
Rice vinegar, 29, 73, 79, 81, 111
Roasted Garlic, 143
Roasted Salmon & Bok Choy, 143, 163
Roasted Tomatoes, 143
Rolled oats, 21, 47, 57, 59, 103, 177, 179
Roma tomatoes, 31, 117
Romaine lettuce, 29
Root Vegetable Soup, 143, 165, 167

S
Saffron, 101
Salad, 4, 7, 9–10, 15, 27, 29, 39, 55, 143, 171
Salmon, 9, 15, 25, 33, 39, 55, 121, 143, 163
Salmon & Egg Toast, 55, 61
Salmon and Kimchi Tacos, 15, 25
Salsa, 99, 127
Sambal oelek, 81
Seared Elk Steak, 55, 79
Seaweed, 6, 43, 73, 159

Second Trimester, 53, 55, 67, 69, 83, 85, 87, 89, 91, 93, 97
Selenium, 5, 87, 123, 167
Sesame Ginger Soba Noodles, 99, 111
Sesame oil, 71, 73, 111, 115, 159
Sesame seeds, 19, 47, 73, 111, 115, 159
Shakshuka, 99, 101
Shepherd's Pie, 99, 123
Shiitakes, 55
Shrimp, 15, 29, 55, 81, 163
Skin health, 5, 77, 81, 87
Smooth Skin Smoothie Bowl, 55, 87
Smoothie, 6–7, 10–11, 15, 31, 51, 107, 143, 151, 179
Smoothie bowl, 55, 87
Snacks, 4, 10–11, 13, 15, 43, 47, 127, 133, 135, 141, 143
Soba noodles, 99, 111
Sockeye salmon, 25, 39, 73
Soothing Miso Ramen, 143, 159
Soup, 4–5, 9–10, 31, 55, 67, 95, 159, 161, 165, 167, 169
Spanikopita, 55, 85
Spelt, 5, 45, 55, 85
Spelt flour, 5, 45
Spelt Phyllo, 55, 85
Spiced Muffins, 143, 183
Spicy Pineapple Miso Shrimp, 55, 81
Spinach, 10, 15, 31, 67, 93, 105, 113
Spirulina, 6, 27, 87, 93, 13
Spring Quinoa Salad, 15
Squats, 77, 97
Sriracha, 81
Steel-cut oats, 4, 10, 15, 17
Steel-Cut Oats with Coconut Cream and Plums, 15
Stew, 31, 143, 151
Strawberries, 87, 99, 125, 179
Stretch marks, 77, 87, 103
Sunflower seeds, 4, 139, 177
Super Digestive Smoothie, 15, 51
Superhero Pancakes, 99, 105
Ssupport system, 139
Sushi, 11, 55, 73
Sushi rice, 73
Sweet potatoes, 15, 23, 155, 165, 169
Swiss Chard, 15, 27, 55, 75, 99, 109, 127

T

Tacos, 15, 25
Tahini, 57, 143, 155
Tahini Dressing, 143
Tarragon, 15, 39, 55, 61, 99, 121
Tarragon Vinaigrette, 15
Tea, 11, 41, 91, 96, 101, 125, 179, 185, 187, 189, 191
Third trimester, 95, 99, 101, 103, 115, 117, 121, 123, 133, 135, 137, 139
Thyroid health, 73
Toxin-free cookware, 35, 105
Tropical Bircher Muesli, 99, 103
Turmeric, 31, 117, 141, 143, 151, 169

U

Uterine lining, 125

V

Vanilla Coconut Custard, 143, 175
Vanilla Coconut Sauce, 99, 105
Varicose veins, 95, 101
Vegan carob chips, 139
Veggie Crust Pizza, 15, 35
Venison Meatballs, 143, 167
Vermicelli Noodle Salad with Shrimp, 15
Vitamin B12, 37, 83, 171
Vitamin C, 6, 10, 33, 63, 69, 87, 95–96, 131, 155
Vitamin D, 61, 109, 175
Vitamin E, 77, 87, 96, 101, 103
Vomiting, 31, 41, 53

W

Walnuts, 4, 15, 21, 43, 45, 89, 135, 139, 147, 181
Watermelon Limeade, 15, 41
Wheat germ, 173
Whole food, 3–4, 6, 41, 69
Whole-Foods Pantry, 3–4, 11
Whole Grains, 4, 10
Wild game meat, 35, 79

Y

Yam and Ginger Soup, 143, 161
Yogourt, 9, 25, 31, 49, 59, 103

www.ingramcontent.com/pod-product-compliance
Lightning Source LLC
Chambersburg PA
CBRC090903080526
44587CB00009B/180